The Cattle Health Handbook

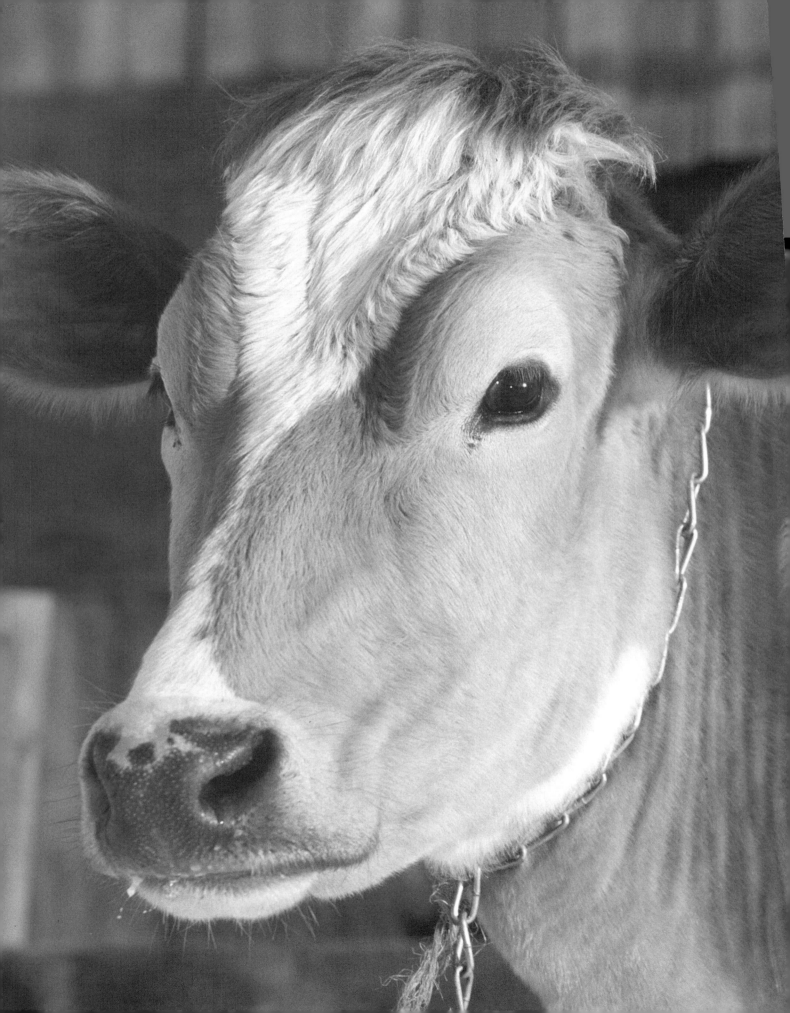

The Cattle Health Handbook

Preventive Care, Disease Treatments & Emergency Procedures

for Promoting the Well-Being of Your Beef or Dairy Herd

HEATHER SMITH THOMAS

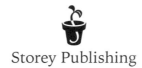

Storey Publishing

The mission of Storey Publishing is to serve our customers by publishing practical information that encourages personal independence in harmony with the environment.

Edited by Rebekah Boyd-Owens, Sarah Guare, and Deborah Burns
Art direction and book design by Dan O. Williams
Text production by Liseann Karandisecky and Ponderosa Pine Design

Front cover and spine photographs by © Lynn Stone. Author's photograph by
    Andrea Hansen
Interior photographs by the author, except for © Lynn Stone, page ii; © Matt Pound, page
    158; courtesy of Dr. Dan Casteel, University of Missouri, page 202 top; courtesy of
    Dr. Marlin Rice, Iowa State University, page 299
Illustrations by © Elara Tanguy
Additional maps and infographics by Ilona Sherratt

Indexed by Christine R. Lindemer, Boston Road Communications

Printed in the United States by Versa Press
10 9 8 7 6 5 4 3 2 1

Library of Congress Cataloging-in-Publication Data

Thomas, Heather Smith, 1944–
    The cattle health handbook / by Heather Smith Thomas.
        p. cm.
    Includes index.
    ISBN 978-1-60342-090-7 (pbk. : alk. paper)
    ISBN 978-1-60342-095-2 (hardcover : alk. paper)
    1. Cattle—Health—Handbooks, manuals, etc.
    2. Cattle—Diseases—Handbooks, manuals, etc. I. Title.
SF961.T46 2009
636.2'089—dc22
                                2009001484

DEDICATION

This book is dedicated to all my cattle — every individual animal I've been privileged to know, starting with my very first cow in 1956 when I was 12 years old. She was a pregnant Hereford heifer in the first group of cows my father purchased after our family bought a small ranch. I named my heifer Bovina and earned her purchase price by working summers for my father, irrigating the fields, digging postholes, and helping to build fences. I kept all of Bovina's heifer calves and their babies (selling only the steers) and had a small herd of cows by the time I went to college.

Later my husband Lynn and I had a dairy for a short time and then began raising beef cattle. Even after raising more than 6,000 calves and watching many of them grow up to be cows, I remember most of them (and their names)! Each one was a unique character; some had very endearing attributes, and others had not-so-endearing traits.

My cattle have been my passion, my addiction, my lifework. Learning how to care for them properly and how to deal with the problems that occasionally arose led me to share that knowledge with others, writing articles for livestock publications and then books about raising cattle. My cows taught me many lessons in life, not only in animal husbandry but also in larger matters regarding things like patience, courage, endurance, determination, and persistence, for it's not always easy to care for them in harsh weather or to save one that suffers from a challenging disease. I am grateful to my cattle for helping to forge the person I've become.

Contents

PART I: Health Management

PART II: Common Diseases

PART III: Body System Disorders

PART IV: Other Ailments, Accidents, and Injuries

Preface

My husband and I both grew up on ranches raising cattle, and together we've been taking care of cattle for more than 40 years. After our wedding in March 1966, we went home to his dairy in southern Idaho to milk the cows — you can't explain time off for a honeymoon to a dairy cow. Lynn had a small dairy herd, as it was easier then for a young person to obtain financing for renting a farm and buying dairy cows than to try to start up a beef-cattle ranch. Our experiences with dairy cows and their calves augmented our youthful knowledge about caring for cattle and keeping them healthy.

At the end of that year we sold the dairy cows, moved back to our mountainous country roots near Salmon, Idaho, and started our own cattle ranch. It was tough trying to make a living and pay for a ranch and cattle on what can only be called marginal land. We have many acres, and it's beautiful country, but it's steep, rugged, high-desert rangeland with very little rainfall and only a few acres that can be irrigated to grow hay for winter feed. But we were persistent. We struggled hard to make it work, developing a hardy, unpampered herd of crossbred cattle that thrive in harsh conditions.

Part of our financial survival depended on not losing any animals; we couldn't afford to lose any. We learned all we could about taking good care of the cattle, and early on we became excellent "cattle doctors," because each animal had to be healthy and producing or fit to sell in the fall. But we also love our animals. Each one is a unique personality — even after our herd expanded to 185 cows, every cow and calf had a name! If one of them was injured or sick, we were diligent in our efforts to treat him and correct the problem. We are poor losers; there's nothing we hated more than losing an animal — partly because we could not afford the financial loss but also because each was a cherished character.

We are poor losers; there's nothing we hated more than losing an animal — partly because we could not afford the financial loss but also because each was a cherished character.

Learning everything we could from each adverse situation and medical case that needed treatment or intensive care, we became excellent cattle caretakers. Over the years, we learned from our local veterinarians and other ranchers and, for unusual cases, sometimes even picked the brains of university veterinary specialists. But our cattle taught us the most.

In my research as a freelance writer, I interviewed many veterinarians and professors for articles that appeared in horse and cattle publications. I've written more than 7,000 magazine articles and now write regularly for about 60 horse, farm, and livestock publications. For 30 years I've written a regular column on ranch life for a Canadian farming newspaper. Much of what I write deals with health care. My goal as a writer has been to learn all I can about my own animals and to share that knowledge with others. After reading my articles, ranchers have been known to phone us from great distances to ask questions about an animal they are treating, and we always take the time to try to help.

After my first four years of college, I planned on studying to become a veterinarian. Instead, I married a rancher, but my education has never ceased. We are forever consulting with veterinarians and utilizing numerous veterinary textbooks. When Lynn and I have a problem we can't handle by ourselves, such as a Cesarean-section surgery or a calf that has a hairball blockage or needs a section of intestine removed, we do not hesitate to call our vet. And if ranchers ask our advice about a condition we can't diagnose or haven't experienced, we always refer them to their own veterinarian. But in many instances our practical knowledge can be of help to others, especially young ranchers or those just starting out who have never encountered certain situations.

Acknowledgments

Much of the information in this book comes from 50 years of experience raising cattle — caring for them in health and illness. My husband and I have always tried to learn as much as we could about taking the best possible care of our cows and calves. This education has included advice and help from a number of veterinarians over the years, and I wish to thank them all — especially Dr. Peter J. South, Dr. Ron Skinner, Dr. Dick Rath, "Doc" Hatfield, Dr. Robert Cope, Dr. Jeff Hoffman, and Dr. Todd Tibbitts.

I also want to thank the many people I have interviewed or quoted over the years when writing articles about cattle health and management for various ranch and livestock publications. My education was furthered by their input: Dr. Don Adams (University of Nebraska); Bruce Anderson, DVM, PhD (Caine Veterinary Teaching and Research Center, University of Idaho, Caldwell, Idaho); Louis Archbald, DVM, PhD (University of Florida); Clell V. Bagley, DVM (Extension veterinarian, Utah State University); George Barrington, DVM (Washington State University); Ellen Belknap, DVM, (Auburn University); Tom Besser, DVM, PhD (veterinary bacteriologist, Washington State University); Steve Blezinger, PhD (nutrition/management consultant, Sulphur Springs, Texas); Anthony Blikslager, DVM, PhD (North Carolina State University); Bob Bohlender, DVM (Nebraska); Keith Bramwell (Extension, University of Idaho); Marie Bulgin, DVM (Caine Veterinary Teaching and Research Center, Caldwell, Idaho); Stuart Burns, DVM (private practice, Paris, Kentucky); Dr. Jack Campbell (University of Nebraska); Robert Carson, DVM (Auburn University); Dr. Peter Chenoweth (Kansas State University); Dr. Bill Clymer (Fort Dodge Animal Health); Dr. Glenn Coulter (Lethbridge Research Center, Alberta, Canada); Dr. Thomas Craig (Texas A&M); Dr. Joe Diedrickson; Ed Duran (Extension animal scientist, Idaho State University); Keith Eberly (professional hoof trimmer, Jeromesville, Ohio); Dr. Floron "Buddy" Faries (Texas A&M); Dr. Bill Foreyt (Washington State University); Clive Gay, DVM (Washington State University); Mike Gaylean, DVM (Department of Animal Science, Texas Tech University); Dr. Jim Gerrish (University of Missouri); Dr. Temple Grandin (Colorado State University); Don Hansen, DVM (Extension veterinarian, Oregon State University); Allen Heath, DVM (Auburn University); Dr. Tim Holt (Colorado State University); Dr. Elaine Hunt (College of Veterinary Medicine, North Carolina State University); Greg Johnson (livestock entomologist, Montana State University); Ray Kaplan, DVM, PhD (veterinary parasitologist, University of Georgia); Bill Kvasnicka, DVM (Extension veterinarian, University of Nevada); Kelly Lechtenberg, DVM, PhD. (Midwest Veterinary Services, Oakland, Nebraska); Dr. Jack Lloyd (University of Wyoming); Dennis Maxwell (McNay Research Farm, Iowa State University); Duane McCartney, Agriculture and Agri-Food Canada Research Station, Lacombe, Alberta; Mike Mehren, PhD (livestock nutritionist, Hermiston, Oregon); David Morris, DVM, PhD (Fort Collins, Colorado); Bob Mortimer, DVM (Colorado State University); Dr. Annette O'Connor (Iowa State University); James Pfister (USDA poisonous plant laboratory, Logan, Utah); Kit Pharo (rancher, Cheyenne Wells, Colorado); Dr. Richard Randle (University of Missouri); William C. Rebhun, DVM (now deceased, Cornell University); Glenn Selk (Oklahoma State University); Geoff Smith, DVM, PhD (College of Veterinary Medicine, North Carolina State University); Don Spiers, PhD (Animal Science, University of Missouri); Patricia Talcott, DVM (Idaho State University); Ron Torrell (livestock specialist, University of Nevada); Dr. Lee Townsend (University of Kentucky); Dr. Tom Welsh (Texas A&M); Doug Whitsett, DVM (columnist for *Cascade Cattleman*); Dr. Jack Whittier (Colorado State University); Dr. Gary Williams (Texas A&M); Milo Wiltbank, PhD (University of Wisconsin); Curtis Youngs, PhD (Iowa State University). My apologies to anyone I've omitted.

A special thank you to Dr. Ron Skinner of Drummond, Montana, for taking time to read through most of my manuscript chapters for this book; I am grateful for his input and advice.

Introduction

This is a book I've wanted to write for a long time. In it I have used simple terms to describe practical health-care methods and offer medical advice we've garnered from others and learned from our own hands-on experience. Although its scope is broad and it contains plenty of detailed information, it is easy to read and sprinkled with anecdotes and a few of our own case histories, and it features real characters of both the human and bovine varieties.

If you maintain a large herd of cattle over a long stretch of time, you will see almost all of the common problems, as well as some very unusual situations. My goal is to help acquaint the reader with the health challenges encountered in raising cattle as well as the treatment methods and options associated with the challenges. The discussions within will also help the reader to determine whether he can handle a condition by himself or must call the vet.

How to Use This Book

Different things cause cattle diseases and ailments, including bacteria, viruses, fungi, protozoa, and parasites. Understanding how these microscopic invaders cause sickness helps the rancher to understand the importance of routine vaccination, sanitation, and a calf's need for immunity-building colostrum. The first section of the book looks at such things as disease resistance, including how cattle develop immunity, and the basics of detecting and treating seasonal and other illnesses and administering medications. For instance, chapter 2 describes basic health maintenance techniques.

The second section of the book covers general disease conditions grouped by the types of pathogens that cause them.

Because it's often easiest for stockmen with sick cattle to research a disease within the category of the body system that is affected, the third section of the book describes symptoms and treatments of specific body systems. So when it's 3 o'clock on a weekend morning, and the veterinary clinic is closed, and you discover a cow with a problem, you can easily flip through chapters with titles like "Respiratory Problems," "Eye Problems," "Foot Problems," and "Skin Problems" to figure out what's wrong.

The fourth section examines other more random types of ailments as well as accidents, and injuries.

I've tried to include all of the diseases you are likely to encounter and some that with luck you'll never see. Because there are so many ailments that can affect cattle, however, some of which are very rare, it is impossible to touch on all of them in this book. A comprehensive look at reproductive diseases, calving problems, and calfhood diseases can be found in this book's companion volume, *Essential Guide to Calving*.

Keep in mind that some conditions are difficult to diagnose without veterinary assistance, and, on occasion, an animal may be suffering from more than one problem at once. When in doubt, you should always consult your vet to help you with proper diagnosis and treatment. It is initially up to you, though, to detect the existence of the problem. The aim of this book is to help you recognize when an animal is sick, so you can identify and treat or get professional help for many of the problems that may be causing the symptoms you have observed.

PART ONE
Health Management

CHAPTER ONE

Preventive Care

Raising a healthy herd of cattle is the stockman's goal. This requires that he or she maintain a clean, healthy environment by avoiding crowded and unsanitary conditions; provide adequate and proper feed; make feed changes gradually; minimize exposure to and vaccinate against common cattle diseases; and avoid stressing cattle, which can lower resistance to disease.

But anyone who has spent any length of time on a ranch or farm knows that even when maintaining optimum health conditions and doing your best to minimize risk for disease, problems occasionally occur. A conscientious stockman is aware of the relationships between stress and disease resistance and between stress and the effects of illness on an animal. An animal's stages of physical development and the various ways immunity is acquired must also be fully understood to appreciate her vulnerability or resistance to disease.

Preventive care means managing the herd's health with an eye to protecting the animals in the future, caring for and observing individuals day in and day out, and having some awareness of the signs and characteristics of various diseases in order to recognize them and keep them at bay.

Disease Resistance and Immunity

Disease is any condition that results in impairment of normal function. We tend to think of a disease as something caused by infection with bacteria or viruses, but poor health can also be a result of parasites, malnutrition, congenital defects, or injuries that interfere with proper body function.

Mammals have many complex mechanisms to guard against constant challenges from disease-causing agents. Survival depends on specific defenses such as antibodies that combat certain pathogens, and nonspecific defenses that include the body's physical barriers against disease. A healthy animal can usually ward off *pathogens* that cause disease, thanks to a strong *immune system*. The immune system's primary function is to recognize and defend against foreign invaders, and it involves several components that work together to maintain health.

Nonspecific Disease Resistance

The body has many ways to protect itself from invading pathogens until it can develop a specific immunity. The first line of defense includes physical barriers such as skin and membrane coverings, mucus on membrane linings, acids in the stomach, and *enzymes*. Helpful *bacteria* on skin surfaces inhibit harmful bacteria. If a cut or break occurs in the skin, bleeding washes away infectious agents. *White blood cells* called *phagocytes* rush to the site to engulf and inactivate debris and any remaining infectious agents.

Mucous membranes line body openings and digestive, respiratory, and reproductive tracts, serving the same function as skin. These membranes create acids and enzymes as protection against invasion. Specialized cells in mucous membranes secrete fluids called *mucus* to wash away irritants. *Antibodies* are secreted to provide specific resistance at the site. The respiratory tract contains cells with small projections called *cilia*. The one-way sweeping motion of these microscopic threads moves mucus and foreign material (dust and pathogens) out of air passages. The body can also wall off some invaders to limit their spread.

Inflammation is the body's response to injury or attack, as part of a local or *systemic* reaction. For example, a splinter creates redness and swelling at the site; white blood cells called *neutrophils* attack and begin digesting the splinter and an *abscess* (an accumulation of dead white cells) forms. Inflammation can cause heat, pain, and swelling, but its purpose is to protect the body from further injury and assist in repair of damaged tissues.

Fever is a defense mechanism that hinders some *viruses* with narrow temperature tolerance. Fever also increases the *metabolic rate* of the body, speeding up all chemical processes. This helps fight disease but also uses up large amounts of energy swiftly. If a fever gets too high, as it does in some diseases, body cells may be damaged, such as those in the brain.

When some pathogens, especially viruses, invade the body, it responds by liberating proteins called *interferons*, which interfere with viral replication.

These are some of the body's resistance mechanisms that can limit invasion, along with the specific protection given by antibodies. Yet this built-in resistance can be overcome by factors that impair the immune system (*malnutrition*, stress, another illness) or by certain types of aggressive disease agents that overwhelm the animal's defenses. *Immunity* is the body's ability to fight off invaders such as bacteria, viruses, fungi, and protozoa. This ability is developed in a complex process in which the body creates specific weapons for fighting specific invaders.

How Immunity Develops

Whether a pathogen enters through a cut in the skin, is drawn into the lungs with a breath of air, is ingested, or takes any other route, the body

Pathogen Preferences

Most pathogens have a preference for certain kinds of tissues and even for specific species. Some human, horse, sheep, and other animals' diseases do not affect cattle, and some bovine diseases do not affect humans or other animals. Cattle do not get West Nile virus, which affects horses and humans. Humans and horses don't get blackleg, bovine viral diarrhea (BVD), or the variety of foot rot that occurs in cattle. All mammals can get rabies, however, and almost all can get tetanus, anthrax, ringworm, salmonella, and other nonspecies specific diseases.

Most pathogens attack specific areas of the body. Some viruses and bacteria invade the nervous system (rabies, tetanus, listeriosis); others prefer the digestive tract (salmonella, coccidiosis). Some attack the respiratory system and cause pneumonia, while others invade the skin to cause ringworm or warts. Some invade and destroy specific body cells, while others produce harmful toxins that circulate through the body, affecting multiple organs and systems. The body must therefore develop numerous ways to protect itself from a variety of attackers.

recognizes it as a foreign protein. These foreign materials — viruses, bacteria, fungi, protozoa, certain *parasites,* or any portion of any of these, such as the cell-wall protein of a bacterium — are called antigens. An *antigen* is a substance that can trigger an immune response in the animal. Presence of an antigen or its toxic products stimulates the body to create an antibody to react with the invading agent and destroy or neutralize it. An animal with a healthy immune system can mobilize a strong defense very quickly, creating antibodies to attack the invader.

The reason vaccination works to protect an animal from a specific disease is that a *vaccine* contains the antigen (inactivated or *killed viruses* or bacteria, for instance), which stimulates the body to mount an immune reaction and create antibodies. Giving a small dose of antigen via vaccine improves the speed and efficiency of the animal's next immune response to the same antigen; the immune system has a "memory" of that antigen. If the animal encounters the disease itself, there are already antibodies in place to fight the pathogens, and more are produced quickly. If enough antibodies are present to inactivate all the pathogens that invade, the animal won't get sick, and the invasion stimulates rapid production of more antibodies for future protection. Most vaccines are given once or twice a year, to keep antibody levels high enough to protect against a specific disease (see Vaccination, page 10).

If an animal is healthy and already has antibodies against a specific disease through natural exposure or vaccination *boosters,* whenever that particular pathogen invades the body, antibodies flock to attack it. One of the most important types of antibody is a serum protein *(immunoglobulin)* that circulates in the blood to seek and destroy a particular antigen. If the animal has encountered the antigen before, there are antibodies lying in wait.

Blood tests can detect the presence of circulating antibodies, which indicate that the animal has been exposed at some time to that specific antigen. The presence of antibodies does not guarantee that the animal is protected against further exposure but does show that the animal has previously encountered that pathogen.

ANTIBODIES ARE ANTIGEN-SPECIFIC

Antibodies are proteins produced in response to an antigen. They bind to that particular infectious agent and help kill it. Antibodies are very specific and can usually bind only with one particular antigen — or one closely associated with it.

Humoral Immunity

There are two types of immunity, both facilitated by a type of white blood cell called a *lymphocyte,* which can recognize anything foreign to the body. The main role of one type of lymphocyte *(B lymphocyte)* is to produce antibodies. Antibody-mediated immunity is called *humoral immunity.* The humoral immune response is developed in the spaces between the cells and in the circulatory system. The antibodies created there can circulate through the body via blood or fluid between cells. A humoral immune response can be a primary response; this means that it is responding to an antigen for the first time, which takes several days to occur. It can also be a secondary response, responding to an antigen encountered previously through vaccination or prior exposure. Secondary response produces a much faster and more effective defense.

Cellular Immunity

Another class of white blood cells *(T lymphocyte)* is involved in *cellular immunity* (cell-mediated immunity). Antibodies from B cells can attach to and neutralize or destroy pathogens in blood, mucous, milk, and body fluids, but can't destroy pathogens within the cell walls. If a cell becomes altered by infection or cancer, the body must recognize that cell as foreign or abnormal and destroy the entire cell to get rid of the pathogen. This is the job of the T lymphocytes, which are programmed to recognize altered cells.

This second type of immunity is stimulated at the cell level in specific body tissues. Viruses, which are smaller than bacteria, live and replicate inside cells, where most antibodies can't find them. A cell-mediated immune response involves finding and eliminating abnormal body cells that contain foreign proteins (viruses). This type of response entails production of T lymphocytes in blood and *lymph.* These lymphocytes send out chemical messengers to communicate with other body cells, directing attack forces to destroy virus-infected cells.

This cell-level immunity is the body's main defense against some types of attack, such as viruses that enter the respiratory system. Cellular immunity generally develops more quickly than immunity via blood circulation and is one reason *intranasal vaccines* against respiratory diseases protect an animal more quickly at the site of attack than does injected vaccine.

The body can also produce a nonspecific immune response to an antigen. Part of this response involves phagocytes (white cells capable of engulfing and absorbing foreign matter). These cells are less specific in what they attack, however, than either the humoral or cell-mediated immune responses.

When Disease Comes Knocking

Immunity results when the body produces antibodies in response to invasion by a foreign protein. In healthy animals, immunity begins to develop whenever an infection occurs. If the invading pathogen is present in small numbers or the animal already has antibodies against it from previous exposure or vaccination, immunity develops fast enough or is already strong enough that clinical disease does not occur. The body fights off the invader and recovers or may not appear sick. But if an animal has no prior immunity or the invader multiplies faster than the body can develop defenses, the result is illness — and death, if pathogens overwhelm the body's ability to fight. It can take two weeks to produce an effective level of antibodies through infection or vaccination.

Exposure to (or vaccination with) one strain of pathogen may result in immunity to that specific strain but not to other strains of the same organism. There are many strains of *leptospirosis* bacteria, for instance, and vaccination against one strain does not give protection against the others. Antibody immunity also depends on the level of exposure. A severe disease outbreak may eventually wear down a healthy animal's immunity and will overwhelm a stressed animal's defenses even sooner.

A cow in a natural environment may not become exposed to many disease-causing organisms, but cattle are often confined in corrals, small pens, or pastures that have been contaminated by heavy cattle use. They may be exposed to contaminated cattle through the fence at a sale yard or feedlot, which furthers the spread of disease. But with vaccination and natural exposure to various pathogens, cattle develop many antibodies and strong immunity.

Passive Immunity from Maternal Antibodies

Young calves are vulnerable to diseases such as *pneumonia* and *scours (diarrhea),* but nature has this loophole sewed up. To help protect calves, antibodies are provided in the cow's *colostrum* (first milk) to give temporary immunity against common diseases. During late pregnancy, a cow's antibodies transfer into the colostrum she produces. Because these antibodies circulating in her body are represented in that first milk, her calf has instant immunity after his first nursing. This colostrum-acquired temporary immunity is called *passive immunity.* Antibodies in colostrum are crucial to the newborn calf because he has very little disease resistance.

Although after 140 days of development a *fetus* can start to produce its own antibodies in response to pathogens that pass through the *placental* wall of an infected mother-to-be, the calf doesn't get any antibodies from his mother's bloodstream before birth because the antibody molecules are too large to cross the placental barrier. A calf can obtain his mother's antibodies only if he drinks her colostrum soon after birth.

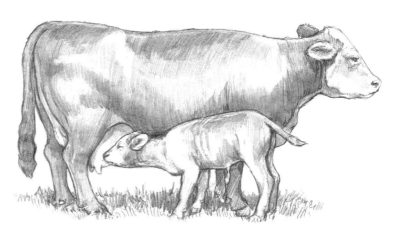

Antibodies in colostrum are crucial to the newborn calf because he has very little disease resistance.

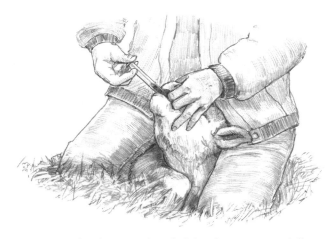

Prevent some diarrhea types by administering a commercially prepared, concentrated antibody source (oral vaccine) soon after birth.

For the first few hours after birth, a calf's intestinal lining is porous enough for large antibody molecules to slip through into his bloodstream and protect him against bloodborne infections. Some types stay in the *gut* to fight pathogens that cause diarrhea. Vaccinating the pregnant cow a few weeks before calving can increase these antibodies, as she can develop the needed antibodies and have peak levels in colostrum at the time of calving.

You can prevent some types of diarrhea by giving the calf a commercially prepared, concentrated antibody source (oral vaccine) soon after birth. There are oral products to protect calves against *E. coli* scours, *rotavirus,* and *coronavirus,* three of the deadliest of infectious diarrhea diseases.

Fetal Immunity

A fetus can also acquire immunity. It can begin to produce antibodies against pathogens such as *bovine viral diarrhea (BVD)* and *infectious bovine rhinotracheitis (IBR)* as early as 140 days of *gestation* and against leptospirosis after 180 days because some of these invaders pass through the placental barrier from an infected mother's bloodstream. Some infections cause the fetus to start making antibodies, but they can also kill the fetus.

Fetal immunity gained via exposure to pathogens doesn't do a calf as much good at birth as it would when he is older because his immune abilities temporarily decrease at the time of birth. For a week or two

before and after calving, the calf's immune system is hindered by his and his mama's high *cortisol* levels, present in their bodies to help stimulate labor.

Passive Immunity

Temporary immunity against disease can be obtained from sources outside the body, such as by ingestion of colostrum or use of injected antiserum (such as an antitoxin). These contain high levels of already-produced antibodies (as in blood serum taken from an immune animal) for immediate defense against certain diseases. This is a mechanical transfer of immunity from one animal to another.

This protection lasts only a few weeks, or in some cases up to six months. Colostrum from a first-calver does not contain as many antibodies as colostrum from an older cow, who has likely encountered more pathogens in her longer life. Maternal antibodies for some clostridial diseases may give a calf protection for four to six weeks, whereas antibodies for IBR may last for four to six months, depending on the level of antibodies acquired through passive transfer and the disease challenge to the calf. A cow vaccinated with killed IBR virus will pass on more immunity to her calf than a cow on a modified live-virus vaccine program will.

If the cow has antibodies for IBR and the calf receives them via colostrum, he will have circulating immunity and probably won't be at risk for fatal newborn IBR pneumonia, but he will still become infected. Most of these calves probably become infected within the first six weeks of life and possibly even in the first few days. If they have received enough colostral antibodies, they will be protected from IBR virus circulating in the bloodstream but not from the nasal infection. Calves with a high level of colostral antibodies don't have a strong immunity of their own if the respiratory illness takes the nasal route; hence, they do not build up their own antibodies. These calves become infected even though their dams have been vaccinated with either modified live or killed vaccines.

Since no antigen is being transferred with passive immunity, the recipient's immune system isn't stimulated; he's protected only as long as transferred antibodies last. Longer-lasting protection must come from his own immune system when it is stimulated to create its own antibodies. After exposure to a pathogen or antigen in a vaccine, it usually takes 7 to 14 days for the immune system to build adequate immunity, whereas passive immunity from an outside source is protective immediately.

Active Immunity

Active immunity is created by the animal's immune system response to an antigen. Active immunity may result from the cycle of natural infection and recovery or from the deliberate exposure of vaccination. It usually takes one to two weeks to develop immunity the first time following natural infection or vaccination, but if the animal is exposed to the same antigen later, a secondary response occurs and the antibodies rise much more quickly to higher levels. This "memory" in the immune system is one reason some vaccines are given in two doses to boost immunity, with an annual dose thereafter.

Duration of active immunity ranges from just a few months to the life of the animal, depending on the type of pathogen. For example, one vaccination against *brucellosis* during calfhood, or one two-shot series against *blackleg,* will confer lifelong immunity, whereas cattle need annual or semiannual booster vaccinations against redwater, lepto, and certain viral diseases causing *respiratory* illness.

Calves lose temporary immunity from colostrum antibodies by the time they're seven or eight weeks old or earlier if they didn't ingest enough colostrum soon enough or if the *dam* had an inadequate level of colostrum. The actual length of protection will also vary depending on the disease type. When this protection wanes, the calf's immune system must take over. If he had high levels of antibodies from colostrum (which neutralizes most invading pathogens), his own defenses are not stimulated to develop until that protection wears off.

Many vaccines for calves should be given at 8 weeks or older and repeated with a booster 2 to 6 weeks later or near weaning time to make sure that the calf's immune system can respond, but there are instances in which calves can be vaccinated at a much earlier age, with good results (see box below). This should be discussed with your veterinarian. Older cattle can be vaccinated any time, but certain vaccines still require a booster to build peak immunity. After that, annual or semiannual vaccination will continue to trigger production of antibodies.

Long-Range Effects of Passive Immunity

Scientists from the U.S. Department of Agriculture (USDA) in Clay Center, Nebraska, monitored health and growth in beef calves to gauge the effects of various levels of passive immunity. Blood samples were collected 24 hours after birth from 263 crossbred calves to determine the amount of passive transfer obtained from colostrum; the health and performance of these calves were then observed throughout the weaning and feedlot periods.

The groups of calves with the lowest levels of passive immunity in that first day of life had a higher percentage of individuals that got sick or died prior to weaning. Calves that were sick during the first 28 days of life averaged 35 pounds (15.9 kg) less at weaning than calves that did not get sick. The risk for getting sick in the feedlot was also three times greater for calves with inadequate early immunity, and this also affected their growth rate.

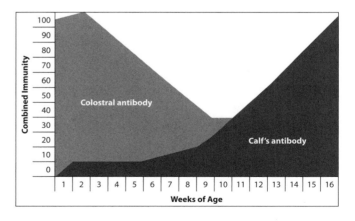

Calves lose their temporary immunity from colostrum by 7 to 8 weeks, but it takes a while longer for the immune system to develop its own antibodies to give the calf strong protection.

Colostrum-Gained Antibodies and Vaccines

If a calf is vaccinated when young, while he still has high levels of maternal antibodies in his blood, his own immune system will not bother to respond to antigens in vaccines because those antigens are being neutralized by maternal antibodies.

Some types of vaccine given to a calf when he's only 2 or 3 weeks old will not give him protection, since they won't stimulate immunity as long as he has maternal antibodies in his blood and lymph. Others can be effective, especially if they are oil-based vaccines, which are slow-release and can dribble into the immune system over a longer period of time.

An example of this is a seven-way clostridial vaccine (Alpha 7, which is an oil-adjuvanted vaccine), given at birth to protect calves against blackleg. Research has shown that calves that were given one shot of this vaccine at birth had more immunity at weaning time than calves that were given one shot of an aluminum hydroxide seven-way vaccine at branding time, with a booster later.

Modified live vaccines are very small viral doses expected to multiply in the body to create a greater antigen and antibody response. This small dose may not always stimulate enough immunity, but a killed vaccine in oil has a large amount of antigen and trickles into the system over a longer period of time. The antigen makes it to the lymph node easier because it is protected from any outside actions by the oil adjuvant.

Some killed vaccines are much more effective than others, and those that are oil adjuvanted can be even more effective than some modified live-virus vaccines. In the past, modified live vaccines were often used because they provided longer-lasting immunity. But some of the killed products do a better job now and may be safer in some instances because there is no risk that the vaccine will actually produce the disease, which occasionally happens with modified live-virus vaccines.

Prevention Practices

Preventing disease is essential for the well-being of animals and productivity. Illness can take a great toll on milk and beef production. A sick cow won't give much milk — not for you or her calf. A young animal that's sick or doing poorly will be slower to reach maturity for breeding purposes or will be a lighter weight at sale time. Severe illness may result in death. If you wait for signs of disease to show up, you may be too late; the disease may be passing through the whole herd by the time you see it. You may spend a lot of time and money on the treatment of some outbreaks, and other diseases may have no treatment at all. It's crucial to the vitality of your animals and your business that you do your best to prevent health problems from cropping up in the first place.

Most stockmen first think vaccination when they think about herd health programs. But herd health has many facets, including nutrition, herd management, parasite control, vaccination, and preventing disease from being introduced into your herd by other animals whose health is questionable.

Nutrition

Nutrition is the cornerstone of cattle health. You can deworm, vaccinate, keep a *closed herd,* and vigorously treat every problem that comes up, but animals may still get sick if they are undernourished or lacking in important dietary elements. For proper body function and optimum immunity, your animals need adequate protein, carbohydrates, vitamins, minerals, and clean water.

Plenty of clean water and good pasture, or adequate forage substitutes if pasture is short or snow-covered, will go a long way toward keeping cattle healthy. Poor nutrition increases susceptibility to disease and interferes with the animal's response to vaccinations. The underlying cause of scours, pneumonia, *foot rot,* or infertility may be poor nutrition — more specifically, a shortage of *trace minerals.*

Minerals are vital to a healthy immune system. Use mineral *supplements* if soils or feeds are deficient. Trace minerals play an important role in the cell replication and enzyme activity crucial to building immunity. Proper levels of copper, zinc, manganese, and *selenium* should be included in a mineral supplement given via feed mix or *salt* mix or by *bolus* or injection if feeds are lacking. Cows may need an additional mineral supplement during pregnancy, and both new mother cows and their calves often need a supplement that complements your soils and feeds. Before your herd encounters disease problems, consult your vet, agricultural extension agent, or cattle nutritionist to examine your feeding program and make any necessary adjustments.

Parasite Control

Parasite control is important. Even if cattle look healthy, internal and external parasites could be robbing them of nutrients and energy, resulting in slower growth, less milk production, and a less-effective immune system. Some types of external parasites carry disease from one animal to another (see chapter 7). Internal parasites (stomach *worms, liver flukes*) and external parasites (flies, lice, ticks) hinder optimum production. Even small numbers of parasites make a difference in the weaning weights of calves, and great numbers can drag an animal down and make him vulnerable to disease.

Biosecurity

To prevent introduction of disease to your farm, maintain a closed herd, if possible. Avoid bringing in new cattle; it's often safer to raise your own *heifers* than to purchase them. If you buy cows, heifers, or a new bull, buy from a reputable breeder rather than an auction, where you may not know the history of the animal. Keep new animals isolated for a while before adding them to your herd, to make sure they're not incubating a disease. If the animal does become sick while in the isolation area, you then have an opportunity to clean up that pen or stall, remove all manure, and use an appropriate disinfectant (see page 10), instead of having the sick animal out with your herd infecting other cattle.

Some diseases, such as BVD (see chapter 5), can be devastating. One infected animal brought to your farm is potentially disastrous, even if your cattle are vaccinated. Vaccinations are *never* 100 percent effective, especially those used to prevent BVD. Always have your vet test a new animal for BVD or *persistently infected* status (see chapter 3) before you add that animal to your herd.

TIDY UP THE WATERING HOLE

Many disease outbreaks begin when cattle imbibe dirty water contaminated by high levels of pathogens. Clean water is important for all animals and is especially crucial for calves. Make sure there are enough tanks so that the babies have access to clean water and don't have to drink out of manure-contaminated puddles. Keep their water-drinking challenges in mind:

- A nice big stock tank may be too tall for a young calf to reach.
- There may not be a chance to drink if cows are fighting over the water because there are not enough tanks.
- Water that freezes makes it even harder for young and timid animals to have access.

Sanitation

Disease control requires a commitment to painstaking cleanliness. Frequent removal of manure and old bedding and disinfecting contaminated barns, pens, calf hutches, and other outbuildings may be the only effective way to break a disease cycle and prevent future cases of disease. If a sick animal has been confined for treatment, the facility should be thoroughly cleaned after the animal has been removed and before using disinfectant. It does little good to disinfectant dirty walls or a barn floor, for instance, since organic matter like straw and manure inactivates many disinfectants and gives pathogens a refuge from germicidal products. Accumulated grime on stall surfaces can be removed by scrubbing or steam cleaning, especially if you use a detergent solution. Soap helps wet the material more completely and breaks organic debris into small particles that more readily wash away. Once the facility has been cleaned out and washed, a chemical disinfectant will be more effective.

Choose a disinfectant most appropriate for the job. In a dairy barn, for instance, it must not have a strong odor or it may taint the milk. A disinfectant strong enough to clean a barn stall may be too toxic for use on feed buckets or water tubs.

Common Disinfectants

Lye and *lime,* both alkalis, have been used as organism-killing disinfectants for centuries, since a *pH* greater than 9 will inhibit most bacteria types and destroy many viruses.

▸ **Lye** is sodium hydroxide. A 2 percent solution can be added to hot or boiling water (1 pound [0.45 kg] of lye per 5.5 gallons [20.8 L] of water) for general use, but it takes a 5 percent solution to destroy anthrax *spores.* Concentrated lye is caustic and poisonous and must be handled with care. It will damage painted or varnished surfaces, textiles, and aluminum.

▸ **Lime** (calcium oxide) in powdered form is inexpensive and can be sprinkled over a barn floor or pen for general disinfection.

▸ **Halogens** include chlorine and iodine and their compounds. Iodine is more effective in the presence of organic matter; chlorine (as in bleach) works well to kill bacteria, fungi, viruses, and most spores, but its effectiveness is greatly reduced unless surfaces are cleaned first. The potency of iodine is related to the amount of free iodine present. Tincture of iodine (2 percent iodine in alcohol) is a very effective *antiseptic,* but 7 percent (strong tincture of iodine) has greater antibacterial action. *Iodophors* are combinations of iodine and detergents. They are nonstaining and nonirritating and are often referred to as "tamed" iodine.

▸ **Coal- and wood-tar derivatives** include phenol (carbolic acid), cresol (such as Lysol) and sodium orthophenylphenate. The latter is effective against *tuberculosis* bacteria.

DISINFECTANT DISPOSAL

Follow label directions for disposal of empty jugs. Do not reuse containers for any purpose. Some product containers, like jugs of Nolvasan, can be rinsed with water and disposed of as trash or recycled with cans and bottles. Iodine containers are quite toxic and should not be recycled.

▸ **Other disinfectants** include alcohols, which are often used for cleaning and disinfecting skin or instruments; chlorhexadine (Nolvasan), which is active against a wide variety of microbes, not inactivated by small quantities of organic matter, and is relatively nontoxic to humans and animals; and formaldehyde solution. The latter can be used as a liquid (Formalin) on surfaces or a gas for fumigating a building. Hydrogen peroxide sometimes used on wounds or cleaned surfaces but is more effective as a cleaning agent than as a disinfectant.

Before using any type of disinfectant, become familiar with its properties and methods for use. Each one has advantages and disadvantages; some are much better for certain purposes than others. When in doubt, ask your veterinarian for advice.

Vaccination

There's a growing movement among stockmen to forego the use of *antibiotics* and other drugs in order to produce *natural* and organic meat and milk. Some people think this means not using vaccines, but this is a dangerous misconception. Vaccination is one of the tools a livestock producer must use to keep animals healthy and to eliminate the need for antibiotic treatment. Maximizing immune response with a carefully considered vaccination program raises the threshold for disease invaders, reducing the need for antibiotics and increasing the percentage of calves that meet criteria for a natural production program. Producing natural or *organic beef* and milk demands a strong emphasis on preventive vaccination programs.

There are some deadly or debilitating diseases that animals may be exposed to even in an isolated and well-managed herd. Some of these diseases are brought onto your farm by wildlife (such as leptospirosis; see chapter 4), or insects (see chapter 7), or bacterial spores that are ever-present in the environment (see chapter 4). Vaccination is the only way to prevent these diseases. Develop a vaccination schedule as part of your total herd health.

The diseases that should concern you depend on your location and your herd's risk for transmission. One or two animals in your backyard, having no contact with other members of their species, may not have as much risk for certain diseases as a large herd that constantly has new animals introduced.

Discuss this with your vet when deciding which vaccines are essential for your animals and work with him or her to develop the best health program for your herd. He or she can recommend the most appropriate products and vaccination schedule for your situation, while maximizing the animals' response. A good preventive health program not only helps to maintain a healthy herd but also serves to reduce the chance of outbreaks that could be financially devastating.

Types of Vaccines

Most vaccines are created from disease pathogens themselves. They contain antigens — proteins from a virus or bacterium — and prevent disease by stimulating the immune system to produce antibodies to fight the pathogen. A vaccine usually contains the pathogen or parts of it in inactivated form; the body recognizes the pathogen and builds a defense, but the pathogen has been previously rendered harmless enough to make it incapable of causing the disease.

There are currently a number of vaccines available, including killed products, modified live products, and *toxoids.*

▶ **Killed vaccines** are generally more stable in storage than modified live products and are safer for pregnant cows, but they usually require two doses (an initial vaccination and a booster) in order to stimulate immunity. Killed vaccines are safer, in general, than modified live vaccines because they do not have the potential for contamination that might cause an outbreak of actual disease, as has occasionally happened with bad batches of *modified live-virus vaccines.*

▶ **Modified live-virus** products generally are administered in single doses (except for IBR, which requires boosters, since this vaccine doesn't give long-lasting immunity) and develop a faster cell-mediated immune response than killed products do. The live organism can replicate; it multiplies the modified virus within the body and produces a subclinical form of disease. This triggers a broad immunity that involves both a humoral and a cell-mediated response. Ideally, the animal

> ## One Piece of the Whole
>
> Vaccination is one part of a total program. Don't expect complete disease protection to come from a bottle of vaccine. Disease prevention for many infections such as scours or weaning-related pneumonia comes from management practices augmented by vaccination. Vaccine is like the cherry on top of an ice-cream sundae; it's the last thing you put on. Yet it's often the first thing people do because it's easiest. You may end up with sick animals if you're expecting too much from vaccination and not concentrating on total herd management.

develops strong immunity without actually getting the disease.

Modified live virus vaccines once were thought to produce the strongest, longest-lasting immunity, but some killed vaccines also generate a strong, long-lasting response depending upon the product's additive (see box on next page). Some killed products provide a complete response, and sometimes, better humoral immunity than modified live virus vaccines.

Modified live vaccines usually come in two bottles: a dehydrated (freeze-dried) product and a vial of *diluent* fluid to insert into the dry product to rehydrate it just before use. Once mixed, it must be used within an hour or the live product may no longer be viable. Modified live products must be handled with great care; they can be inactivated by sunlight, heat, and chemical disinfectants.

▶ **Toxoids,** a third type of vaccine, are created for diseases in which the lethal component is a *toxin* produced by bacteria, rather than the bacteria themselves. The vaccine (toxoid) protects against the effects of the toxin. Examples of the toxoid vaccine are the *tetanus* and the seven- and eight-way *clostridial* vaccines.

New vaccines are becoming available that take advantage of technology that allows more fine tuning of killed or modified live-virus products.

- **Subunit vaccines** contain only the immunological components necessary to trigger protective immune response without the actual infection.
- **Gene-deleted vaccines** use technology that isolates and removes disease-producing genes in bacteria or virus, while keeping components that stimulate immunity.
- **Virus-vectored vaccines** are products in which immunity-producing genes of a pathogen are placed in a transport virus that takes this material into the body. The transporting virus is harmless but serves as a route to get immunizing material into the vaccinated animal. As science progresses, safer, more effective vaccines will become available. Your vet can advise you on what's best to use for your situation.

Handling and Using Vaccines

To be effective, vaccines must be properly handled — not only by you but also by wholesalers and retailers. Because they must be shipped in a cool, well-insulated container, be sure to buy from reputable suppliers so you know they're fresh and have been kept at proper temperature. Keep vaccines in a cooler with a cool pack while traveling home.

- **Follow label directions** for storage, mixing, and injection. Check expiration dates; buy only what you need right away. Vaccines kept beyond their expiration date may lose potency. Some medications have a long shelf life and may be effective beyond expiration dates, but most vaccines have a short storage life. Always use a vaccine before its expiration date, and when you buy it, make sure it has an expiration date that won't go by before you use it. Plan far enough ahead so you can purchase or order the product you need and won't have to settle for something at the last minute that's not ideal for your vaccination program and schedule.
- **Keep vaccines refrigerated** until use, within temperature ranges stated on the label. When using them, keep them cool and out of the sun. Direct sunlight (heat, ultraviolet rays) may inactivate modified live-virus vaccines. Keep the vaccine and syringes in the shade, in a Styrofoam chest, or in a cardboard box with an ice pack or a plastic jug of frozen water in one corner to keep it cool. An insulated cooler is also wise on a cold day to keep vaccine from freezing. If it's really cold, put a jug of warm water in the insulated picnic box. Then if your needle freezes up between uses, you can stick it in warm water to thaw it.
- **Don't mix different vaccines;** one may have ingredients that inactivate the other. Combo products that protect against several diseases at once work well, but don't mix two different products yourself.

VACCINE ADDITIVES

Since a killed vaccine does not stimulate a strong immune response, adjuvants and immune stimulation compounds are usually added. An adjuvant is a substance that holds the antigen at the injection site and slows the breaking down or removal of the vaccine. If antigens are absorbed over a longer period, the body continues to produce protective antibodies.

There are several types of adjuvants, but the most common are aluminum hydroxide and oil. An aluminum hydroxide gel absorbs the antigen and holds it on its outer surface, keeping it at the injection site for about two weeks. Vaccines that contain aluminum adjuvants include toxoids, whole-culture bacterins, and inactivated viral vaccines, all of which are relatively stable when cool or at room temperature, but when they are frozen, the hydrated structure of the gel can be destroyed.

Oil emulsions are also used; oil absorbs some of the antigen, holds it on the outer surface, and keeps it there for about a month. Oil-based vaccines often produce longer immunity and provoke a greater immune response because the oil acts as an immunostimulant. As long as the antigen is continually presented to the immune system, it continues to stimulate immunity. The drawbacks to oil-based vaccines are a higher incidence of temporary swelling at the injection site and *cyst* and small nodule (*granuloma*) formation. Some vaccines also contain an immune stimulant that helps rouse the immune system into a stronger, quicker response following vaccination.

If you are giving two or more vaccines at the same time, use different syringes or needles for each, to make sure you never mix them up or fill the wrong one with a different product. If traces of a *bacterin* are left in a syringe later used for a modified live-virus product, the bacterin can destroy effectiveness of the vaccine. Color code syringes or mark them to make sure you know which one you are filling and using to avoid accidental mixing or giving the incorrect dose.

▶ **When giving multiple injections,** use different locations at least 4 inches (10.2 cm) apart. If different products are injected too close together, they may react with one another and hinder proper response or cause tissue damage. To avoid contamination, make sure injection sites are clean and dry. Don't use the same needle for injecting and for filling a syringe or you may contaminate contents of the vaccine bottle. When filling a syringe, remove any air trapped in it. Hold the syringe with the needle straight up and push the plunger until all air is out, or pump a little vaccine back into the bottle in this upright position so you won't waste any vaccine as you are pushing the air out. Air in the syringe interferes with giving the correct dose and increases the chance that it may not stimulate immune response.

▶ **If a product must be reconstituted,** use a sterile transfer needle to make the process easier and cleaner. Place one end of the needle into a bottle of sterile diluent and the other end into the bottle of freeze-dried vaccine so that the diluent will flow down into the dried vaccine. A vacuum in the freeze-dried portion immediately pulls diluent into the vial. If not, this may be a sign the vaccine is contaminated or no good. Discard it. Keep the transfer needle in a clean place in your box between uses.

▶ **When using large vials containing multiple doses,** shake and mix thoroughly before use, and take time to shake the bottle now and then as you use it. Otherwise the product may settle, giving an inconsistent amount of antigen in each dose.

▶ **To clean the syringes and needles,** use hot water (at least 180°F [82.2°C]) or boiling water to sterilize them. Don't use disinfectants in syringes that

will be used for modified live-virus vaccines. Don't use mineral oil to lubricate them. Hot water is really the only safe option for cleansing and lubricating. When using killed-vaccine products, keep a sponge nearby and wipe the needle with disinfectant between animals, but don't use a disinfectant with modified live vaccines or it may destroy the effectiveness of the vaccine. Use clean, disposable needles (a new one for each animal) or change needles after 10 to 15 uses. Keep plenty of new needles on hand.

▶ **Use a needle of proper size and length** for the job. A needle that's too small in diameter may bend or break. An overly large needle damages more tissue and increases the risk that vaccine will leak out. If a needle bends or gets dull or blunt, discard it, or it will tear tissue and create more risk for injection-site problems. Neck shots can be difficult to give in many squeeze chutes. If

Is Your Refrigerator Working?

It's okay to use an old refrigerator to store vaccine, but make sure it still works efficiently; some old units freeze the items placed near the cooling unit. If the door doesn't seal well, items stored in the door may get too warm in summer.

A refrigerator in an unheated barn during an extended cold spell may freeze your vaccine even if the unit is working properly. Also, in a refrigerator that's seldom opened, the temperature may creep downward, just as the temperature will creep upward if the door is opened frequently. Vaccines stored in the door will be warmer, while vaccines placed near the freezer compartment will be colder.

Freezing or warmth can destroy the potency of most vaccines; they are meant to be stored between 35 and 45°F (1.7 and 7.2°C). Vaccines usually contain an adjuvant to enhance the immune response, and freezing may cause it to separate from the antigen in the vaccine. In some instances freezing may also increase the amount of free endotoxin in a bacterin, increasing the potential for an adverse reaction.

an animal moves, there's risk of ramming the syringe against the chute, which could bend or break the syringe or needle. Your chute may need to be modified for vaccinations.

▶ **Don't keep partially used vials** unless they were opened in a clean manner, were touched only by a sterile needle, were kept refrigerated, and are *not* live-virus vaccines. Empty live-virus vials should be burned. Keep records of all vaccinations and the date they were given. For more information on giving injections, see chapter 2.

Immunization Considerations

Vaccination is no guarantee an animal will be protected from a specific disease. To be effective, vaccines must be given to healthy animals of proper age,

Why Vaccines Fail

Your vaccination program may fail if:

- You use a vaccine with the wrong strain or wrong antigens for the disease you are trying to prevent

- You give the vaccine via the wrong route, such as giving an intramuscular product subcutaneously or a subcutaneous product between layers of skin

- You store the vaccine improperly, expose it to heat, rehydrate it too far ahead of being used, or expose it to chemical disinfectants

- The animal suffers from malnutrition, mineral deficiencies, parasites, or other disease, or has been mistreated or stressed during handling

- A booster was not given as directed; many vaccines require two injections a few weeks apart before immune response is stimulated

- Maternal antibodies from colostrum interfere with development of active immunity in calves

- The animal was already exposed and incubating the disease at the time of vaccination or shortly after; there may be a lag time of one to two weeks before the immune system starts producing antibodies

with healthy immune systems capable of mounting a response to the vaccine and creating antibodies. The immune system can produce an immune reaction to thousands of different antigens, but each animal is limited by heredity regarding the number of antigens it can react to and the extent of reaction to each antigen. If you vaccinate a thousand calves of similar size, age, and physical condition, each will react differently. Some will produce extremely good immunity, a few will produce no immunity, and the majority will range somewhere in between.

Immune failure can result if animals are too stressed at the time they're vaccinated. Anything that hinders the immune system — wet, cold, or hot weather; extreme fluctuations in temperature; being weaned, dehorned, *castrated,* or shipped at the same time you vaccinate; malnutrition; trace-mineral deficiency; *dehydration;* illness; infection with BVD; parasites; fatigue — may thwart the animal's ability to develop immunity.

In some instances vaccinated animals may still get the disease if faced with an overwhelming level of pathogens, as in a contaminated environment. Sanitary conditions are necessary or vaccination may be ineffective. Vaccination should be given well ahead of exposure to a disease, since it takes about two weeks for a protective level of antibodies to be produced. Vaccines to protect cows from diseases that cause *abortion* should be given at least two to three weeks prior to breeding. Vaccines to protect calves during the stress of weaning should be given two to three weeks before weaning.

When killed vaccines are used, it generally takes two doses given several weeks apart to provide protection. If the first dose is given at or before weaning and the second two weeks later, calves won't have full protection until three to four weeks after the first dose and may not be protected during weaning stress. If you vaccinate *after* a disease appears in the herd or vaccinate newly acquired animals exposed to the disease before you got them, it won't kick in soon enough to prevent illness or halt an outbreak.

The key to keeping cattle healthy is to keep the level of resistance (immunity) above the level of the disease challenge. Immunity acquired through natural exposure or vaccination gradually diminishes.

How long it lasts depends on how high the level was initially, and the nature of the antigen. Some produce stronger and longer-lasting immunity. Once a calf is properly immunized against blackleg, for instance, he may be safe the rest of his life. By contrast, animals vaccinated against lepto may be susceptible again in 10 months.

Usually after an animal has been immunized against a certain antigen he responds more quickly and effectively to subsequent exposures. Repeated booster shots maintain immunity if given at proper intervals. Outbreaks of disease occur when immunity levels are dropping as the disease challenge is rising. Acquired immunity is never absolute; resistance developed via vaccination can be overcome if the challenge is great enough. A calf with immunity can still become ill if exposed to a large number of potent pathogens.

If there are vaccines for a certain disease, use them to maintain high resistance. For diseases with no vaccines, your main defense is to reduce the challenge level by cattle in a clean environment and preventing exposure to that disease if possible. Reducing the challenge through application of other arms of disease management is always necessary, since high exposure to disease can still overwhelm an animal's resistance if vaccination is the only tool used.

Vaccination Reactions

Sometimes an animal has an allergic reaction to an antigen; this can be serious or fatal. The first sign is difficult breathing, followed by collapse. The animal goes into anaphylactic shock (which affects the whole body) and needs immediate treatment with *epinephrine* and steroids to help reverse that condition. These should be kept on hand when you vaccinate, since there usually isn't time to call your vet. Some animals recover spontaneously without treatment, some recover if treated, but a few die even with treatment because the reaction is swift.

More commonly, a reaction is a local response to the *adjuvant* — a substance added to vaccines to slow absorption and increase immune response. Oil-based vaccines, for instance, often produce longer-lasting immunity than vaccines using other adjuvants but may cause swelling, and sometimes permanent lumps, at the injection site (see chapter 2).

VACCINATE ONLY THE HEALTHY

When giving vaccines, vaccinate only healthy animals that are not under stress. Anything that hinders the immune system's ability to mount a strong response to vaccine — severe weather, weaning, heavy parasite load, illness — may result in inadequate protection for the animal. In young cattle, especially, it's important to give vaccinations before they are stressed, such as two to three weeks ahead of weaning or shipping.

Vaccination for the Adult Cattle

There are basic vaccines every stockman should use once or twice a year to protect cows. These include vaccines for IBR-BVD and leptospirosis because they are encountered in every geographic region and can cause abortion. You should also vaccinate against other diseases found in your area. You may need to give pregnant cows a scour vaccine so newborn calves obtain antibody protection via their dams' colostrum. Work with your veterinarian to customize a vaccination program for your individual herd. The time of year to vaccinate may depend on whether you calve in spring or fall.

Don't forget to vaccinate bulls and steers. In most instances, they need the same vaccinations as your cows and heifers, except for pre-calving scours vaccines.

Several important vaccines should be given to cows a few weeks before breeding; vaccinating at that time provides maximum protection during early pregnancy, when these diseases are most likely to affect the fetus. Keep in mind that modified live-virus IBR-BVD vaccines should not be given to pregnant animals, making the period before breeding ideal for administration of those vaccines. A five-way leptospirosis vaccine should also be given at that time. If your farm has conditions that make lepto a concern — ponds, areas of stagnant water, or plentiful wildlife — you may need to vaccinate for lepto two or three times a year.

If your cows are all calving at a certain time of year, this makes a vaccination program easier; they can be vaccinated at the same time because they're all at the same stage of pregnancy or between

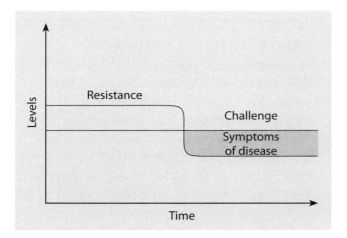

Disease symptoms occur when the resistance level of the herd is lowered and falls below the line of challenge.

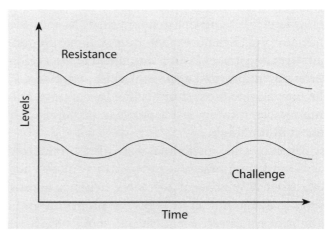

A healthy herd exists when the resistance level of the animals remain above the disease-challenge level.

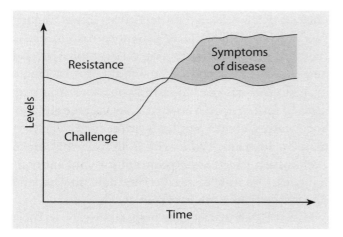

Symptoms of the disease occur when the level of the disease challenge is raised above the level of resistance.

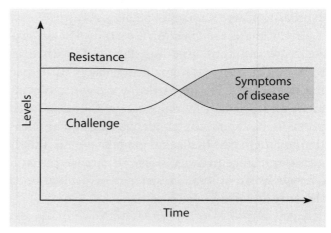

Disease symptoms occur when the resistance level is lowered and the disease challenge is raised simultaneously.

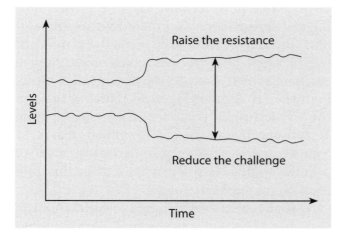

Herd health programs provide a comfortable spread between the resistance and the disease-challenge levels.

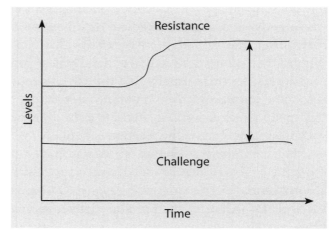

Rise in resistance due to vaccination helps widen the spread between resistance and disease challenge.

pregnancies. If you calve year round (as in some dairies), this makes it harder to maintain a schedule for herd vaccinations. You must keep records on each cow and vaccinate her at the proper time.

You may need to vaccinate twice a year for *redwater*, a highly fatal clostridial disease, depending on the region. If there is a possibility that shared bulls will breed cows on public ranges or in pastures where cattle from multiple ranches are all run together, vaccinate the cows against sexually transmitted diseases such as *vibriosis (campylobacteriosis)*. You don't always know the vaccination status or disease risk of your neighbor's bulls. Information on vaccination for specific diseases is found in later chapters under each type of disease.

Combine Vaccination and Regular Checkup

A good time to vaccinate cows is while they are in the chute being tested for pregnancy. They can also be treated for lice, worms, *grubs*, and liver flukes (see chapter 7) at this time, if your vet recommends it. It's best to find out if a cow is pregnant before you administer these products; there's no point in wasting money on vaccines and other treatments if she'll soon be sold because she is open or has some other problem. She should not receive vaccines or *pesticide* treatments if she'll be sold for slaughter before their *withdrawal times* (number of days before all traces of residue have left the body) are past.

While the vet is there, have your heifer calves vaccinated for brucellosis if this is required in your state. This is also a good time to check cows for problems that might affect future health or production. As they go through the chute check:

- Eyes for injury, *pinkeye,* or signs of early cancer (see chapter 9); most eye problems can be successfully treated in early stages
- Face and jaw lumps to see if they're bony infections or soft tissue abscesses that can be drained (see chapter 13)
- Teeth on older cows that seem to be losing weight; a cow that's lost some teeth may not be able to chew feed properly and won't be in good condition for breeding or *lactating*
- *Body condition* to see if cows ended the summer fat or thin; this helps you decide whether to wean calves early so cows can regain weight before cold weather

A checkup gives you a chance to make management decisions that will improve herd health and affect profit or loss. You can have "hands on" every cow and have a better sense of what's happening with the herd. This is also the time to make culling decisions if cows have bad teeth, *bony lump jaw,* bad eyes, bad *udders,* or other undesirable traits.

SAMPLE VACCINATION SCHEDULE FOR COWS

VACCINE	WHEN TO ADMINISTER
IBR-BVD	Modified live virus vaccine is given after calving and at least 3 weeks before breeding. Killed virus vaccine can be given any time during pregnancy and may be needed twice annually.
Lepto (5-way)	Can be given any time of year. Cows in some regions need 2 or more boosters annually.
Clostridia	Not needed for adults that had calfhood vaccinations unless redwater is a problem; in those regions cattle need 2 or more boosters annually.
Scours prevention	Needed only if there's herd history of rotavirus, coronavirus, or E. coli scours in baby calves. Vaccination given to pregnant cows 2 to 4 weeks before calving. Some products require initial 2-shot series (with last dose just before calving) and annual booster thereafter.
Vibriosis	Needed only if there's a herd history of disease. Given 2 to 4 weeks before breeding, though some products have a longer window of protection.

Vaccination Tips

Do not give modified live-virus injected vaccines to pregnant cows; the risk of abortion is lessened with intranasal vaccines. They are safe for pregnant cows, newly weaned calves, and yearlings experiencing a respiratory-disease outbreak. Immune response begins in 18 to 36 hours, whereas most intramuscular or subcutaneous vaccines take 7 to 21 days for protective immunity. Be aware that a disadvantage to intranasal vaccines is shorter-lasting immunity.

Killed-virus vaccines are beneficial if cows were not vaccinated before breeding. Give clostridial vaccines subcutaneously, because there's often a local reaction and inflammation at the injection site. Give all vaccines at the side of the neck; that way, if there's any tissue damage, abscess, or scarring, it can be easily trimmed out of the carcass at slaughter, without sacrificing better cuts of meat, such as the rump (see chapter 2).

Vaccination for Calves

Age is an important factor in calfhood vaccination. A calf less than 3 weeks old may not be able to develop immunity to clostridial disease if he got antibodies via his dam's colostrum because the cow was vaccinated, unless he's given an oil-based vaccine (see above). A calf less than 6 months old may not develop antibodies against IBR if his dam was vaccinated and had antibodies in colostrum. Those antibodies do protect the calf temporarily from disease, but they can also neutralize antigens in the vaccine if you vaccinate him when he's too young.

In many instances his immune system does not bother to mount a response (to make antibodies against the injected antigen) because he's already protected via passive immunity from the colostrum. A calf vaccinated when he's very young should be revaccinated a few weeks later. Most calfhood vaccinations should be repeated after the calf is 6 months old (such as a few weeks before weaning) to boost immunity. Follow label directions, and also ask your vet for advice.

The most important vaccine to give every calf is for blackleg (see chapter 4), because these clostridial bacteria may lurk anywhere and this disease is almost always fatal. With blackleg, the first dose is routinely given between 8 and 16 weeks of age (though it can be given earlier if you have a problem with this disease on your farm), with a booster at weaning time. Some stockmen also give another booster to heifers before they are bred for the first time. These calfhood vaccinations usually give lifelong protection.

Most stockmen vaccinate calves against IBR and BVD. If you wean calves before you sell them, they

Palpation, Ultrasound, or Blood Test?

For many years, rectal palpation was the only way to see whether a cow or heifer was pregnant. Then ultrasound came into use, and though it's more expensive, it has the advantages of being less invasive and detecting pregnancy sooner.

Now there's a blood test. A small sample (2 or 3 cc) of blood is taken from a vein under the tail and sent to a lab to check for the presence of a hormone produced by the placenta. The samples can be taken by the stockman, the test is cheaper and more accurate than ultrasound, and it can be done earlier in the pregnancy than palpation.

There are also health advantages to the blood test: There's no risk to the embryo/fetus, which is sometimes bruised or killed by palpation, and no risk for diseases transferred from one female to another. Rectal palpation always carries the risk of spreading diseases (such as BVD, lymphosarcoma, and others), unless the person completing the procedure changes gloves for each female — a precaution most people don't have time to take.

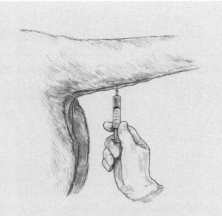

Draw a small blood sample from a vein under the tail, and send it to the lab to determine if a cow is pregnant.

may also need vaccination against various respiratory problems, such as PI3 and *Pasteurella*. In some instances, you may need to vaccinate calves against respiratory diseases as early as 8 weeks of age for adequate protection. Most stockmen use respiratory vaccines a few weeks before weaning to give calves more protection during weaning stress, with another booster at weaning time to maximize protective immunity.

It's a common practice to give boosters, because maternal antibodies from colostrum still circulating in the body and the immature immune system of young calves can hinder a calf's ability to respond to vaccines. A good rule of thumb: If an animal has not been sold by 12 months of age, he should be boostered with vaccinations for all common diseases. This would be the case if you keep calves to sell as yearlings or if you are keeping replacement heifers.

In some instances and states, you should vaccinate all heifer calves against brucellosis *(Bang's disease)* between 2 and 10 months of age. Even if your state does not require this, vaccinating all heifers may make them more valuable and is a good marketing strategy; you and your buyer have more options for where they can be sold. This vaccine must be given by a veterinarian; consult with him or her about the requirements. In certain regions you should vaccinate all calves against lepto, but usually this vaccine is only necessary for replacement heifers.

Carefully timing initial shots and boosters to produce maximum immunity is key to a successful vaccination program. Try to protect calves when they are at greatest risk, bolstering their immune system before they are exposed to that risk. For the young animal it is especially crucial that you follow vaccine label directions regarding timing and number of boosters.

Talk with your vet about all vaccinations. Unless you are familiar with the vaccine, you may not know when to use which products. You need to understand the vaccine, what it is supposed to do, and how to use it.

Minimizing Stress

Stress is a hidden enemy when raising animals. It can interfere with feed consumption and feed efficiency (ratio of pounds of feed to pounds of weight gain), weight gain, reproduction, and immunity, increasing the risk for disease. If susceptible animals with little disease resistance are highly stressed at the same time they're exposed to a disease challenge, they usually become rapidly and severely sick.

Many things stress cattle physically, including bad weather, inadequate nutrition, and more. Weather stresses are discussed at length in chapter 3. Nutritional stress occurs when the animal does not receive proper nutrients in adequate amounts for normal body function. Psychological stress occurs when cattle experience overcrowding, disruption of normal social patterns, weaning, or the fear and anxiety that result from improper handling.

The immune system is a complex mechanism that protects the animal from most diseases under

SAMPLE VACCINATION SCHEDULE FOR CALVES

VACCINE	WHEN TO ADMINISTER
Blackleg or eight-way clostridial	The first dose is given at 8 to 16 weeks of age (or earlier if needed), with the second dose at weaning.
Brucellosis (Bang's disease)	This is for heifers, 2 to 10 months of age.
IBR, BVD, PI3, BRSV	Killed vaccine can be used if given preweaning. Modified live virus can be used at weaning or after, though there are now a few products that have been approved for use on preweaned calves.
Lepto (5-way)	This vaccine is needed only if there's a herd history of calves sick or lost from lepto. Vaccine can be given at the same time as blackleg vaccine to young calves or after weaning.

ordinary circumstances. But stress can hinder normal workings of the immune system. One of the body's defenses against stress is production of a *hormone* called cortisol (a *corticosteroid*). During the short term, this hormone changes the body's *metabolism* in several ways to help it function better under stress. It temporarily increases *blood glucose,* for example, which can be used as energy by the animal.

But over a longer period of time, the extra production of cortisol can be detrimental and has negative effects on the immune system if stress is prolonged. Excess cortisol hinders the creation of antibodies and white blood cells — part of the body's defense against pathogens. *Steroids* such as cortisol in high doses also keep white blood cells from leaving the bloodstream and having contact with viruses and bacteria at the tissue level. The lungs are especially vulnerable to effects of stress and lower resistance to disease, since harmful organisms are a natural part of an animal's environment, and some pathogens are always present in the respiratory tract, just waiting for an opportunity to invade the tissues.

One of the most common causes of stress to livestock is human handling. We have an agenda we need to meet; we move, drive, work, vaccinate, brand, dehorn, tag, castrate, deworm, wean, and transport cattle. That's a lot of work for humans and animals, and it can be stressful for both.

It's important not to double up stresses. Calves should not be dehorned, castrated, or branded at the same time you wean them, for instance. The least stressful time to castrate and dehorn is when calves are young, horns buds are small, and there is little blood supply to testicles. If calves are weaned and transported at the same time, stress is compounded. Stressed calves that are not completely immunized against respiratory viruses before being transported are three times more likely to develop pneumonia than fully vaccinated calves.

Low-Stress Cattle Handling

One of the best ways to reduce stress is to adopt a program of conscientious cattle handling while gathering, treating, and processing them. Understanding how your cattle respond to various situations will reduce stress on both you and your herd.

One way that animal behavior affects cattle production lies in an animal's learned response to a negative experience. If your cattle have been in a situation where they are fearful or highly stressed, they will remember it vividly, and that memory will affect their reactions to the same or similar experiences later. For example, if you had to run them all over the place to get them into the corral or beat them with a stick to make them go down through the chute, they will be more fearful and reluctant the next time they see or hear you or find themselves faced with that or a similar situation.

By contrast, if they are treated gently and with patience, they become more at ease. Feedlots that have schooled their cowboys and pen riders in low-stress cattle-handling methods and proper techniques for cattle-checking have cut their death losses in half.

Ways to Reduce Handling Stress

▶ **Use properly designed facilities.** Make sure all corrals and chutes are designed to ease movement and sorting of cattle. Eliminate square corners where cattle crowd up and may be injured. A long chute should be curved to help keep cattle moving forward; if they can't see what's up ahead

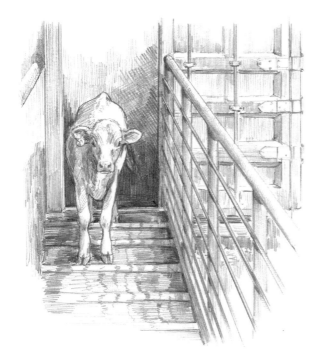

Transportation stress after a long trip can result in illness.

they aren't so apt to balk. The chute should not be too narrow or too wide or cattle will try to turn around. The chute and squeeze chute should have good footing and traction, so animals won't slip and be injured. If those areas are concrete, they should be deeply grooved to keep animals from slipping.

- **Keep things quiet.** Make sure all moving parts of the squeeze chute are lubricated for smooth operation and lower noise level. Don't shout. If you use dogs to gather cattle, keep them away from the cattle once they are in the corral. Barking dogs or even the presence of a dog when you are working cattle can make them more unruly and stressed.

- **Train your herd.** Have a training session for heifers that you plan to keep as cows. Bring them quietly into working facilities, and move them through the chute without doing anything to them. This helps them get used to the process with minimal bad memories — and they'll know what to expect when you put them through for actual vaccinating, tagging, and other procedures, and will be less fearful. Bring them into the corral a few times just to feed them, so they'll be at ease with coming in.

- **Make travel safe and calm.** Transportation stress at any age can result in illness, especially if cattle

must be in trucks or trailers for a long time. A short haul is always less stressful than a long one. Stress can be reduced if gathering is done quietly and trucks are ready to load once cattle are corralled.

Don't overcrowd trucks and trailers, and make sure trucks have nonslip floors to provide traction and minimize falling. If an animal does fall down, there should be enough room for him to get back up again. An overcrowded truck may make it impossible for a downed animal to rise. On the other hand, cattle also travel better

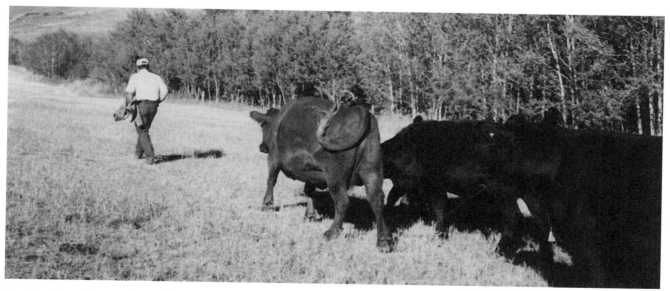

Gentle cattle can be moved or gathered with no stress at all. The easiest way to move cattle is to lead them. If they trust you, they will follow when you call them.

if they cannot move around too much. If loaded too loosely, they may constantly mill about and risk injury.

▶ **Spend time with your cattle.** Get them used to your walking through them or riding among them. This gentling process greatly reduces any stress associated with having humans close by, and they will be easier to handle.

The most important thing — even more important than chute designs — is learning how to work cattle properly. If they are handled correctly, they will simply follow one another right through any chute.

Gentle Cattle Are Less Stressed

Developing a herd of easy-handling, easygoing cattle involves genetic selection as well as gentle handling. It's typically easier to handle cattle and keep them stress-free if they've been selected and bred for mellow temperament. Some breeds and some individuals within breeds are more high-strung and flighty than others; they are more excitable and susceptible to stress. When you are selecting a new bull or heifers to keep as cows, evaluate each individual's disposition and the disposition of the sire and dam before you make your decision. If a cow in your herd is a problem to handle, don't keep her offspring, because you may find them to be hard to handle and more readily stressed as well.

Cattle, like horses, can be trained, and mellow ones are easier to train than flighty ones. If you always handle your cattle in a quiet, understanding way and avoid yelling and hurrying, the cattle become more at ease rather than more fearful. They'll go willingly into the corral and stay calm in the chute rather than trying to run in the wrong direction. Acquaint cattle to new things in a gradual and nonconfrontational way, and they will do what you want them to with minimal resistance.

An excitable animal may find a new experience frightening, whereas a calmer individual may tolerate it. Reactions are forged by a combination of genetic predisposition and previous experience. All animals remember rough handling and are more fearful and stressed during future handling, but thoughtless methods are especially detrimental to

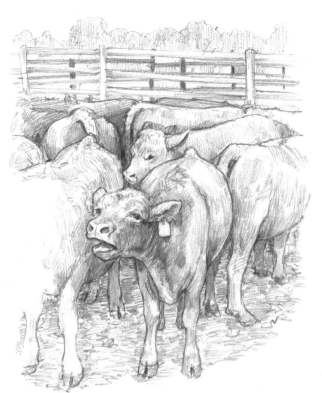

Traditional corral weaning is stressful for calves; they pace the fence or stand by the fence and bawl for their mothers.

cattle with an excitable temperament and can make calm individuals wild.

Although an extensive discussion of the topic of low-stress handling is beyond the scope of this book, there are many resources for the interested reader. Animal handler Bud Williams teaches stockmen proper, efficient, and stress-free ways to handle cattle. He wins the acclaim of many a rancher by modeling effective ways to influence single animals or a herd to do what the rancher wants them to do with little effort and minimal stress to the animals.

Temple Grandin, Colorado State University professor of animal science, has also helped pave the way for the movement toward low-stress handling. Over the past two decades, she's completed many scientific studies and designed scores of low-stress animal-handling facilities in her efforts to better understand animal behavior and to make humane animal handling the norm internationally.

Weaning

When cattle were wild, weaning was a gradual transition that took place when the cow's milk production diminished late in the season after grass was no longer green. Eventually she dried up or kicked her calf off, but he still tagged along with her and had the emotional security of Mama and the herd. In some instances a calf might continue nursing until the cow was nearly ready to give birth to her next calf, at which time she'd kick off the big calf. But he always had her nearby for companionship and security and was not emotionally stressed.

Today, weaning is a stressful time for calves. Unless care is taken to make this transition as easy as possible, they're vulnerable to disease. Traditional corral weaning — locking calves in a corral and taking their mothers away — is probably the most stressful way to wean. They pace the fence and bawl, often running frantically back and forth trying to find a way out to find their mothers. If corrals are dry, this churns up dust that irritates respiratory passages and opens the way for respiratory infections. If you haul the calves to a different place or sell them and leave cows in the pasture, the cows are not as stressed (they're still in familiar surroundings), but the calves will be very stressed. Transport with weaning at the same time is very hard on calves, and they're more likely to get sick.

A weaning calf is doubly susceptible to illness because stress hinders proper functioning of the immune system. Hot, cold, and wet weather are physical stressors, but the psychological stress of losing Mama also puts calves at risk for illness. A calf that's old enough to have a functional *rumen* and is able to digest forages can manage fine without milk; the nutritional stress of weaning is minimal. The larger problem is his emotional dependence on his mother.

The least stressful weaning enables calves to have the comfort of adults during the transitional period. This can be accomplished by taking only some of the cows out of the herd at once or by fenceline weaning on pasture. With fenceline weaning, cows and calves are put in adjacent pastures where they can still see and smell one another through the fence, but calves cannot nurse.

Calves are traditionally weaned at 6 to 9 months old. If they are weaned early, due to drought or some other situation, more care must be taken. Calves have a functional rumen by 4 months and can get their nutritional needs met without milk, but the emotional stress of being weaned this young can be very traumatic.

Pasture Weaning

A small pasture with lush grass is the best place to wean calves. Grass is a feed they're used to; they don't have to suddenly adjust to hay or grain. A green pasture is not dusty, so lung irritations are avoided. If pasture isn't green it can be supplemented with a little high-quality *alfalfa* hay.

Leaving calves in their familiar pasture and hauling the cows far enough away so their babies can't hear them bawling is one way to wean; calves continue to graze and aren't as stressed as if they can hear the cows. They go back to the spot they last nursed, looking for Mama and bawling, but soon give up. Since they don't know where she is, they're less likely to try to crawl through a fence to go to her. By contrast, if a calf can hear his mother, he'll try very hard to get through the fence to go to her. Cows may pace the boundaries of their new pasture wanting to go back to their calves, but if they're far away from them and don't know where they are, they soon settle down to graze. Some will return periodically to the fence and bawl, but after 2 to 4 days they usually resign themselves to the loss of their calves.

Another method entails taking a few mamas at a time away to graze where they can't see or hear their babies. The calves being weaned are left in familiar pasture with the rest of the herd for security. If the calf last saw Mama with the herd, he usually won't look any farther because he doesn't know which way she went and soon resigns himself to her absence. The last group to be weaned no longer has adult cows for security but has the calm, already weaned calves for company.

If all calves must be weaned at once, you can reduce stress by leaving a few babysitter cows with calves in the pasture. This gives calves security and companionship until their emotional crisis is past.

Fenceline Weaning

If the pasture is enclosed with a net-wire fence that calves can't crawl through (or any good fence with two electric wires along it on both sides so cattle won't press it), calves can be weaned in a pasture next to their mothers. They walk the fence for a day or so, looking and sniffing at each other, but green grass is available whenever they are hungry. The cows stay close to the fence for a while but also go off to graze.

Cows and calves both leave the fence to eat but come back to one another. As soon as they sniff noses through the fence, they settle down and are not so anxious; they have each other's company. They lie next to one another on opposite sides of the fence, chewing the *cud*. After a couple of days, fewer cows come to the fence to check on their calves, and soon the calves realize that they don't need Mama. After the third or fourth day you can move cows or calves to new pasture and they won't be stressed. Having their mamas next to them on green pasture for the first several days reduces the frantic pacing, running, and bawling behaviors typical of corral weaning.

Nose-Flap Weaning

Some stockmen wean calves using antisucking devices called *nose flaps*. This method allows contented calves to stay with their mothers while the milk dries up. Studies at the University of Saskatchewan and Montana State University in 2005 showed

SORTING TIP

When separating pairs for weaning, use adjacent pens so you can let cows exit through a gate into the next pen. Then if a calf slips past, he's not out in a big field where he can get away. If the cow pen gets too full before you are done sorting, periodically release groups of cows.

that this two-step process resulted in less stress on calves than did traditional weaning.

Calves are fitted with a nose flap made of flexible plastic, which keeps them from getting a teat in their mouths but does not interfere with grazing, eating, or drinking. Nose flaps (sold by Villa Nueva S.A., Villa Maria-Cordoba, Argentina) cost less than $1 each and can be reused (disinfect them between calves). They can be placed (and removed) in seconds once a calf is chute-restrained. Nose flaps should be left on for no longer than four or five days. Calves can then be removed from their mothers with little stress.

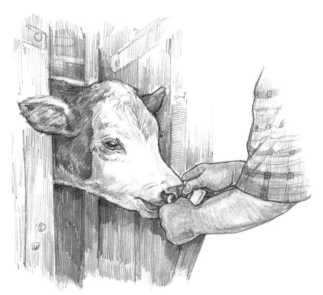

The rancher puts in the nose flap, which is made of flexible plastic and is used as an antisucking device.

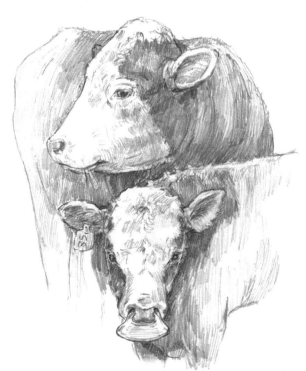

While wearing the nose flap, a calf cannot nurse his mother, but he can eat grass or hay and drink water — and still be with her for a few days as he adjusts to not having any milk.

Corral Weaning

If you have no alternative to weaning in a corral, there are ways to minimize stress and illness. First, plan ahead, and vaccinate calves against weaning-related respiratory diseases two or three weeks beforehand, while they're still with their mothers. This gives calves a chance to build stronger immunity before the stress (see pages 111–112). If you don't have an opportunity to vaccinate before weaning and are vaccinating calves at weaning that will be in a corral next to their mothers (nose-to-nose contact) or if any vaccinated calves will still be with pregnant cows, use killed vaccine that will not cause a pregnant cow to abort.

If calves will be weaned in a corral, inspect it ahead of time and make any necessary fence or gate repairs so they can't crawl out or injure themselves. Provide shade and a windbreak; if the pen is dusty, sprinkle it with water to settle the dust. Use a small pen to cut down on frantic pacing and running. If calves have lots of room to run and pace, they wear themselves out. Placing a few large bales of hay or straw along the fence will slow them down; they'll be more apt to stand and bawl instead of running frantically back and forth. Locate feed and water along the fence so they'll find it as they pace around; they may not go to the center of the corral because they're too busy trying to find a way out.

If the water supply is a trough or tank rather than a ditch or stream, make sure calves already know how to drink from this type of water source. If calves

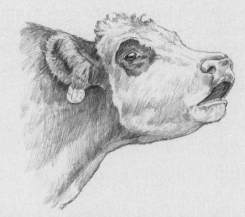

don't know how to drink from a trough, let it run over, as long as the overflow can drain away from the corral and not make a mud hole. Make a little ditch, if necessary, to take the flow out of the corral. The trickling water helps calves find the source and also keeps the water cleaner. A calf with a runny nose often leaves mucus in the water when he drinks; the snot floats on the water and can infect other calves. If you let it continually run over the tank, this infective material is flushed away.

Feed small amounts of hay several times a day rather than in one or two large feedings. Calves are attracted to fresh feed, so this way they'll eat more and waste less. They won't eat hay that's been slobbered on, walked on, laid on, or contaminated with manure and urine. They waste hay if you feed on the ground; they will be walking around a lot and trampling it. Use bunks or feeders to keep them from walking in it.

Take time to turn the hay over in the bunks between feedings, so there's always fresh hay on top. Your actions will stimulate calves' curiosity; they'll come to see what you are doing and will eat again. Calves that are already gentle and used to you wean with less stress than wilder ones not accustomed to people. Gentle ones come to you at feeding time and are more willing to eat. Wild calves run off when they see you and are upset at being confined; the combination of added stress and poor feed consumption makes them more likely to get sick.

Feed hay that's fine and palatable, not coarse or stemmy. Calves are fussy eaters and during times of stress eat even less. You want every mouthful to be nutritious. If they're not used to eating hay, put a babysitter cow or yearling with them. They'll feel less alone and frantic, and she'll show them the feed and water and encourage them by her example.

Corral Weaning Is Hard on Cows, Too

When you are sorting cows and calves in the corral for weaning purposes, even if you put cows back into their familiar pasture, they are stressed because they last saw their calves in the corral and will try to go back to them. If calves are still in the corral and the cows can hear them, they'll stand by the fence and bawl if the corral is adjacent or try to come through any fences that are in between. To save wear and tear on fences it's best to have the cows right next to the corral, even if calves have been hauled away, since cows will try to come back to where they last saw their calves. If they come back to the corral but do not find their calves or stand next to the corral and bawl but can't get to their calves, they give up and go back to grazing after a few days. If the calves are still in the corral, however, the calves may spend all their time bawling by the fence, trying to get to their mothers, instead of eating. They may continue to do this until the cows are finally taken away.

Even if you lock up the calves and drive the cows far away to where they can't hear one another, it's still stressful for both. The cows don't want to leave their calves and can be hard to drive. Calves will settle down in a few days because they don't know where their mothers went, but the cows are very upset because they know where their calves are and will try very hard to go back to them. Even if you drive them several miles, they remember the way. They'll stand by the gate or fence corner losing weight and trying to come through the fence instead of grazing. Unless it is a really good fence, some cows will get through it and come back to the corral. Every time a cow comes back home, all the calves hope it's their mama and will start bawling and pacing again.

CHAPTER TWO

Treatment Fundamentals

BEFORE YOU CALL A VETERINARIAN or decide to treat a sick animal yourself, you first need to determine that something is not right — that the animal has a problem. The best way to become a good judge of health and illness is to spend time with your cattle. If you know each animal as an individual, or at least observe her enough to have a feel for how she normally behaves, you'll have a much better chance of being able to recognize any abnormalities. Early detection and treatment often can make the difference between quick recovery and prolonged convalescence, and sometimes between life and death for the sick animal. Having an understanding of basic medications and how to properly administer them using restraint methods that ensure safety are also crucial to successful treatment.

Detecting Signs of Illness

Regularly seeing the herd when milking and feeding them, or when just walking or riding through, enables an observant stockman to recognize signs of health and detect subtle clues of early disease. Close observation and attention paid to small details are important. Not only will this help you become more proficient at assessing the health of your animals, but it can also be beneficial if you need to describe the symptoms of a sick animal to your veterinarian.

Alert or Dull?

A healthy cow or calf is bright and alert, has a good appetite, and comes eagerly at feeding time or is out grazing with the rest of the herd when they are foraging. Cattle generally graze in the morning, late afternoon, and evening, and lie down to chew the cud in the middle of the day, especially during hot weather. If an animal is slow to come to feed, or spends more time than her herdmates lying around instead of grazing or eating hay, this is a signal for you to take a closer look.

Unless it's a pregnant cow that leaves the herd to deliver her calf, a lone animal should be cause for concern. A sick or lame animal often leaves the group to find solitude, to avoid the jostling and pestering of bossier individuals. Curious herdmates, or subordinate animals that ordinarily defer to that individual, may take advantage of the ailment to chase the compromised individual around. Unable to defend herself, she goes off by herself.

A sick animal may be dull, with ears drooping instead of alert. If she's not chewing her cud, she may have pain, fever, or some type of digestive problem that halts rumen activity. An animal with a high fever will not chew her cud.

Any animal lying down when the rest of the herd is grazing or eating hay should be cause for suspicion. If she seems healthy and normal in other aspects, make her get up and walk a few steps to see if she's injured or suffering foot rot.

How Does She Move?

An animal that feels good will usually stretch when she gets up, and has an interest in her surroundings. She responds with curiosity to sounds and motion. She is alert and perky, and spends time licking and grooming herself. When traveling, she moves freely and easily, with energy.

By contrast, a sick animal may be dull, show a decreased interest in and response to things around her, and may look more tuned in to her own internal misery. She may stand with eyes closed and head drooping. If she has been lying down, she gets up slowly or with effort and may not stretch. She's usually too preoccupied with discomfort to lick herself. Movement may be slow and methodical with sparing effort or may appear pained. If you make her move, she may walk slowly rather than with her usual energy or friskiness. An animal experiencing pain, discomfort, or fever doesn't move "right" and doesn't have the sparkle of vitality and health exhibited by a normal animal.

A sick animal won't expend any more effort than necessary. If you're moving the herd from one pasture to another, the sick individual tends to end up at the rear, traveling more slowly. The more serious the illness, the more indifferent the animal may be to her surroundings and the more reluctant to move.

At the other extreme is an abnormally excited animal. If she is overly alert, abnormally anxious, constantly looking around or restless, this may be a sign that she's in constant pain or discomfort. This happens when a cow is in early labor or is suffering from some other condition that causes pain or distress. Abdominal pain may cause her to be restless, kicking at her belly or switching her tail, looking around at her *flanks*, or lying down and getting up repeatedly.

An animal bothered by flies may be restless, even to the point of running, tail in the air. She may stop suddenly and kick at her belly or swat at it with her head, trying to knock flies off. You may need to spend several moments observing to determine whether flies or internal pain are causing the restlessness and anxiety. A calf with *acute* gut pain from a toxic intestinal infection may run wildly and then throw himself to the ground or stop suddenly and kick at his belly. Excitability and running (along with abnormal behavior or running into walls or fences) can also be due to serious diseases like *rabies* that affect the brain and cause nervous disorders.

Respiration Rate

In the resting animal, respiration rate is a clue to sickness or health. On a hot day it may be hard to tell if a fast-breathing or panting animal is ill or merely hot. Cattle don't have as many sweat glands as horses or humans and must breathe faster or pant with an open mouth. They use air exchange in the lungs to cool themselves in hot weather; they draw the cooler outside air into their lungs when they inhale, and rid themselves of some of their body heat when they exhale. A hot animal will pant when traveling long distances, moving uphill, or after running.

You can compare respiration rates of nearby cattle to determine if there's a problem. Are the cows lying next to the panting one also breathing fast? Keep in mind that black cattle suffer more than lighter-colored cattle on a very hot day because black absorbs more heat. Previous exertion will also elevate a respiration rate. Appearance of the animal (dull or alert, ears up or down, nasal discharge) can give clues as to whether the animal is ill or is merely hot. If in doubt, restrain her and take her temperature, or check her later to see if her respiration rate slows after the heat of the day is past.

Abnormal breathing may be audible if the animal is struggling to draw air into the lungs through narrowed airways (wheezing) or is having difficulty forcing it out (grunting) due to compromised lungs. A respiratory problem may also cause the animal to make exaggerated flank movements.

OBSERVE WITHOUT BEING OBSERVED

To get a true picture of any animal, watch her before she's aware of your presence or she may become alert and focused on you. Instinctively, a sick animal that senses danger or feels challenged will attempt to look alert and might mask signs of illness. An animal that's very dull, with ears hanging down, may perk up as you approach, and you might not realize how sick she is. Stop and look at the herd before you get close, and before they notice you or feel challenged by your presence.

Eating Habits and Digestion

Scrutinizing an animal's eating habits is another way to determine health or sickness. Observe the animal to see if she is exhibiting any of the following behaviors that might signify illness:

▸ Does she chew and swallow properly, or is swallowing painful?

▸ Is saliva drooling or feed dropping from the mouth?

▸ Is she unable to belch up and chew the cud?

▸ Is cud spilling from the mouth?

▸ Is she coughing up food or regurgitating stomach contents out the nostrils?

▸ Is there difficulty (such as grunting or effort) in belching up the cud?

▸ Is she grinding her teeth?

▸ Are defecation and urination normal?

▸ **Teeth grinding** and overactive "chewing" are generally signs of belly pain, especially in calves. A calf with a digestive problem or gut pain will often grind his teeth, making a disagreeable grating sound.

▸ **Constipation** occurs with some digestive problems. Passing manure may be difficult, with straining and pain evident. Manure may be firm and dry or absent if there's gut blockage. To check for constipation, try to get the cow up, make her walk, and follow her to see if she passes manure. If she doesn't, there may be a problem.

▸ **Diarrhea** is common for a number of cattle ailments. Severe diarrhea in some cases may cause so much irritation to the rectum that the animal strains continuously and eventually the rectum prolapses.

▸ **Scant or absent urination** may be a result of dehydration due to diarrhea, or may occur when an animal has not been drinking enough. Urination may be difficult if there's obstruction or partial blockage of the urinary tract (such as by a *bladder stone*) or inflammation of the bladder or *urethra*. The animal may dribble small amounts of urine, remain in urinating position a long time, kick at the belly in pain, or stand stretched.

Posture

Abnormal posture in animals should be noted.

▸ **Resting a leg or sticking it out to the side** instead of putting full weight on it indicates a sore foot or leg and lameness.

▸ **Arching the back** with all four legs bunched under the body usually indicates abdominal pain or chest pain due to pneumonia.

▸ **Downward arching of the back** may mean the animal has severe abdominal pain.

▸ **Splayed out front legs** could mean chest pain or difficulty breathing.

▸ **Standing with the front end of the body uphill,** with front feet higher than hinds, allows for easier belching of gas and might be a sign that the animal is bloated.

▸ **Lying down in an abnormal or awkward position** may mean a sore or dislocated leg or an attempt to ease internal pain.

▸ **Lying on the breastbone** allows an animal with pneumonia to breathe easier.

▸ **Lying with the head tucked around** toward the flank is a common sleeping position of healthy animals, but it may mean she's not feeling well, especially if she's not sleeping.

▸ **Lack of desire to get up when approached** is usually a clue that an animal is sick, unless she's a pet and has total trust when people approach.

Don't Miss Small Clues

Much information can be gleaned from observing an animal's general attitude and behavior from a distance while she's preoccupied with her problems and before she becomes distracted and focuses attention on you. When checking cattle, try to get an overview of the group before you distract them by coming closer. Unobtrusive observation will allow you to take note of hints of problems. You can see if an animal is off by herself or acting in an abnormal way, is dull, or is in an unusual posture or position that might indicate pain or distress. Keep in mind that symptoms are not always typical. Uncommon presentation of common diseases are more often observed than common presentations of uncommon diseases.

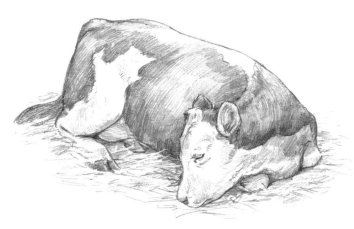

A sick animal may spend more time than usual lying down and may lie with the head tucked around to the side.

There is usually something different about a sick animal that brings her to your attention. These small clues should lead you to take a closer look at a specific animal to try to determine what might be wrong. It's this kind of awareness and careful checking that will help you discover early sickness, lameness, or some other problem that might need your attention and care.

There's no substitute for knowing your cattle well. And it helps to be tuned into bovine behaviors that can tell you about well-being. A head count or a once-over-lightly look at the herd without "seeing" each one as an individual won't do the trick. By the time the next day's observation rolls around, a sick

VITAL SIGNS

Many diseases affect pulse, temperature, and respiration. The first signs of illness may be mild and may go unnoticed, but with close attention paid to vital signs (taking the animal's pulse, respiration rate, and temperature, if need be), clues may be found.

A normal temperature for cattle ranges from 100.5 to 102°F, though 103 might be normal on a hot day. Unlike humans, ruminants have a wider range of normal temperatures because their digestion requires fermentation, which produces heat. A ruminant's body can safely accumulate heat up to a point (see chapter 3).

Fever is a temperature above normal; hypothermia is a temperature below normal. The temperature of cattle varies depending on the amount of physical activity, stage of pregnancy, time of day, and environmental temperature. In cattle, body temperature of 103.1 to 104.6 is considered a mild fever; 104.7 to 105.8 is a moderate fever; and 105.9 to 107 is a high fever. Usually temperature does not exceed 107°F in cattle, even in severe illness, except in heat stroke — in which the animal's temperature may get as high as 110 degrees.

A normal pulse rate in adult cattle is 40 to 80 beats per minute (100 to 120 for young calves).

A normal respiration rate for adult cattle on a cool day is 10 to 30 breaths per minute and up to 50 per minute on a moderately warm day. Higher rates are normal on a hot day; lower rates are normal on a cool day. Pulse and respiration rates also vary with age (young animals have faster heartbeat and respiration rates), the animal's activity, and the time of day.

TIPS FOR TAKING VITAL SIGNS

The pulse can be found with your fingers by pressing on certain areas of the body where superficial arteries are in soft tissue and can be pressed against the bone beneath them. To check pulse and temperature, a small calf can be held, but a larger animal should be in a chute.

TO CHECK RESPIRATION RATE:

- Watch flank or chest movements; each in-and-out movement counts as one breath
- Count the total number of breaths the animal takes in 15 seconds

Multiply by four the number of breaths that you counted in 15 seconds to figure the animal's respiration rate (breaths per minute)

TO CHECK TEMPERATURE:

- Tie a string to a rectal thermometer so you'll never lose it in the *rectum*
- Shake it down well below a normal reading before you insert it
- Spit in your hand and lubricate the thermometer with saliva or use a small dab of petroleum jelly

animal may be worse (or dead), or the ailment may be more difficult to treat or reverse. Cattle checking is an art, and you can be the artist, if you learn to read your cows' subtle behavior changes.

Treating Sick Animals

Effective treatment for any condition depends on an accurate diagnosis and proper medication — both given early in the disease. If the animal has inadequate immune defenses, most pathogens multiply at a very high rate and quickly overwhelm the body. If there is a delay in treatment, the damage done may be beyond repair; the animal may die.

A bacterial infection may require appropriate *antimicrobial* drugs. Blackleg, for instance, rapidly overwhelms body defense but if caught early can be reversed with *penicillin*. This drug is effective because blackleg (a clostridial bacterium — see chapter 4) has a well-defined cell wall that is ruptured by penicillin. In contrast, penicillin is useless against organisms like *anaplasmosis* or other disease microbes that lack a well-defined cell wall.

There are dozens of antimicrobial drugs. You have to know which ones will work against certain diseases, based on chemical properties of the drug and vulnerabilities of the pathogen. A fungus infection needs treatment with a *fungicide*. A disease

- Hold the animal's tail to one side, and slide the thermometer into the rectum gently with a slightly upward and twirling motion so it will go in easily
- Insert it fully, leaving just the end sticking out. Pay attention! Make sure the animal doesn't expel the thermometer with manure. Drape the string over the tail head or hold onto it so you don't lose it with passing manure.
- Leave the thermometer in for about three minutes to get an accurate reading

If the temperature is elevated above 102.5, this is usually an indication of heat stress or infection. If the temperature is subnormal (below 101), the animal may be very cold or very ill and going into shock.

TO CHECK PULSE:

- Check the pulse with a stethoscope over the heart (on the left side of the ribcage, just behind the elbow); you can often feel the heartbeat of a young calf with your hand
- Or feel the pulse on an animal by pressing your fingers against the middle artery on the underside of the tail, about 6 inches (15.2 cm) down from the animal's tail head

- Or under the lower jaw, where a large artery crosses the lower edge of the jaw just in front of the big cheek muscle. If you place your fingers flat on the cheek in front of that muscle and move them back and forth, you can feel the artery. Once you locate it, hold it steady with your fingers and apply gentle pressure to feel the pulse.

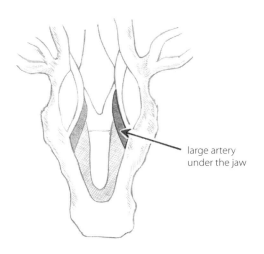

large artery under the jaw

Check the pulse rate by feeling the big artery underneath the jaw.

caused by *protozoa* may need treatment with something that hinders these parasites. Your veterinarian knows which drugs are best for various types of infections; enlist his or her help when making these choices. Use of appropriate drugs gives the animal time to build a defense by holding an infection in check and by preventing any *secondary infections.* Antimicrobials are often very beneficial, especially for preventing secondary bacterial infections, but are not effective against viruses.

How Are Antibiotics and Antimicrobials Different?

We often use the term "antibiotics" loosely, applying it to any pathogen-hindering drug. The proper all-inclusive term is "antimicrobial." Antibiotics are compounds produced by living organisms (usually bacteria) that impede the growth of other organisms. Antimicrobial drugs include antibiotics as well as synthetic and semisynthetic compounds that have the same effects.

Using Antimicrobials

Ever since the 1930s when *sulfa* drugs were found to stop the growth of bacteria and penicillin was isolated from certain strains of fungi in the soil in 1941, stockmen have been treating livestock infections with antimicrobial products. Newer classes of antimicrobials have come into use in more recent years.

Bacteria cause a wide variety of cattle infections and illnesses, making treatment with antibacterial drugs the proper choice, especially since many of these drugs are not toxic to the sick animal. Some protozoa, *rickettsia,* and *fungi* are also hindered by certain antimicrobials. These drugs do not affect most viral diseases, however. The only reason your veterinarian might prescribe an antibiotic in these instances would be to prevent or control any secondary bacterial infection that might crop up. In many cases the initial viral infection weakens the animal's defenses and allows opportunistic bacteria to invade and multiply. It is important to prevent this, since

the bacterial infection may be more deadly than the initial viral infection.

The antibiotics in use today include several types and classes. Different drugs have different actions. For example, penicillin and the *cephalosporins* affect the cell walls of certain bacteria. *Tetracyclines* inhibit bacterial protein synthesis. The *sulfonamides* and the *fluoroquinolones* inhibit the DNA function of certain bacteria. Some of these drugs kill bacteria outright *(bacteriocidal)* while others merely inhibit or arrest their growth *(bacteriostatic)* without actually killing them, giving the sick animal a chance to fight them off more readily. It is important to know about the various classes of drugs and whether they are bacteriocidal or bacteriostatic.

Bacteriocidal and bacteriostatic drug types generally should not be mixed together or used at the same time. Bacteriostatic products such as tetracycline and long-acting sulfa are often used effectively together for treating pneumonia or foot rot because they are synergistic and work better together than separately. But typically, if you try to use a bacteriocidal and a bacteriostatic drug at the same time, they cancel each other out. If the bacteria are growing very slowly or not at all, due to the use of a bacteriostatic drug, the use of the bacteriocidal drug won't work to kill them. Know what products are effective when used in conjunction with another. When in doubt about proper usage, consult your veterinarian.

Which Drug Is the Right Drug?

The choice of drug when treating cattle should always be made on a case-by-case basis. Because there are no specific guidelines as to what will work best, you'll need a proper diagnosis in order to target the troublemaking pathogen. Most of the older over-the-counter drugs (penicillins, tetracyclines, tylosin and some sulfas) list uses on the label. But it's best to ask a vet to examine the animal or guide you through such an examination in order to select or prescribe the most effective drug in each situation.

All of the newer drugs require a prescription because it's impossible to cover in a label list all the things they might be used for or all the stipulations regarding proper use. Your vet is the best judge. He or she may legally sell you the drug to treat the animal yourself, however, as long as there is a proper diagnosis to begin with, and a valid doctor-client-patient relationship — which means the vet knows what ails the animal being treated and is confident that you know how to administer the drug properly. Otherwise, these drugs are not legal for stockmen to use.

Treatments for specific disease conditions will be discussed in later chapters. Keep in mind, however, that new treatments become available from time to time, and some of the "old reliables" are sometimes taken off the market. While some veterinarians prefer one type of treatment or drug over others for certain illnesses, they will also be aware of new products that might be more effective than what's been used in the past. Get advice from your vet regarding treatment of a disease condition, especially if it's a situation you have not experienced before.

Newer Drugs

Some of the new drugs are longer acting than older medicines, decreasing the need for a repeat dose in many instances. For example, one dose of Draxxin (tulathromycin, which is a macrolide) is effective for up to 10 days and is very useful for treating respiratory disease because there will still be therapeutic levels in the lung tissue for this length of time. You rarely need to retreat the animal unless it does not respond, in which case your vet may suggest switching to a different class of drugs. For respiratory disease your vet might choose instead to prescribe the older drug Micotil (tilmicosin), which is another macrolide and also very effective, but he or she will have considered that it is not as long lasting (three to four days).

Many of the commonly used drugs today, including all of the newer ones, are prescription drugs and should be used only following a consultation with the veterinarian. These newer drugs include Draxxin (made by Pfizer), Nuflor (Schering-Plough), Excede (Pfizer), Baytril (Bayer), Micotil (Elanco), Tetradure 300 (Merial), and Naxcel (Pfizer). Many of them are low-volume products, which means they are more potent, can be given in smaller doses, and do not irritate the animal's tissue as seriously as a high-volume treatment might. They are often less painful to the cattle and also more efficient to ship and store.

The only drugs you can legally purchase without a prescription (from a feed store or catalog supply company) are penicillin, sulfa, tylosin, and most of the tetracyclines. There is some indication that this may eventually change, but at this time they can still be purchased over the counter.

The Old Reliables

Most stockmen continue to use traditional antimicrobials: sulfa boluses, injectable *LA-200* and other tetracyclines, penicillin, and injectable tylosin. On many farms and ranches these are still effective. For instance, the combination of LA-200 and sulfa still work well to combat respiratory disease, if the targeted bacteria have not yet developed resistance.

In feedlots, however, some of the newer drugs are more effective because in situations where cattle are continually brought in from many sources there is more frequent exposure to a variety of pathogens and a greater risk for the development of antibiotic resistance. Feedlots contain many more and different pathogens than you'd have on your home farm. The feedlot animal is also more stressed. Many of the newer drugs, such as the long-acting ones, were developed to combat these problems and to enable the stockman to treat the animal only once instead of multiple times, thereby minimizing the animal's stress from handling.

If the older, less expensive products still work on your farm, however, there's no reason not to use them. If they don't work very well, then you could switch to one of the newer, more expensive drugs — upon diagnosis and recommendation by your veterinarian. If cattle respond well to an inexpensive treatment, however, and have a low relapse rate, there's no need to change just because there's a newer antibiotic available.

The FDA regulates drugs used to treat the animals we use for food. Unless your vet gives you different instructions for treating your animals, the dosage for all medication must be given in accordance with label directions. Pay close attention to instructions regarding the interval between administering the drug and slaughter of the animal for meat or sale of her milk (withdrawal time) to avoid getting any residue from the drug into the meat or milk. This withdrawal time varies with certain drugs, so always read the label. If you raise natural or organic meat or milk, any animal that requires antibiotics cannot be sold as such and its meat or milk must be marketed a different way.

Residue Avoidance

When using any microbial, check the label for withdrawal time. It is important to allow the proper length of time before the treated animal is sold or butchered. Different products have different withdrawal times, and the length of time is also dependent upon dose. If you overdose the animal, the withdrawal time must be extended to longer than stated on the label. It is illegal to sell an animal before an adequate withdrawal time has elapsed.

The first beef quality-assurance program in the United States began in 1986. The National Cattlemen's Association developed it in response to consumer

---

Penicillin Allergies

Even though penicillin is nontoxic, it is also one of the most common allergenic antibiotics. It is often used in human medicine, and some people are allergic to it and its derivatives. Since it is usually administered into the muscle (rather than IV), if you give an animal five times the labeled dosage to effectively treat pneumonia or foot rot and only observe the normal label withdrawal time, there will be some residue in the muscle if the animal is butchered too soon. If the neck muscle where you injected the drug is ground into hamburger and contains a residue, someone who is allergic may eat that meat and go into anaphylactic shock. Some cattle may also have an allergic reaction to penicillin.

Even though this drug can be very effective against foot rot and some types of pneumonia, in order to get tissue levels high enough to do the job, you have to use so much penicillin that it's almost cheaper to use one of the newer, more expensive drugs. There are many more options today than we had 30 years ago and more choices for selecting a product that fits a specific need. In earlier times when we had only penicillin, sulfa products, and tetracyclines, they were often used extra-label, or a veterinarian might compound something to address a particular problem. But this is not as acceptable anymore, since the compounded drug or extra-label use might not be any better than what is currently available. Always work with your vet to diagnose and treat various conditions, to know which antibiotics (and dosages) are most appropriate.

concerns about cattle health issues, growth hormones, and potential residues of hormones and medicines in meat. Since then, the U.S. Department of Agriculture Food and Drug Administration's guidelines and rules have been established, with withdrawal times for each medicinal and growth-enhancing product. Detectable residue at slaughter is a violation that results in condemnation of the carcass and a complete loss for the stockman. Studies and reports on residue violations have shown that most residues are seen in *cull cows* (especially dairy cows) and calves that were treated shortly before market. Stockmen need to be more careful and wait an appropriate length of time before selling a recovered animal or a cull cow that received vaccinations or delousing products at the time of pregnancy checking. This is a good reason to wait and see if cows and heifers are pregnant or open before administering or applying products. If you'll be selling *open cows,* it's crucial to observe proper withdrawal times for each product. So plan ahead!

Questions about Antimicrobial Resistance

Antimicrobial use in food animals is a controversial issue. There is growing concern that overuse of these drugs in humans and animals may be leading to resistant strains of pathogens that may not be readily controlled in the future. During the latter half of the twentieth century, use of antibiotics had a dramatic effect on improving the health and longevity of humans and animals. Sulfa was first used in human patients in 1936 and penicillin by the 1940s. But it was soon discovered that not all bacteria were susceptible to penicillin, and some that were earlier susceptible developed resistance. Many new drugs were found or synthesized, however, and people became optimistic that we could eventually control infectious disease with drugs.

People became complacent about antimicrobial resistance. Pharmaceutical companies shifted research efforts to other challenges like human cancer and heart disease. Development of new or more effective antimicrobials has thus lagged behind the development of antimicrobial resistance. Some people feel that indiscriminant use of these drugs is hastening development of resistant strains.

It's important for livestock owners to use antimicrobial drugs responsibly, and to realize they are just one weapon in the fight against disease. Rather than looking to antimicrobials as a cover-up for poor management, we need to look at preventing disease in the first place. All too often people just grab an antimicrobial drug to treat a sick animal, rather than doing what it takes to prevent that disease by having a clean environment or a closed herd (preventing exposure to the disease) or keeping a vaccination program up to date to optimize immunity.

Yet, no matter how meticulous your disease management, there will still be times you need antimicrobial drugs or you may lose an animal or have a severe illness go through a group of calves. Properly used, these drugs keep animals healthy. Without use of drugs, there are many instances in which the meat or milk would be less safe because the animals were stunted or sick. If you can keep calves healthy as they grow up, not stunted by *coccidiosis,* a low-grade *salmonella* infection, a heavy parasite load, or damaged lungs due to pneumonia, they will provide a more desirable food product. An unhealthy animal cannot produce top-quality meat.

Proper use of antibiotics, for instance, can turn a disease situation around and enable the animal to recover more quickly or completely. Intervention with immediate and proper treatment when an animal first starts showing signs of illness can greatly shorten recuperation. With a shorter course of treatment, there is less total medication in the body that must be eliminated. Keeping close track of your animals, being in tune with signs of health and sickness, and immediately treating any that become sick can often help minimize the risk of losing that animal and the risk of spreading the disease to others in the herd, as well as shorten the recovery time for that animal. Proper use of all antimicrobial drugs can help us minimize their use and is definitely a case of "a stitch in time saves nine."

Off-Label Drug Use

Using any animal health product in a way that is not specified on the label, without a vet's prescription, might be harmful to an animal or to humans consuming the meat or milk from that animal.

BACTERIOCIDAL PRODUCTS AND USAGE

These drugs kill bacteria outright.

Penicillin

Brands/Formulations: Procaine penicillin G, Durapen, and benzathine penicillin (long-acting Dual Pen or BP-48). IV formulations (potassium penicillin and sodium penicillin)

How It Works: Affects the cell walls of certain bacteria

Drug's Properties: Broad-spectrum antibiotic. This class of drug is absorbed very quickly from the injection site into the bloodstream.

Commonly Used for: It is the most effective drug for treating clostridial diseases such as blackleg, malignant edema, and tetanus, and is very effective for septicemia if the causative pathogen is susceptible to penicillin. But it is also often used for pneumonia, pinkeye, foot rot, and other infections caused by susceptible pathogens.

Withdrawal Period/Precautions: Pen G — 5 days; Penicillin G Procaine Solution — 10 days; Procaine Penicillin G with Benzathine Penicillin (BP-48) — 30 days

Usage Notes: Penicillin is still available over the counter and is used for many things. One drawback, however, is that it generally needs to be given in a higher-than-labeled dosage to be effective for conditions such as pneumonia, pinkeye, or foot rot. Even though it is labeled for treating pneumonia, in order to use it effectively for this illness, you must use it at higher doses than listed on the label, and you need to obtain a prescription from your veterinarian or you will be acting illegally.

The label dosage was determined early on by what would be effective against septicemia. This class of drug is absorbed very quickly from the injection site into the bloodstream. A calf with pneumonia, however, needs it in the lung tissue, not the blood. In order to get effective treatment for pneumonia, foot rot, pinkeye, etc., you need very high blood concentrations, so there will be some spillover effects into these tissues. Penicillin is safe and nontoxic, so there is no problem with giving high doses, but this also increases the withdrawal time. And since this is extra-label use, someone must be responsible for any residues. Work with your veterinarian to determine proper withdrawal time for the higher dosages. IV formulations are not commonly used; they are more expensive and should be given by a vet.

Cephalosporins

Brands/Formulations: Naxcel, Excenel, Excede (all various formulations of ceftiofur)

How It Works: Affects the cell walls of certain bacteria; inhibits cell-wall formation

Drug's Properties: Related to the penicillins in structure and mode of action but are much more potent and have a broader spectrum

Commonly Used for: Respiratory disease and foot rot

Withdrawal Period/Precautions: Naxcel — none for meat or milk, if used in accordance with label directions for dosage and route of administration; Excenel — 48 hours; Excede — 13 days for slaughter; no withdrawal for milk

Usage Notes:

Naxcel is very short acting (1 day) and might need to be repeated, but it has the advantage of a very short withdrawal time. You don't need to worry about drug residues in the animal. If you are treating a cull cow for foot rot or some other susceptible infection before you sell or butcher her, Naxcel may be a better choice than LA-200, Nuflor, or one of the other drugs labeled for treating foot rot, since those drugs have a much longer withdrawal time. Using a cephalosporin keeps your slaughter options open for adult animals; you won't have to wait so long after treatment. For instance, foot rot usually clears up quickly with treatment, but if you used LA-200 you'd have to wait at least 28 days after the final treatment before you could sell or butcher the animal.

Excenel has 2 days of effectiveness.

Excede is a different formulation in a different carrier and has a longer duration of effectiveness than the other ceftiofur drugs (10 days). But it is different from the mechanism in Draxxin or Micotil, which are absorbed rapidly and then concentrate in the white cells of the body. Excede is absorbed more slowly, so it's like giving a continuous slow-release dose.

Draxxin and Excede are both excellent as long-action drugs, but your choice of which one to use will depend on what you are treating, since Draxxin is bacteriostatic and Excede is bacteriocidal. Draxxin is effective against Micoplasma bovis, for instance, but Excede doesn't work at all for this one. Bacteriocidal drugs like Excede inhibit the formation of cell walls but don't work for M. bovis because Micoplasma bacteria do not have a cell wall.

Aminoglycocides

Brands/Formulations: Gentimycin, Streptomycin, Neomycin

Drug's Properties: Given orally, these drugs stay in the GI tract.

Commonly Used for: Diarrhea-causing pathogens

Withdrawal Period/Precautions: Neomycin sulfate solution — 1 day; Neomycin soluble powder — 30 days

Usage Notes: Cattle injections are not legal for these drugs, but they can be used orally, since they stay in the gut and are not absorbed into the body. They do not affect the meat or milk, but some of them still have withdrawal times listed on the label.

Trimethoprim

Brands/Formulations: SMZ/TMP

Drug's Properties: Broad-spectrum antibiotic

Commonly Used for: Respiratory disease, GI tract infections, calf diphtheria

Withdrawal Period/Precautions: Variable. Check labels or ask your vet.

Usage Notes: This product is closely related to pyrimethamine (a human antimalarial drug) and is given orally in combination with a sulfonamide because the two together are much more effective than either one alone (the one instance where a bacteriocidal and a bacteriostatic drug are combined).

Fluoroquinolones

Brands/Formulations: Enrofloxacin (Baytril) and danafloxacin (A-180)

How It Works: Inhibits the DNA function of certain bacteria

Commonly Used for: Respiratory diseases

Withdrawal Period/Precautions: Do not use in cattle intended for dairy purposes. Withdrawal time for slaughter — 28 days

Usage Notes: These two drugs are different variations of this class and are both very potent and effective against certain pathogens. The parent compound is ciprofloxacin, a human antimicrobial drug that is effective against some strains of bacteria that have developed resistance to penicillins and cephalosporins.

Baytril and A-180 both have some restrictions for use and carry warnings on the label stating that it is illegal to use them in any extra-label fashion, such as for baby-calf diarrhea. Even though they are very effective against salmonella and *E. coli,* they are illegal for treating these intestinal infections because there is public concern about development of antibiotic-resistant gut bugs (enteric pathogens) that can infect people. These drugs can be used for baby-calf pneumonia (and are labeled for this use) but not for scours.

Example of Label Directions

- **Indications:** For treatment of Bovine Respiratory Disease

- **Dosage:** 3 ml per 100 lbs of body weight

- **Timing:** Dose may be repeated after 48 hours

- **Route of administration:** IM in neck muscle

- **Warnings:** Not for use in female dairy cattle over 20 months of age

- **Withdrawal period, if any:** Do not use within 28 days before slaughter

- **Storage:** Store at 36 to 86°F (refrigeration is not required)

- **Shelf life:** Expiration date

The package insert for an antibiotic will also contain such things as data regarding safety and the effectiveness of the product, possible adverse effects, and more details on dosage administration.

BACTERIOSTATIC PRODUCTS AND USAGE

These drugs inhibit or arrest bacterial growth.

Sulfonamides (sulfadimethoxine, sulfamethazine)

Brands/Formulations: Albon (effective against coccidiosis protozoa, as well as certain bacteria), Sustain, Calf-span boluses, soluble powders, and injectable sulfadimethoxine

How It Works: Inhibits the DNA function of certain bacteria

Drug's Properties: Broad spectrum

Commonly Used for: Pneumonia, scours, foot rot, calf *diphtheria*, *mastitis*, and metritis; some types are used for coccidiosis

Withdrawal Period/Precautions: Some of these products can be used in lactating dairy cows. Read labels or consult your vet for withdrawal and milk-discard times for various products.

Usage Notes: There are many types of sulfa products (oral solutions, soluble powders, boluses, injectables), used for many different diseases.

Tetracyclines (biosynthetic antibiotics, including chlortetracycline and oxytetracycline)

Brands/Formulations: LA-200, Biomycin-200, Duramycin, Aureomycin, Terramycin, and Tetradure 300, among others

How It Works: Inhibits bacterial protein synthesis

Drug's Properties: Effective against a wide range of diseases, with a wider spectrum of action than that of penicillin. The intramuscular products that call for high-volume doses are irritating to muscle tissue, so are often given subcutaneously.

Commonly Used For: Diphtheria in calves, pneumonia, foot rot, pinkeye, scours, *wooden tongue*, leptospirosis, and metritis

Withdrawal Period/Precautions: For most injectable tetracyclines — 28 days if given IM, 36 days if given subQ; Duramycin soluble powder given orally — 5 days

Usage Notes: Some of these products are injectable, and some are given orally. Several of the older tetracycline products are still used, and the long-acting forms are often given in combination with a long-acting sulfa to give 3 to 4 days' worth of coverage.

LA-200 can be given IM, sub Q, and IV.

Tetradure 300 is one of the newer formulations of oxytetracycline. A prescription drug, it contains 300 milligrams per milliliter, compared to Biomycin 200, LA-200, and generic equivalents. It is not longer lasting; it is just more potent — you can give a smaller-volume dose, with decreased risk for tissue irritation. It was created to give vets the option of prescribing the same amount of drug in less volume. It is less painful to cattle than its higher-volume counterparts. Still, it should not be given IM in the neck muscle of small calves because it may cause painful swelling.

Macrolides

Brands/Formulations: Tulathromycin (Draxxin), tilmicosin (Micotil), tylosin (Tylan), and erythromycin

How It Works: Inhibits growth of bacteria

Drug's Properties: Some of the newer formulations in this class tend to concentrate in lung tissue and are thus very effective against respiratory disease.

Commonly Used for: Draxxin, Micotil, and erythromycin are used for respiratory disease. Tylan-200 is used for pneumonia, metritis, mastitis, and foot rot.

Withdrawal Period/Precautions: Micotil — 28 days for beef animals. It cannot be used in female dairy cattle 20 months of age or older. Tylan-200 — 21 days; not for use in lactating dairy cattle. Draxxin — 18 days; not for use in female dairy cattle 20 months of age or older, nor for calves that will be processed as veal

Usage Notes:

Draxxin is one of the longest-lasting formulations, similar in length of effectiveness to Excede, but it has the advantage of being highly effective against the pathogen Micoplasma bovis.

Micotil has been in use longer and is not as long lasting (3 to 4 days) as Draxxin but is also very effective against respiratory disease. Both of these drugs are absorbed rapidly and then concentrated in the white cells of the body. A big disadvantage of using Micotil is that it can be fatal to humans if accidentally injected. For this reason, your veterinarian should administer it unless you are very experienced in giving injections and your vet is confident that you can do it safely. Make sure the animal is properly restrained when using Micotil so that you don't accidentally poke yourself with the needle.

Tylan-200 (tylosin) is still available over the counter. It must be given daily, but when given intramuscularly it is very irritating to the tissues. IV treatment is better, but this is extra-label use and must be prescribed by a veterinarian.

An oral preparation of tylosin is commonly used in feed to prevent liver abscesses. It is also sometimes used in a salt/mineral product to help control pinkeye.

Phenicols

Brands/Formulations: Nuflor

How It Works: Inhibits bacterial function

Drug's Properties: A unique class of drugs that has both bacteriostatic and bacteriocidal properties

Commonly Used for: Respiratory disease

Withdrawal Period/Precautions: If given IM — 28 days; if given subQ — 38 days. Not for use in female dairy cattle 20 months of age or older, or for veal calves

Usage Notes:

Nuflor is the only drug in this class that is approved for use in food animals (chloramphenicol is a related drug but is no longer legal in food animals). Nuflor is effective against respiratory disease and lasts about 4 days. This class of drugs is very effective and broad spectrum, but some veterinarians do not prescribe it for calves less than 30 days of age, since it may give them diarrhea.

Time to Treat Again?

Most of the newer drugs are effective with just one dose, as when treating respiratory disease. If the animal is not making progress before the time window of effectiveness for that particular drug has elapsed, it may indicate that the animal is suffering from more than one ailment or that the first diagnosis was incorrect. You may need to reevaluate the diagnosis and change antibiotics.

For example, a calf may be diagnosed with pneumonia, but he may also have septicemia, which affects body systems and organs other than the lungs. Or he may have a viral infection that causes the problem, and while the antibiotic may prevent a secondary bacterial infection, the real problem is the viremia. In that instance, changing antibiotics won't help. Or if the animal has a chronic condition in the lung, the antibiotic will not be effective.

When a drug appears to be ineffective, you need to have your veterinarian reexamine the animal and reconsider the treatment.

Antimicrobial Resistance

Antimicrobial resistance is a natural process that can occur in three ways:

1. In any group of bacteria, there are some that are naturally stronger than others and may survive treatment. They live to reproduce more of their kind, creating a resistant population.

2. A small percentage of bacteria may be naturally resistant to certain antimicrobials.

3. Antimicrobial resistance can be transferred from one type of bacteria to another through genetic material called plasmids.

Giving a higher or lower dose, administering it in a different location or via a different route, using it on a different species from that for which it is intended, or administering it at more frequent intervals is called *extra-label* or *off-label* drug use, and it is illegal. Even if the treatment is not harmful to the animal, there may be more risk for the drug's residue to appear in the animal's meat. For example, a drug used on beef cattle that was prescribed for animals not raised for food may leave a residue in meat, as withdrawal times have not been determined by researchers.

There are situations, however, when veterinarians prescribe a product for off-label use for certain purposes or to treat an unusual condition. According to the Food and Drug Administration, this is acceptable if there is no approved drug already labeled to treat the condition, if treatment at the recommended dosage or location would not be effective, or if a certain off-label vaccination protocol would be more effective. The law also stipulates that there must be a valid veterinarian-client-animal patient relationship. This means the vet has a good working relationship with the client, has seen and diagnosed the animal, and agrees to take the responsibility for making a judgment regarding the health of that animal, and the client agrees to follow the veterinarian's instructions. Finally, a record of the animal's off-label treatment must be kept, and the withdrawal time before marketing for slaughter must be extended in the case of some products or overdoses. The veterinarian determines the necessary withdrawal time.

Giving Injections

Most vaccines, antibiotics, *anti-inflammatory* drugs, and some vitamins and minerals are given to cattle by injection, so it is very important to know how to administer these correctly and in the proper locations. Most cattle must be vaccinated once or twice a year against certain diseases, and young cattle need a series of booster vaccinations to begin building adequate immunity.

If an animal becomes ill with pneumonia, foot rot, pinkeye, or some other disease caused by bacteria, your vet may recommend an antibiotic injection. Always follow his or her advice, along with label or package-insert directions (unless your vet is

---

SUPPLIES NEEDED FOR INJECTIONS

Obtain the tools listed below from your veterinarian or veterinary-supply catalog.

☐ Disposable needles (18 gauge — 1 to 2 inches [2.5 to 5 cm] long for calves; and 16 gauge — 0.5 to 2.5 inches [1.3 to 6.4 cm] long) for adult cattle

☐ Disposable syringes of various sizes (3 to 20 cc)

☐ Pistol-grip multidose syringe (for vaccinating multiple animals at once)

☐ Pliers for removing a bent, dull, or broken needle from a multidose syringe

☐ Transfer needle for transferring sterile diluent into vials of dried modified live-virus vaccines for reconstitution

☐ IV kit with needle and tubing

☐ Antidote (epinephrine) for allergic injection reaction

---

prescribing a drug for a specific off-label use) for *any* injectable product.

Dosage and Timing

Make sure you give the correct dosage for the sick individual, in the proper injection site, and at the correct intervals. Some antibiotics may be repeated after a certain number of days, for instance. Improper use of any injectable vaccine or drug may render it ineffective or even life threatening, so learn how to administer it properly. If you are inexperienced at giving injections, have your veterinarian or an experienced stockman show you the basic techniques.

Route of Administration

Most vaccines and antibiotics are given intramuscularly (IM) or *subcutaneously* (SubQ). Some medications are given *intravenously* (IV). Your vet should do this unless he or she has shown you how to do it properly and you feel confident following through. The animal should be adequately restrained (see pages 56–57) before you administer any type of injection. If she moves, you're at risk for injury, and the product may be incorrectly injected or partially wasted, resulting in improper dosage. Needle movement during IM (intramuscular) injection due to inadequate restraint of the animal increases muscle damage. Part of the dose may end up entering the body subcutaneously or even via a *vein*. Movement during a subcutaneous injection may lead to accidental IM injection. The improper site, in either case, may affect efficiency or withdrawal time.

Intramuscular Injections

Use a needle that's long enough to go deep into the muscle and large enough in diameter to cut through tough skin when giving *intramuscular* injections. Needle diameter is determined by gauge size; the smaller the number, the larger the needle. For example, a 14-gauge needle is too big for IM and SubQ injections, and a 20 gauge is too small for cattle.

Location, Location, Location

For vaccines, both IM and subQ injections should be given in the triangular mass of muscle on the neck (see pages 43 and 44). The acceptable area for subQ injection starts three fingers' width behind the ear, extending down to the front of the shoulder. The acceptable area for IM injection is slightly smaller. Take caution to avoid the top of the neck, which contains a thick ligament, and the bottom portion of the neck where the bones, windpipe, and jugular vein are located. An alternate choice for subQ injections is the area just behind the shoulder blade. If more than one product is injected, be sure the sites are separated by at least 4 inches.

For antibiotics, the neck is a preferred location. Split the total dose if it is more than 10 mL (0.3 oz), and inject those portions no closer than 4 inches (10.2 cm) apart for adequate tissue absorption. If you make the mistake of putting a large volume into one site (IM or SubQ) the medication may be absorbed too slowly to have adequate concentration in the area of the infection, and the necessary withdrawal time before slaughter will be increased. If large doses must be given, use both sides of the neck. If there's still not enough area on the neck to absorb the injections, an alternative site for IM injections is the back of the thigh.

IM needle specifications for an adult cow:

▸ Use a needle at least 1.5 inches (3.8 cm) long for vaccines.

▸ Use a needle at least 2 inches (5 cm) long for antibiotics, which are often larger doses.

▸ Use a 16-gauge diameter, which is large enough to go through the animal's tough skin without bending or breaking.

▸ Don't use anything larger than 16-gauge needle or there may be tissue damage and leaking of the vaccine. Even in cold weather when some products may be thick, it's better to keep the product warm enough to flow freely rather than resort to a larger diameter needle.

IM needle specifications for a calf:

▸ Use a needle 1 inch long for vaccines, 1.5 inches (2.5 to 3.8 cm) long for antibiotics.

▸ Use a smaller diameter needle than you would for an adult; one with an 18-gauge diameter is best.

Use sterile disposable needles to ensure the needle will be clean and sharp. Needles should not be reused unless they have been boiled to sterilize them between uses. The exception is when a large number of cattle is being vaccinated at once. In that case, care must be taken to make sure the needle stays clean and sharp during multiple uses.

A new, sharp needle always goes in easier and causes less pain and tissue damage. If a needle gets dull or dirty after use on several animals, exchange it for a new one. Needles are designed to cut into the skin, not puncture it. After you've used a needle on 10 or more animals, it begins to dull and develop a burr on the tip. Once it's dull, you need to use more force; instead of cutting through the skin, it punctures it and folds a small piece underneath, possibly carrying dirt or bacteria with it. If a needle starts to get dull, exchange it, even if you've used it on only a few animals.

Always change to a new needle if the one you are using becomes bent. Bending weakens it, and it may break. You don't want it to break off in the animal. Whether you are giving IM or SQ shots, change needles frequently when vaccinating large numbers of animals, especially if a needle becomes bent, dirty, or dull, or if the tip is blunted by accidentally bumping on the chute. Try to reduce the chance for tissue trauma or an infection. Never thrust a needle through wet, dirty, mud- or manure-covered hide, or the needle will pull the contaminating matter in with it, leaving the animal at risk for abscess development at the injection site. Never inject an intramuscular product into a vein.

Most injections should be put in the neck to avoid injecting into parts of the body that will eventually become important cuts of meat. If there's any long-term tissue damage, it can be more readily trimmed from the neck than the rump, for instance. Also, if there is scar tissue (*gristle*) in the neck it's not as critical; neck muscle is usually made into hamburger.

Today there are some new antibiotics that can be injected under the skin on the back of the ear, to completely avoid damage to any future meat.

The rump area is no longer acceptable as a place to receive injections, even though these thicker muscles are better for absorbing an injection. Many types of injections occasionally create a scar or an abscess, which would damage one of the best cuts of meat if put in the rump. It's better to put an IM injection into the neck, splitting a large dose into two or more sites if necessary. If an animal needs multiple injections at one time, or repeat treatments at a later date, vary the injection sites on subsequent treatments.

Sometimes it's a trade-off between what might be ideal from a carcass standpoint and what's practical or best for the animal. Due to the high volume of some antibiotic injections or a need for multiple treatments in the course of severe illness, it may not be feasible or humane to put all injections into the neck. That area can become so sore the animal can't raise or lower his head to eat and drink. The stress of discomfort may diminish the effectiveness of the treatment, making the animal slower to recover. Your first concern is to save the animal. If both sides of the neck won't adequately absorb all IM injections, use the back of the thigh, putting the injection at right angles to the leg where there is less risk of hitting nerves that run along the back of the muscles.

Abscesses and Scars Affect Meat Quality

Never inject medicines or vaccines through dirty skin; avoid risk for infection. An abscess will usually show up a few days later as a lump, which may grow larger and then break and drain. If it does not break on its own, it must be lanced and drained or flushed, and the animal may need antibiotics. An abscess deep in the muscle that may not be detected until the animal is slaughtered is an even greater problem, affecting a larger area. Although an abscess is rarely a risky medical problem, scar tissue from a surface abscess can result in significant amount of carcass trim. A deep abscess may contaminate the meat around it and must be trimmed even more.

Even a poke into muscle with a clean needle without injecting anything leaves a scar and a tough area in the meat. Sterile scar tissue in the muscle after a shot can still be there months or years later. Injections given to a calf may create lesions that must be trimmed at slaughter even a dozen years later when she goes to market as a culled cow. These lesions contain more connective tissue and fat than normal muscle, and the meat may be less tender in an area up to 3 inches (7.6 cm) around the lesion — a piece of meat the size of a grapefruit.

HOW TO GIVE AN INTRAMUSCULAR INJECTION

1. Make sure the area for injection is clean and dry.
2. **If using a trigger-type syringe,** thrust the needle into muscle and pull the trigger.

   If using a smaller or disposable syringe, detach the needle from the syringe to make it easier to insert without breaking the syringe. Thump or press firmly against the skin with the side of your hand in the area where the needle is to enter in order to desensitize the region and keep the animal from flinching. Thrust the needle in quickly and forcefully so it goes through the skin and all the way into the muscle. If the animal jumps, wait till he settles down before attaching the syringe to the inserted needle to give the injection. If the needle starts to ooze blood before you put the syringe back on it, you've hit a vein. Take it out and try a slightly different spot. Do not inject an IM product into a vein.

3. To reduce the chances of medicinal leakage, keep the needle inserted for at least two seconds after the injection, or pull the skin taut across the injection site with one hand while you inject with the other, then release the skin after you remove the needle. The skin will move over the hole and close it up.

4. Rub the injection site afterward to help distribute the product within the muscle and to reduce the pressure so it is less apt to ooze back out.

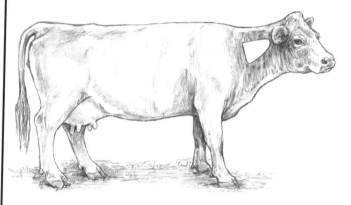

The best place for an IM injection is in the middle of the neck, neither too high nor too low.

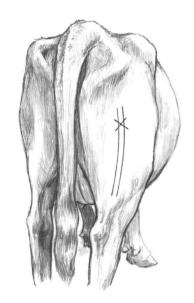

The back of the thigh is the alternative site for an intramuscular injection. The needle should go in at right angles to the animal, from the side.

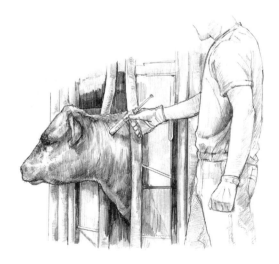

Intramuscular injections are put straight into the muscle tissue, preferably in the neck.

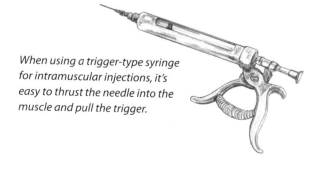

When using a trigger-type syringe for intramuscular injections, it's easy to thrust the needle into the muscle and pull the trigger.

Subcutaneous Injections

Originally, subcutaneous (subQ) injections were used because a particular product was highly irritating to muscle tissue or designed for a slower rate of absorption. Today, however, due to concerns over carcass quality and trying to avoid IM shots, more and more vaccines and antibiotic treatments are being approved for subcutaneous injection and no longer must be given intramuscularly. When label directions give you a choice, it's best to avoid tissue damage and administer a product under the skin rather than into muscle. A serious abscess due to a dirty needle is more likely to develop with IM shots than with subQ injections; an infection induced by a subcutaneous injection is just beneath the skin and more readily breaks open to drain.

Some of the automatic gun-type syringes have flexible ends to help keep needles from bending. Make sure a trigger or squeeze-type syringe gun is easy to use and well lubricated, especially if you have small hands. The easier and more quickly you give an injection, especially if the animal has any room to move around in a chute, the less likely you'll end up with bent or broken needles.

Always be aware that the animal may lunge when being injected. Make sure you have access to the injection site and that your hand and the syringe or needle won't be jammed into the bars or front of the

---

HOW TO GIVE A SUBCUTANEOUS INJECTION

1. Make sure the area for injection is clean and dry.
2. **If using a small or disposable syringe,** lift a fold of skin on the neck (or shoulder if you are treating a small calf) where skin is loosest, and slip the needle in between the skin and muscle. **If using a trigger- or squeeze-type syringe gun,** aim the needle alongside the animal's neck or shoulder — nearly parallel to the surface — so it goes just under the skin and not into the muscle.

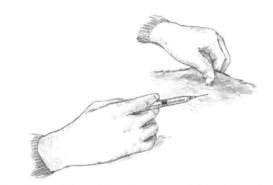

To inject medicine subQ, pull up a tent of skin with one hand and slip the needle under the raised skin.

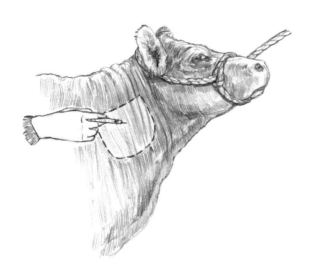

The best location for a subcutaneous injection is in front of the shoulder where the skin is loose.

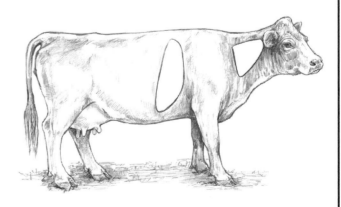

An alternative site for the subcutaneous injection is the area just behind the shoulder blade.

SLOW-RELEASE INJECTIONS INTO THE BACK OF THE EAR

Some of the newer antibiotic products can be injected subcutaneously at the back of the ear. This site will not affect any meat and is a way to avoid tissue reactions, scarring, and other problems that might otherwise affect the carcass when the animal eventually goes to slaughter.

Take care to restrain the animal adequately and give the ear injection correctly to minimize the health risks of accidentally going too deep or injecting into a blood vessel. Sudden death of the animal may occur if you inject into an artery.

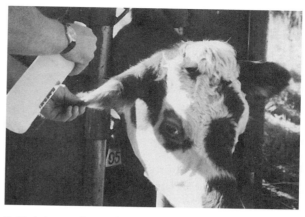

1. To inject a slow-release antibiotic under the skin at the back of the ear, first clean the skin after shaving the back of the ear.

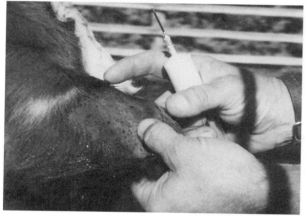

2. Determine the proper location for the injection, to be sure to miss the blood vessels.

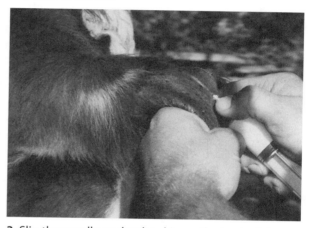

3. Slip the needle under the skin on the back of the ear.

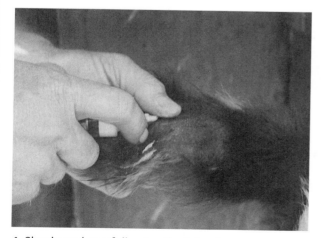

4. Slowly and carefully give the injection.

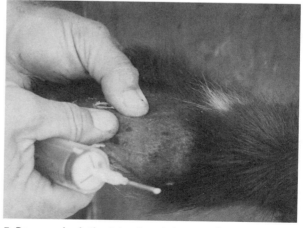

5. Press and rub the injection sight to make sure none of the antibiotic leaks back out before the hole seals off.

chute if the animal jumps. Many of the new squeeze chutes have access doors at the neck area or a neck extension that holds the animal's head and neck still so he can't ram forward and backward while you are trying to give an injection. Try to insert the needle at an angle so you can use a one-handed technique with a syringe gun, rather than using both hands to pull up the "tent" of skin to slip the needle into for a subQ injection. There's less risk of getting your hands injured (jammed between the animal and the chute) or accidentally hitting yourself with the needle if you can do it with one hand.

SubQ Needle Specifications:

▸ Use a needle 0.5 to 0.75 inches (1.3 to 1.9 cm) long if using a gun-type syringe one-handed.

▸ Use a needle up to 1 inch (2.5 cm) long if you are using both hands and can pull up a tent of skin to slip the needle under, so it is less likely to bend or break.

▸ Use a 16-gauge needle for adult animals and an 18-gauge needle for calves. This type of injection is usually given in the neck, but for a small calf it may be easier to give the shot under the loose skin of the shoulder. Also, if there is any local reaction, it won't make his neck sore. A calf with a sore neck may be reluctant to nurse his mother.

Intravenous (IV) Injections

Some medications act faster, are more effective, or are more readily absorbed if given intravenously. Some drugs are very irritating to muscle tissue and are best given by IV, and others can only be given by IV. If an animal is in *shock* or the gut is severely compromised by disease and can't absorb fluids, fluid therapy and any necessary antibiotics must be given by IV.

It's not difficult to give IV injections, but you must know which treatments can be given via IV and how to administer them properly. Chances of problems, such as adverse reactions if some medications leak into tissues surrounding the vein, or reactions associated with administering the product too swiftly, are greater with IV injections, as is the speed with which

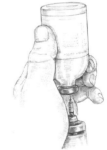

Always use a sterile needle to fill your syringe. Do not insert a used needle into the bottle; it may contaminate the contents.

a serious problem can develop if given incorrectly. Large volumes of fluid given too swiftly can put too much load on the heart, and some drugs speed up the heart. Heart rate should be monitored when giving IV medications or fluids. It's best if your vet or another experienced person shows you how to do it. Giving an IV requires more precision than other injections, and administering IV fluids takes time.

The most common problem is pushing the needle too far, clear through the vein and out the other side. Sometimes the animal moves and the needle slips out of the vein. Don't assume it's in the vein just because you see a little blood; blood will flow steadily from the needle if it's actually in the vein. Make sure it stays in the vein as you give the injection or administer the fluid. Injecting some drugs

---

HOW TO GIVE AN INTRAVENOUS INJECTION

Any large vein will work for an IV, including the major veins under the tail and the big milk vein ahead of the udder on a dairy cow. For ease of administration, most people use the large jugular vein on the side of the neck, located in the groove above the windpipe and esophagus. A large needle, at least 16 gauge and at least 2 inches (5 cm) long, works best for adult animals.

1. Sterilize the needle and the syringe or tubing to be used or use a new disposable kit.

2. Restrain the animal.

3. Find the *jugular vein;* clean and dry the area if necessary.

4. Press down on the vein with your fist or fingers to build up pressure between your hand and the head and so the vein stands up and is more accessible.

5. While still pressing on the vein, hold the needle aimed toward the head and parallel to the vein. Push the needle through the skin and on into the vein at a point between your hand and the animal's head. Then move the needle forward its full length (inside the vein) parallel with the neck.

6. If blood flows steadily and freely from the needle, it's in the vein. Attach your syringe (or tubing, if giving fluid).

7. Inject the medication from the syringe, or, if giving fluid, allow the tubing to fill with fluid before attaching the tube to the needle. Hold the bag or bottle above the animal so gravity will take it down through the tubing and into the vein. Flow rate can be adjusted using needle size or a regulating device on the tubing.

8. If no blood appears when you attempt to insert the needle, this may mean the needle is clogged or embedded in the wall of the vein. Pull it out and start over again.

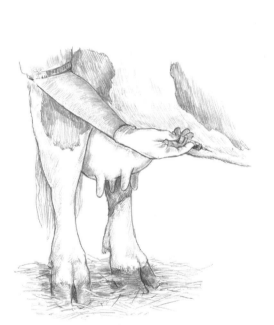

It's common to administer an intravenous (IV) injection into the jugular vein. Press the vein down with one hand, and insert the needle between your hand and the animal's head with your other hand.

You can also use the large milk vein on a lactating cow for an IV injection.

into tissues around the vein can cause severe irritation and stress and sometimes death. If the needle slips out of the vein while giving fluid, tissues around the vein will start to swell. If the needle slips out of the vein, take it out and start over. If you are giving the animal fluids, the needle must be in the vein for a while. In that case, it's best to use an IV *catheter*, which is longer and more flexible than a needle and stays in the vein with less difficulty.

Tips on Needles

For all injections, use good-quality needles that stay sharp. Disposable needles are generally best, but avoid those with plastic hubs because they are more likely to break. Use the proper size. If the needle is too large, it allows leakage; if it's too small, it may break or slow the procedure because more pressure is needed to inject the material through it. If it's too long, it may bend and break; too short, and it may deliver the product into the wrong location. If the needle's bent, discard it.

Make sure the needle is still attached to the syringe when you finish the injection. On the rare occasion that a needle breaks off in the animal, it's usually sticking out, and you can grab it. Otherwise, mark the site so your vet can surgically retrieve it, and contact your vet as soon as possible. A needle shaft can migrate several inches within an hour (either going deeper or moving laterally under the skin). When working cattle, have a container by the chute for disposal of used needles. After use, clean all nondisposable needles and syringes with hot water, then boil them for 15 minutes.

In the future, stockmen may not need needles. There are new devices being tested that will administer injections through intact skin by use of compressed air. Even now, some of the newer injectable products are also being designed for injection or implantation in locations that won't affect meat quality. One example of this is an antibiotic implant in the ear that provides slow-release coverage for a much longer time than that of traditional antibiotics.

By injecting medication in areas that don't enter the human food chain, the effects of the drugs on meat quality and human safety become less of a public-health issue. And injections become easier for the rancher and safer for all involved, including the cow. This technique

will prevent scarring, abscesses that develop as a result of the introduction of contaminants, and the breaking off of needles in animal tissue. New vaccines may also be genetically engineered in such a way that they require fewer irritating adjuvants, which can cause reactions at the injection site.

Reactions to Injections

When you give any kind of injection, always keep in mind that an animal may react adversely to the product being injected. Reactions are most common if you give an overdose or administer a product in an inappropriate location. For instance, a medication might be safe when given subcutaneously but fatal if the same dose is injected into a vein. But an individual may be extrasensitive to a particular product and will react to it even if it's given in the proper dosage and location. The reaction may be as mild as local swelling that subsides in a few days or serious enough to be life-threatening if the animal goes into shock.

Swelling

Temporary, mild swelling at the injection site is usually nothing to worry about, but if you inject the neck too close to the shoulder blade, the swelling makes it hard for the animal to walk. It's impossible to move that shoulder forward without discomfort, and she may be lame and sore for several days. Some types of vaccine (such as clostridial products) are notorious for causing swelling. Individual animals may react more than others to certain products. To avoid making the animal lame and sore, put a neck injection well ahead of the shoulder; give the shot closer to the head than to the shoulder.

Allergic Response and Shock

A more serious type of reaction occurs when an animal is very sensitive to the product being injected and experiences a severe allergic response called *anaphylaxis*. This may result in difficult breathing, and the animal may go into shock, collapse, and die. Hypersensitivity reactions sometimes occur following administration of vaccines or drugs, with signs developing within 10 to 20 minutes or sometimes longer. *Ruminants* may show acute breathing problems, extending the head and neck and panting open-mouthed or slobbering. The back of the throat and voice box may swell, creating a loud wheezing. There is sudden *edema* in tissues, especially the lungs; they fill with fluid and the animal suffocates.

Oral Medications and Fluid Therapy

Fluid therapy and many medications can be given orally. Pills and boluses can be given with a *balling gun* — a long-handled tool with a cylindrical "cup" on one end to hold the bolus while you place it into the mouth and throat. Maneuver it carefully so as not to injure the mouth or throat tissues. Once the pill is past the back of the tongue (so the animal can't spit it out), the plunger on your end can be gently pressed, pushing the pill out the other end so the animal must swallow it. Small tools for young calves are sometimes made of hard plastic, but a larger one for adults is usually metal so it won't be crushed if the animal grabs it with her teeth while you're trying to push it to the back of the mouth.

HOW TO GIVE CALVES FLUIDS ORALLY

1. Fill a syringe with the fluid.
2. Restrain a small calf by backing him into a corner and straddling his neck. Have a helper on hand for a larger calf and put a very big calf in a chute.
3. Hold the calf's head up toward you, and stick the syringe into the side of the mouth, aiming the tip toward the back of the mouth.
4. Push the fluid in a little at a time to give the calf time to swallow before giving him more.

Whenever you give fluids by mouth, there's always a risk of getting some in his windpipe if the calf doesn't swallow it or if you give him so much at once that he can't swallow it fast enough. If he gets fluid in his lungs, he may develop pneumonia.

When giving large volumes of liquid medication, it's best to use a tube, bypassing the mouth and throat and putting the fluid directly into the stomach.

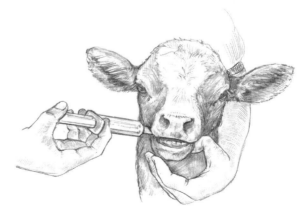

Liquid medication can be given to a calf by syringe. This is called drenching. Dose syringes work best for drenching. Extensions allow you to put the fluid to the back of the throat where the calf must swallow it.

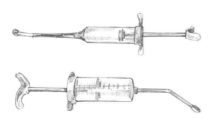

Drenching

Drenching is the term for giving fluid by mouth. If you hold the calf's head up, he generally can't spill or spit out the fluid. A special *dose syringe* works better than a regular syringe because it has a stainless steel probe with rounded tip that goes into the side of the mouth and toward the throat, putting the material farther back where the calf has to swallow it. Also, he can't chew up the syringe, since only the metal probe is in his mouth.

SUPPLIES NEEDED FOR GIVING ORAL MEDICATION

Obtain the tools listed below from your veterinarian or veterinary supply catalog:

☐ Balling guns (calf and cow sizes) for administering boluses
☐ Dose syringe for administering liquids to calves
☐ Esophageal feeder for baby calves
☐ Nasogastric tube (small and large diameters)
☐ Larger-diameter tube or hose for adult animals

Fluid Therapy

When administering fluids in large doses, use a tube that will deliver the hydrating liquids directly into the stomach. The easiest method for baby calves is to use an esophageal feeder — a long plastic or stainless steel probe attached to a bag or container that holds the fluid, with a rounded ball on the end of the tube that goes down the throat.

Nasogastric Tube

A nasogastric tube is a long, small-diameter tube with a smoothed end that goes into the nostril, down to the back of the throat, where the animal swallows it. Use a tube with a ⅚ inch (2.1 cm) outside diameter for baby calves and a tube ½ to 1 inch (1.25 to 2.5 cm) for adults. With this simple tool you can give a quart (0.95 L) of fluid to a sick calf, a gallon (3.8 L) of *mineral oil* to a cow, or several gallons of water, medication, and/or nutrients to an adult animal that's dehydrated or not eating or drinking.

A nasogastric tube or a tube down the throat can also be used to let gas out of the rumen if an animal is bloated. See chapter 8 for a complete discussion of this condition.

HOW TO GIVE PILLS OR BOLUSES

Pills and boluses can be given with a long-handled balling gun. The pill is inserted into the mouth with the balling gun and aimed toward the back of the throat. Once the balling gun is pushed to the back of the throat, the pill is ejected or pushed out of its holder so that the animal must swallow it.

1. Restrain the animal so you have easy access to her head and she can't move it away from you.
2. Place the bolus in the cup of the balling gun.
3. Insert the balling gun gently into the side of her mouth where there are no teeth, then aim and move it straight back toward the throat, so she can't grab it with her teeth. Do not ram it forcefully, or the throat tissues may be injured.
4. Make sure the cup containing the pill is at the back of the throat, where the animal cannot maneuver her tongue to spit out the pill, then eject the pill.

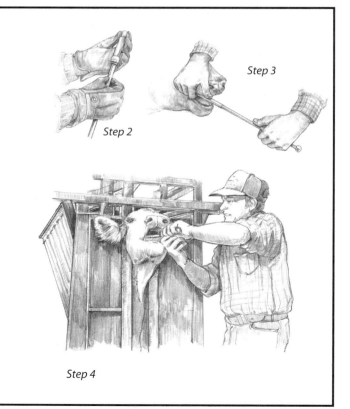

Step 2

Step 3

Step 4

Tube Down the Throat

Although it is often easier and safer to use a nasogastric tube, fluid or mineral oil can also be given to an adult animal with a large diameter tube put down the throat into the stomach. This can be hard to do because the animal tries to grab the tube with tongue and teeth to avoid having it put down the throat, and she may chew up the tube. A metal *speculum* is often used; this is a round metal tube that the flexible tube goes through, protecting the softer tube where it goes through the cow's mouth. If you don't have a speculum, put a block of wood between her jaws so she can't bite down. Once you get the tube started down the throat, however, you can usually keep it going straight down and out of reach of the molars. Make sure it is in the stomach before pouring fluid down the tube.

HOW TO GIVE CALVES FLUIDS WITH AN ESOPHAGEAL FEEDER

1. If working by yourself, restrain the calf by backing him into a corner or sitting him on his haunches with his head held between your knees. If you have a helper, that person can hold the calf.

2. The calf's mouth should be held up toward you and his neck extended, creating a straight line with his mouth and throat and on down to his stomach.

3. Gently set the probe in the side of the mouth and then aim it straight back, sliding the probe gently back and forth over the tongue and then down the throat, and into the *esophagus*. The rounded ball helps keep the probe from going into the slightly smaller windpipe.

4. Test to see if the probe and tube are entering the esophagus rather than the windpipe by feeling the outside of the neck (just behind the head) as you push it down. Keep in mind that the esophagus is above the windpipe. If the calf coughs you may need to try a different angle.

5. Once the probe is in place in the esophagus, with the end of it pushing into the stomach entrance or nearly to it (depending on the size of the calf), you can tip up the feeder bag or container or open the valve and let the fluid flow down the tube into the stomach.

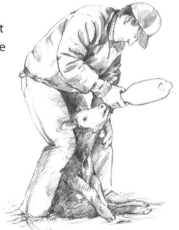

Using an esophageal feeder

HOW TO GIVE ANIMALS FLUIDS WITH A NASOGASTRIC TUBE

1. Restrain the animal. A calf can be held; a cow should be walked into a chute. The animal's head should be slightly tucked with the nose down rather than up. If the head and nose are straight out, the tube is more likely to go into the windpipe rather than the esophagus when it gets to the back of the throat.

2. Insert the smooth end of the tube into the nostril and push it to the back of the throat where the animal must swallow it. Don't ram it forcefully or it will probably end up in the windpipe. Give the animal a chance to swallow it, while also providing the momentum to get it down the esophagus.

3. As you push the tube in, make sure it's in the esophagus and not the windpipe. If it enters the windpipe, the animal will cough. If he coughs, take it out and start over.

4. Once it's in proper position heading into the esophagus, push the tube on down into the stomach.

5. Blow on it to make sure it's in the right place. If you hear burbling noises, it's in the stomach. If blowing makes the animal cough, it's in the windpipe.

6. Once it's in the stomach, attach a funnel to your end of the tube and administer the fluid.

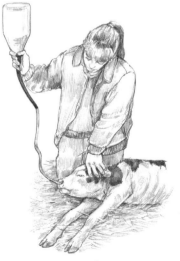

Using a small nasogastric tube for a calf

Restraints

To examine an animal closely or treat it, some kind of restraint is usually necessary. Dairy cows can often be restrained in a *stanchion,* since they are already accustomed to this type of restraint. For a beef animal, some other method is usually needed.

Halter

If the animal is gentle, a halter may be an adequate restraint for some medical procedures. It's always good to have one around, and it can be made easily, using a long, strong, soft, and flexible rope. Don't use a hard-twist or nylon rope that will burn your hands if the animal tries to pull away while you are handling or tying her.

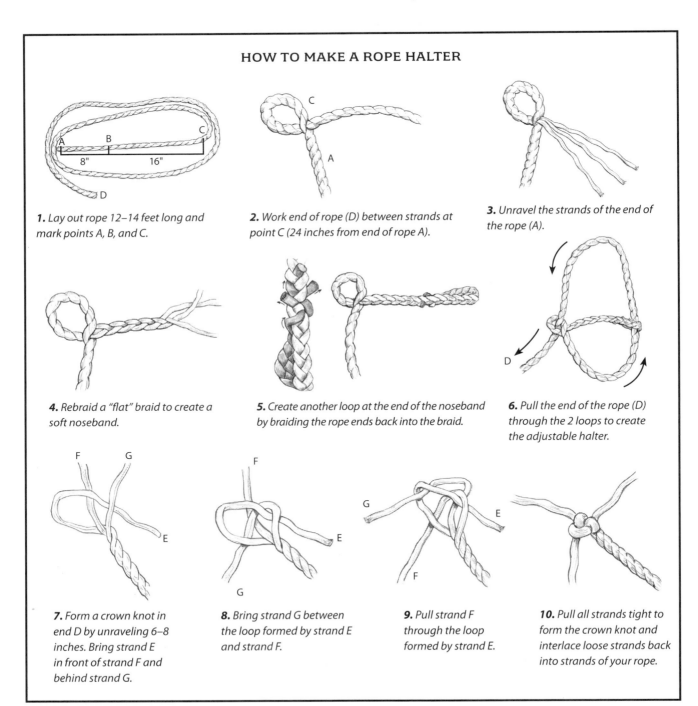

HOW TO MAKE A ROPE HALTER

1. Lay out rope 12–14 feet long and mark points A, B, and C.

2. Work end of rope (D) between strands at point C (24 inches from end of rope A).

3. Unravel the strands of the end of the rope (A).

4. Rebraid a "flat" braid to create a soft noseband.

5. Create another loop at the end of the noseband by braiding the rope ends back into the braid.

6. Pull the end of the rope (D) through the 2 loops to create the adjustable halter.

7. Form a crown knot in end D by unraveling 6–8 inches. Bring strand E in front of strand F and behind strand G.

8. Bring strand G between the loop formed by strand E and strand F.

9. Pull strand F through the loop formed by strand E.

10. Pull all strands tight to form the crown knot and interlace loose strands back into strands of your rope.

Once you've found the right rope, simply create a permanent and adjustable headstall with a nose band at one end (see How to Make a Rope Halter). You can create an instant, make-do halter starting with a rope tied loosely around the animal's neck or by using a rope with a ring installed at one end (see Instant Halters). A halter is very handy if you halter train your cows at an early age; they will always be easy to tie up.

Even when restraining an animal in a *head catcher* or squeeze chute, there are times when you need to immobilize the head, and a halter will be needed. With a halter you can tie the head around to one side to keep the animal from slinging her head when you are examining or treating an eye, dehorning, or performing other procedures to the face or head. A *nose lead* can also be used for this purpose (see page 58).

When tying with a halter, use a knot that is secure, yet easy to untie in a hurry, even if the rope has been pulled very tight. For instance, if the animal fights and pulls back or falls down in her struggles, the knot may be very tight. If the animal is on the ground with her head held up and hanging by the halter, you must be able to untie the rope quickly. Never use a slipknot.

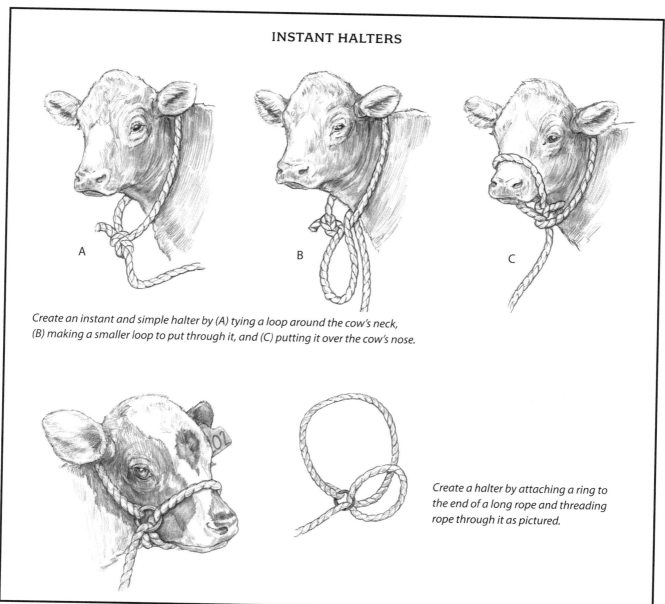

INSTANT HALTERS

Create an instant and simple halter by (A) tying a loop around the cow's neck, (B) making a smaller loop to put through it, and (C) putting it over the cow's nose.

Create a halter by attaching a ring to the end of a long rope and threading rope through it as pictured.

Kick Restraint

To work with the udder or hind legs on a standing cow, you must be able to keep her from kicking. Cows are very good at kicking forward and to the side, making it dangerous for anyone trying to work at the rear end of the cow. To keep a gentle cow in a stanchion from kicking, an assistant can hold the tail head firmly straight up. This does two things: It affects the leg nerves, making it harder for her to kick, and the pressure of holding her tail in this position tends to stimulate release of endorphins in the body, which have a calming effect.

Care must be taken, however, not to push the tail forward too strongly, or you may break the tail. The tail should be held very close to the tail head, lifting it from the underside. Another gentle-cow method requires a strong helper to hold up a front foot on the same side on which you are working. Then the cow can't pick up that hind leg to kick because it puts her too much off balance.

A flank rope can keep a cow from kicking while being treated or milked or when you are suckling a calf on an uncooperative cow. This can be used in conjunction with a halter, stanchion, or head catcher to restrain a cow. Always have her head restrained before applying a flank rope. For beef cows, it's generally simpler just to tie the hind leg on the side on which you are working back to something behind her, such as the back part of the chute. The rope should have enough slack so she can stand comfortably on that leg but can't bring it forward to kick.

A dairy cow in a stanchion may not have anything at the rear you can tie her to, in which case it's easier to use a flank rope. The rope is put around her flanks just ahead of her udder and behind her hip bones and pulled snug. Mild pressure just ahead of her udder makes it more difficult and uncomfortable for her to bring a hind leg forward to kick. Make sure the rope is not too tight or it may cause discomfort or damage the milk vein. Most cows tolerate a flank rope, but some try to jump around, defeating the purpose.

For examining or trimming feet, a rope is often necessary to hold up the foot being worked on. Cows can't balance themselves very well on three legs. When working on a front foot, tie up the animal or confine her in a stanchion or head catcher, and hold the front leg up with a rope around the *withers*. When working on a hind foot, the hind leg must be similarly held up and restrained to keep the cow from bringing it forward to kick, especially if you need to hold the foot up and to the rear to examine or treat the sole of the foot.

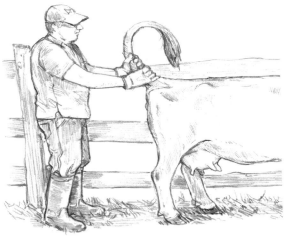

Hold the tail up firmly to keep a cow from kicking.

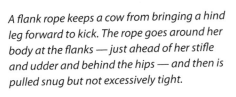

A flank rope keeps a cow from bringing a hind leg forward to kick. The rope goes around her body at the flanks — just ahead of her stifle and udder and behind the hips — and then is pulled snug but not excessively tight.

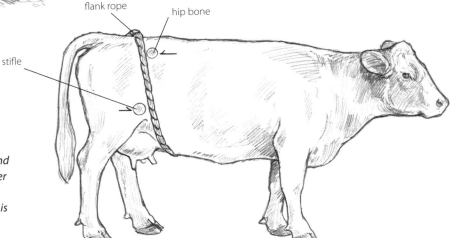

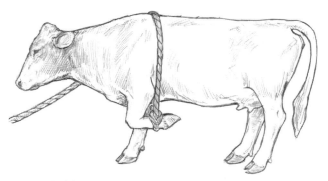

Hold up a front foot with a rope over the withers.

One way to do this is with a *lariat* with a *quick-release honda* (loop): Put the loop around the hind *pastern*. Put the long end of the rope over an overhead beam, part of the chute, or whatever is available above the animal, then bring it down to create a half hitch around the *hock*. An assistant can hold the end of the rope or *dally* (loop) it to something behind the animal. When the foot is picked up, slack can be taken out of the rope to support and suspend the leg in whatever position you need it for working on the foot. The dallied rope should always be held, not tied, so it can be released instantly if the animal struggles and falls. If it's tied, it will put too much strain on the leg and may injure the animal if he goes down.

Chutes and Head Catchers

Restraining animals in a chute is the easiest way to keep them still for vaccination and treatment. Most stockmen have a running chute — a narrow alleyway about 28 inches (71 cm or 0.7 m) wide, with tall, secure sides at least 6 feet (1.8 m) high — leading from a funnel-shaped holding pen and ending in a squeeze chute with a head catcher. Many procedures such as vaccinating or applying a pour-on for lice can be done very quickly in the running chute (going down the line of restrained cattle and giving each one an injection or treatment) without having to restrain each animal in the head catcher.

A 28-inch chute width is adequate for most adult cattle, yet narrow enough so they can't turn around. Sides should be tall enough to keep them from climbing over even when they are rearing up over the back of the animal in front of them, the way some nervous cattle do. Many running chutes are built with a slight curve so the animals can't see that the far end is blocked, so they will enter it more readily. A

catwalk along one side, partway up, enables a person to walk along and easily reach over the side to administer vaccine or pesticide products.

The length of the chute depends on how many animals you plan to work at one time. It's handy to be able to put 10 to 12 adult cattle in the running chute. You don't want it much longer than that, however. If you get too many animals in the chute, it takes more time to process them. The longer you have them in the chute, the more risk there is that they'll become uncomfortably jammed or injured. Animals in a chute for an extended period often become stressed and panicky and will push forward or try to climb over one another. Sometimes they fall down and are walked on by herdmates.

For more meticulous procedures the animals can be caught individually in the squeeze chute/head catcher at the end of the running chute. A good squeeze chute is the best way to restrain an animal for medical procedures. A smaller chute can be used for calves for branding, vaccinating, castrating, or dehorning; a *calf table* can be tipped once the calf is caught by the head, putting him on his side at a level easy for you to work on him.

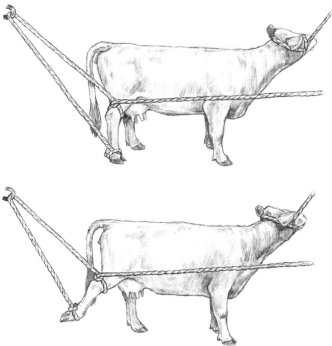

Preparing to lift a hind foot (top). After the foot is lifted off the ground, slack is taken up in the rope so the foot can be held at the desired height (bottom).

Restraining an Animal against a Post

One way to restrain a fairly gentle animal if you don't have a chute or head catcher is to hold the head and neck against a sturdy fencepost (next to a board or pole fence, not a wire fence), using a rope with a loop in it. The adjustable loop should be large enough to put over the top of (and around) the post, then under the cow's neck and back over the top of the post again before you tighten the loop to hold her neck against the post.

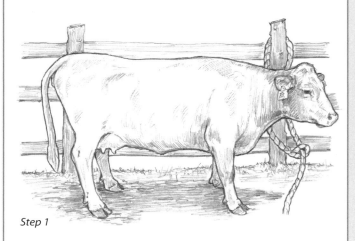

Step 1

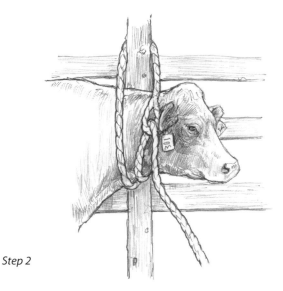

Step 2

Restraining a Cow, a Large Calf, or Yearling on the Ground

A long rope is useful if you need to put a large animal down on the ground for treatment. This can be handy if you don't have a squeeze chute and need the animal completely immobilized or if you need to have the animal lying down rather than standing, as is the case with some surgical procedures.

1. Put bedding down where you intend the cow to be restrained, or choose an area with soft ground so there's less risk of injury if she collapses and goes down hard.

2. Using a nonslip knot, tie a long rope around the cow's neck and one front leg.

3. Tie two half hitches around the body — one around the girth or withers area and one around the flanks, ahead of the udder.

4. After making the second half hitch around the flanks, pull the free end of the rope from behind to squeeze the cow's body. This tends to numb and paralyze the nerves going to her legs, and she lies down.

5. Once she goes down, someone can sit on her head and neck; she can't get up if she can't raise her head.

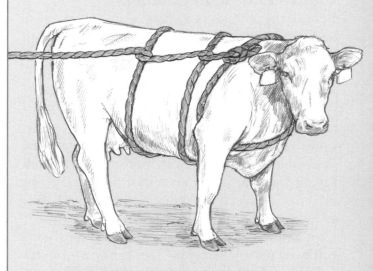

Using a long rope to get a cow off her feet

Restraining a Bull on the Ground

1. Put bedding down where you intend to restrain the bull, or choose an area with soft ground so there's less risk of injury if he collapses and goes down hard.

2. Drape the middle section of a long rope over the animal's withers.

3. Bring the free ends back between the front legs and up to the back.

4. Cross these ends over the back, and pull them down to the flanks and between the hind legs from front to back.

5. Pull on the ropes behind the animal to squeeze his front end and flanks. This puts the animal on the ground.

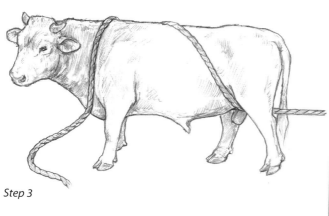

Step 3

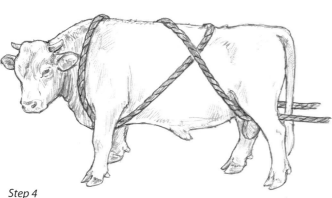

Step 4

This method is best for a bull because a rope pulled tight around his flanks could seriously injure his penis. Whatever method you use, remember that adult cattle can't be flat on their sides or on their backs for very long. Do the necessary procedure quickly, and get them up again.

Tying method to keep the animal on the ground

If legs must be restrained while the animal is down, the free end of the squeeze rope can be used for tying the uppermost rear leg (so the animal can't kick, as shown in A, B, and C). A short piece of extra rope can be used to restrain the uppermost front leg, if necessary, as shown in D and E.

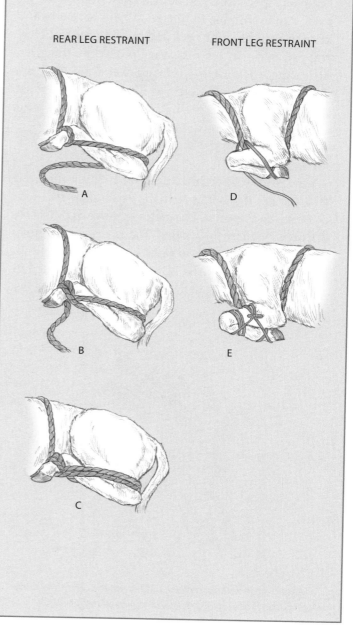

REAR LEG RESTRAINT   FRONT LEG RESTRAINT

A

D

B

E

C

Restraining a Calf

If you don't have a calf chute or table, an easy way to restrain a calf is to put him flat on the ground. Even a fairly large calf can be put down by *flanking*—putting him off balance by taking his legs out from under him. This is done by standing alongside him, leaning over and grabbing the front leg and flank skin on the side away from you, and then quickly lifting. This tips the calf toward you instead of away from you, so you can help break his fall with your legs and kneel on his neck to hold him down.

A calf can be held down easily if he can't get his head up, especially if you flex the uppermost front leg so he can't scramble to his feet. If you have a helper kneeling on the calf's neck and holding the front leg, you can perform the necessary procedure (tagging, castrating, vaccinating) leaning over from the back side, out of the way of kicking hind feet. If you must work by yourself, tie the calf's hind legs to his head and neck so he cannot rise.

Nose Lead

A nose lead is sometimes used for holding the head still, though it is not as humane as a halter. The nose is tender, so the animal hesitates to move or pull away once the metal lead is applied. The easiest way to apply it to a very gentle cow is to stand beside the cow's head, facing the same way she is, while she is restrained in a stanchion or head catcher. Put your arm over her head and neck to slow down her head movement, and then quickly slip the nose lead in place with your other hand. Your body helps block her vision so she can't see the nose lead coming and avoid it.

This is not a safe way to apply a lead to a suspicious cow, however, because if she slings her head (which she may do just because you are close to her), she may bruise your chest or crack a rib. The safest way is to stand in front of her and very quickly snap the tongs into her nose before she has a chance to move. If you are not quick enough, however, you'll have lost the element of surprise, and she'll dodge the tongs on your next attempt.

Because the metal pincers put pressure on tender inner tissues of the nostrils if she jerks her head, she will generally hold still once the tongs are in place. The rope attached to the nose lead can be dallied around a post, a stanchion frame, or the side of the head catcher, and held by an assistant. Don't tie the rope; you must be able to let it go slack immediately if the cow falls or goes down on her knees, or she may tear her nose.

It's less stressful and much safer to use a halter.

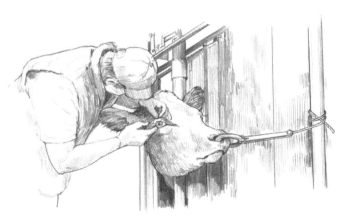

Nose tongs can help hold a cow's head still when certain procedures need to be done, such as treating this cow's early cancer growth on her eye.

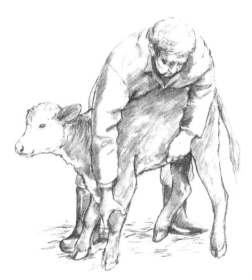

To restrain a calf without a chute, put him on the ground by flanking him, then kneel on his neck to keep him on the ground.

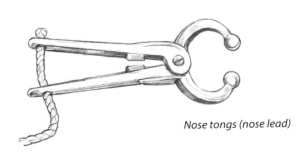

Nose tongs (nose lead)

CHAPTER THREE

Seasonal Health

As with humans, daily weather affects the health and well-being of cattle. A hot, humid spell can cause cattle to overheat. Heat-stressed cattle are uncomfortable and do not eat well; cows give less milk and calves don't grow as well as expected when it's too warm. In extremely hot weather cattle may die.

Bitterly cold or extremely wet weather is just as stressful. Cold or stormy weather conditions can lead to pneumonia, frostbitten teats and ears, and an increased need for calories just to stay warm. If cattle can't eat enough food to maintain body temperature, they use up fat and muscle tissue to generate needed energy and in the process lose weight, becoming more vulnerable to stress-related diseases.

Hot-Weather Problems

Summer and hot weather can create a number of serious health problems for cattle, especially in climates with a combination of high temperatures and high humidity. Problems range from infertility to death. For example, in July of 1995 more than 3,750 cattle in one feedlot in Iowa died in a 24-hour period because of high heat and humidity. Although these cattle were properly cared for and had access to water, several days of extreme heat and high humidity culminated in lethal heat overload.

Cattle in hot weather may lose weight because they don't eat as much and because it takes more energy to pant and try to keep the body cool. Air temperatures that hover around 68 to 70°F (20 to 21°C) are ideal *(thermo-neutral)*, with no additional energy needed to heat or cool the body. If air temperature drops or rises significantly from this level, however, more energy is needed to maintain normal body processes. How well an individual handles heat depends on breed, hair-coat length, age, health (sick animals or those with lung damage can't handle heat), body condition, nutrition, stage of pregnancy, and acclimation.

Some Breeds Tolerate Heat Better

Along the Gulf Coast and most of the southern part of the United States, stockmen often choose animals with *Brahman* or *zebu* breeding because *Bos indicus* cattle (those from India, Asia, and Africa) have more heat tolerance and less risk for problems. They have more sweat glands and also some metabolic differences that help them handle higher temperatures. *Bos taurus* (British and European) breeds are stressed more readily and to a greater degree in hot environments unless crossed with *Bos indicus* cattle.

Crossbred cattle that are one-half or one-quarter Brahman are better able to handle heat and humidity. On a hot, humid day cattle with zebu breeding (such as Brahman or Senepol) will usually be grazing, while British or European breeds are seeking shade or standing around panting. The farther south you live, and the less zebu breeding in your cattle, the more important shade becomes.

The upper limit of the comfort zone for cattle is about 75°F (24°C), but this depends on breed, size, and color of the animal. Light-colored animals have an advantage over dark animals, as reflection reduces the amount of heat they absorb, though they may have a higher incidence of sunburn.

Dark colors absorb more heat because they have less ability to reflect it. If you have dark-hided cattle, such as black Angus, they tend to have a higher body temperature — up to 104°F (40°C) during hot weather — whereas lighter-colored cattle have normal temperatures of 101.5 to 102°F (38.6 to 38.9°C). Studies of deaths in feedlot cattle during hot weather have shown that 70 percent are due to heat stress in animals with dark hides.

If body temperature rises to the critical point of 107°F (41.7°C), the animal may have circulatory collapse, and the heart will stop. Once the animal's temperature gets this high, heat stroke occurs, especially if the animal can't get enough water to maintain his proper blood pressure.

Large cattle also suffer more heat stress. Cattle with lots of muscle mass generate more heat than cattle with less body mass. The bulky muscles have more heat to dissipate and less body surface per pound of weight, so it's harder to get rid of the heat. Smaller, lighter-muscled animals do significantly better in hot weather.

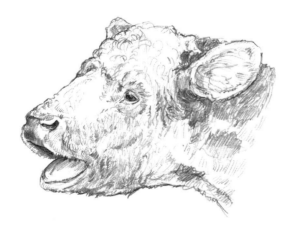

On a hot day cattle may pant open-mouthed to try to cool themselves, especially after exertion.

Humidity

Degrees of humidity make a difference. Even in hot weather, a dry climate is easier on cattle than a climate with high humidity. In the desert, for instance, cattle that have access to adequate water and shade generally do not suffer heat stress because they can dissipate body heat at night when the air temperature drops. In Arizona, New Mexico, and some parts of Texas, most cattle do fine because they can cool off at night.

By contrast, hot weather in a moist climate can lead to heat stress in any animals that are not genetically programmed to handle it, because air temperature generally doesn't cool down much at night. In a dry climate, any moisture on the body (sweat, saliva slung over the back and sides) evaporates quickly and helps cool the animal, whereas in humid conditions, moisture on the body cannot evaporate very well and has little cooling effect.

Heat Wave

Nighttime air temperatures are crucial to a cow's ability to cool herself. Because humidity tends to be higher at night than during the day, if it doesn't drop below 80°F (26.7°C) at night, this is a major problem, especially if it continues for several days or nights. Cattle can rid themselves of body heat accumulated in the daytime if night temperatures drop below 75°F (23.9°C). They have a window of time for heat loss and can often drop down to normal. But if nighttime temperatures stay in the upper 70s (25 to 26°C) or higher, cattle don't have that means of dissipating heat and start to accumulate it. If a heat wave lasts three days or more, cattle may die. They accumulate a little heat the first day, and if they can't get rid of it at night, they are a little hotter the second day. By the third day it becomes critical.

In 1993 thousands of cattle in Nebraska died due to lack of nighttime cooling combined with high humidity. Thousands of dairy cattle perished in California during the summer of 2006 when temperatures stayed above 100°F (37.8°C) for many days. Even though the California weather was not as humid as Nebraska's, the cumulative effect of such a long hot spell did not allow cattle to lower their body temperature enough.

To prevent fatalities, especially in dairy or feedlot cattle, you must create a break in the heat before they get to that third day, which seems to be the time it takes to accumulate a lethal load of extra body heat. You must break that cycle, if it doesn't break naturally, by cooling cattle with water or fans (see below).

If cattle are outdoors you can hope for clear nights with no clouds to facilitate heat dissipating from the body surface into the cooler air (*radiant heat* loss). The sky is a "heat sink" on a clear night, letting warm air move up into the atmosphere. If it's cloudy, air temperature does not go down as much, as the cloud cover holds the warmth close to the earth. It's especially difficult to get rid of heat if humidity is high at night, and it tends to be higher if there's cloud cover or there's been a recent rain. The air is full of water, and evaporation is next to impossible.

How Cattle Respond to Heat Overload

Ruminant animals handle heat differently from the way that humans or dogs do. Cattle generate a lot of heat during digestion of forages in the rumen via fermentation and don't sweat as much as humans. But they can handle high heat load by being able to allow their core body temperature to rise. They don't have to maintain a temperature within a very narrow range like humans or dogs must in order to survive. Things that affect bovine body temperature include metabolism, body processes that produce heat, and the heat of digestion, which can be affected somewhat by the type of feed eaten (see page 64).

A cow's core body temperature can safely rise several degrees before she is in trouble. Only when it reaches high levels will she begin to pant. Respiration rate can be an indication of heat stress. Cattle can increase evaporation heat loss by increasing their respiration rate and exchange of air through the respiratory passages, thereby creating more evaporation in the airways. Breathing with the mouth open, however, is an inefficient way of cooling and also creates metabolic problems (if panting continues) because of the loss of hydrogen ions out of the mouth via saliva.

Though many people think that cattle can't sweat, they do have sweat glands — and zebu cattle have the most. When an animal gets hot, blood vessels in the skin dilate to take more blood to the surface and extremities and to transfer more heat to the environment in order to cool off. Sweat glands open and excrete moisture from the blood vessels onto the skin. Cattle hair is water repellent, so moisture from sweat tends to condense on the hair and be pushed back down to the skin to evaporate, which has a cooling effect on the body. The cow's body may not look wet, but the skin is damp and is evaporating the water so fast that you often won't see it. There may only be a slight dampness on the hair.

Four Cooling Methods

There are four ways that cattle cool themselves — evaporation, *conduction* (movement of heat from the animal to a cooler solid structure like the ground she's lying on), *convection* (movement of air over the animal that takes heat with it), and radiation (radiating heat out from the body into the air). In order to be effective, all these factors except evaporation require the surrounding temperature to be cooler than body temperature. When air temperature gets close to body temperature (101 to 103°F [38.3 to 39.4°C]), the only route for heat loss is evaporation. Since cattle don't sweat as efficiently as horses or humans, their body temperature tends to rise during periods of hot weather.

Evaporation is facilitated when air is dry enough for moisture on the body to dissipate into the air and take some of the heat with it. A breeze helps speed evaporative heat loss. Convective cooling also works best if there's a breeze and some air movement between animals (because they are not bunched together and overcrowded).

Cattle slobber more in hot weather and sling saliva over their backs in an effort to induce evaporation. This can help cool them, but because saliva contains bicarbonate and sodium, excess saliva production and loss means that they are losing bicarbonate that's needed in the rumen to buffer digestive acids. They are also losing body fluid, so must drink more water when it's hot.

If cattle are losing a lot of saliva to try to cool themselves, this puts them at greater risk for acidosis if they are on a high-grain diet, or for bloat if eating fermentable feeds such as alfalfa.

People tend to think cattle are hottest in midday when air temperatures are highest, but this isn't true. Their bodies accumulate heat, so there's a delay of several hours in the rise of body temperature when cattle are exposed to heat. If they've been eating, there is also an increase in metabolic heat produced. Cattle don't reach peak body temperature until four to five hours after they finish eating. This is why they graze very early in the morning and late in the evening during hot weather, resting and chewing their cuds during the middle of the day. During very hot weather they'll do most of their grazing at night.

If cattle are not accustomed to hot weather or if it comes on suddenly, it takes a while for them to become acclimated and make functional and behavioral changes. The body needs time to adjust to the heat; it may be several days before a cow's metabolism drops to lower levels so she's not producing as much body heat.

Signs of Heat Stress

You can tell when cattle become too hot by observing their behavior. They quit eating and spend all their efforts trying to stay cooler. They breathe faster and sling saliva, crowding into shady areas or around a water tank or standing in a pond. When her respiration rate rises above 100 breaths per minute, the animal is lethargic and does not want to move, and it's hard for her to eat.

If body temperature continues to rise, the animal becomes nervous and anxious, unable to be comfortable. If respiration rate rises above 100 breaths per minute and cattle are breathing heavily and drooling or panting with their mouths open, they're too hot. If they're panting with a respiration rate of 120 or higher, with head and neck elevated, this means they are having trouble breathing. If this alarming situation is not resolved soon and they become hotter, they may die.

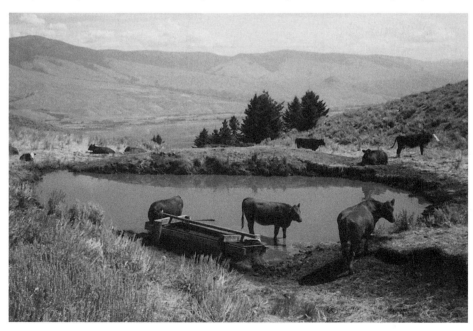

If cattle depend on a pond, make sure it doesn't dry up.

Heat Effects on Reproduction

In hot climates, avoid having cows bred during the hottest months. The impact of high heat, *thermal loads* (heat accumulation in the body), and a high *heat index* (the combination of high humidity and high temperature) can have a detrimental effect on the survival of the embryo after the cow is bred. Cows may become pregnant and then lose the embryo. Dairies in hot southern regions generally don't try to breed cows during the hottest seasons because of this adverse impact on fertility. The most common time for embryonic loss due to heat stress is the first week after conception, when the embryo fails to attach to the uterus, but losses can also occur through the first month of gestation.

Heat stress can also cause infertility in bulls. Under normal conditions, the testicles are kept a few degrees cooler than the body, since heat interferes with sperm development. But during hot weather the body's methods for keeping testicles cool may not be adequate. A bull may be temporarily infertile because sperm that were developing during hot weather were adversely affected.

Calving during hot weather can result in calf losses. Young calves don't have much body reserve and can easily dehydrate. If it's so hot that they don't feel like nursing, they dehydrate quickly, especially if they are sick. Shade and water are very important for them. Dark-colored calves have the most trouble handling heat.

Effects on the Immune System

Heat stress adds to other stresses (such as weaning, transport, and parasite loads) and may make cattle more vulnerable to disease. Stress of any kind causes the *adrenal glands* to secrete more cortisol, which depresses the immune system. If part of the maintenance energy is being used to cool the body, other requirements, such as that of the immune system, may not be met. A high respiration rate (panting) to try to cool the body may increase susceptibility to respiratory disease, especially if dusty or smoky conditions irritate the airways and lungs.

Water, Water Everywhere

Plenty of sources of water and shade are crucial for cattle during hot weather. If there's not enough water,

---

HOT AND HUMID? MORE WATER!

In temperatures up to 70°F (21°C), cattle may drink more than 2 gallons (7.6 L) per 100 pounds (45.4 kg) of body weight daily.

In temperatures over 95°F (35°C), cattle need more than 4 gallons (15 L) per 100 pounds of body weight daily.

In a feedlot, cattle may need more than 2 gallons per hour for each 100 pounds of body weight, if temperature is above 80°F (26.7°C).

If a cow is lactating, she needs even more water in order to keep producing milk (the actual amount depends upon how much milk she is producing). Her metabolism is also higher when lactating, so she's at greater risk for heat stress than a dry cow or a steer.

---

an animal's body tries to conserve it. Hormonal changes take place to reduce sweating, urination, and saliva creation. If cattle have enough water available so they can drink all they want, however, they get rid of some body heat through these same body processes. If they can keep replenishing water loss, everything they can get rid of takes heat with it. Some dairies and feedlots have found that providing chilled drinking water during hot weather can help prevent heat stress, keeping cattle body temperature within safer limits.

Make sure ponds don't dry up. If pond water gets low, it may become muddy, dirty, and stagnant from trampling, and there's more risk for contracting disease if cattle drink it. If water quality is poor, animals drink less, which may put them at risk for dehydration and heat stress. They also eat less if they are not drinking enough water; young animals won't gain much weight, and cows' milk production drops.

If animals are bunched together or crowded around a water trough trying to drink or stay cool, they reduce any beneficial effects of a breeze. During hot weather dominant animals hog the troughs, and others can't get to the water. The more watering areas (with fresh clean water) you can provide, the better.

Hot-Weather Water Checklist

Go through this checklist each day during hot weather to make sure your herd is getting the proper amount of good quality water:

▸ Make sure the streams and ditches that cattle depend on for water are running, and supply the animals with another source if the waterways dry up

▸ If water is supplied in troughs or tanks, make sure there are plenty of them, that they are always working, and that smaller, passive animals can get to them

▸ If cattle are in pens, make sure they are not over-crowded and that they all have access to water

▸ Make sure ponds are not too low or stagnant

Shade and a Breeze

During hot weather, cows often seek shade if it's available. Shade is extremely important in an environment without cloud cover. Animals constantly exposed to direct sunlight get much hotter than those with access to shade. A naturally shady area may or may not be the most comfortable place for cattle, however. Natural shade along a brushy creek, for instance, may be swarming with biting flies, and cattle will avoid it. Shade may be stifling hot in thick brush that obstructs wind movement. If there are no open-air trees or brush to provide natural shade, build shade structures in pastures.

Man-made structures should have high roofs, at least 10 feet (3 m) or more off the ground, to allow air movement over the animals. Crowding and lack of airflow reduce the beneficial effect of shade. At least 40 to 50 square feet (3.7 to 4.7 sq m) of space per animal is recommended. Even more space is necessary if you depend on trees, since too many cattle crowding around the trees may kill them.

When constructing a shade roof, use materials that can handle the weight of snow if you're in a northern climate. Put insulation under a metal roof to minimize the heating effects of the sun — otherwise it will produce radiant heat and be like an oven underneath. Strong mesh shade materials are inexpensive, needn't be taken down in cold weather as they are fairly durable in wind and snow, and reduce up to 95 percent of radiant heat.

Cattle often prefer to be on a high spot or ridge with a breeze (and away from flies) rather than in shade that acts as a windbreak with no ventilation. If cattle spend energy fighting flies or group together in an attempt to evade biting flies, they are more at risk for heat stress. In a summer pen or pasture, cattle prefer shade from tall trees or structures that don't hinder air flow. You don't want windbreaks; cattle need all the air movement they can get. It usually takes at least a 3- to 5-mile(4.8 to 8.1 km)-per-hour breeze to remove the heat and water they are evaporating, so the best shade is something that does not obstruct airflow.

In feedlots or dairies, fans are sometimes utilized to help cool cattle. Research has found that nighttime fan use is generally more effective than daytime cooling if you have a choice; you get more benefit from air movement when air temperatures are cooler. There are times during summer when it may get so hot you must cool cattle continually, but in spring and fall it's usually better to turn on the fans when air temperature drops to a cooler level.

Feed Makes a Difference

If cattle are fed hay or grain (as in a feedlot rather than at pasture), what you feed them can be a factor in how hot they get. When feeding forage, such as hay, green chop, or silage, use high-quality forage that is easily broken down and digested quickly. It generates less heat during digestion than the fermentation breakdown of low-quality roughages such as coarse hay, straw, or any type of forage that contains a lot of fiber.

Salt and Minerals

Salt should always be supplied in ample amounts during hot weather. If cattle can't replace sodium, potassium, and other electrolytes lost through sweat and other body fluids, they are more stressed in the heat. Trace minerals like copper and zinc are also depleted during heat stress and must be replaced. Put salt, mineral, or supplement feeders close to shady areas so cattle won't have to walk far to get to them or be out in the heat for very long. They'll use them more often.

It also makes a difference what time of day you feed them. Cattle always eat more when they are comfortable and cooler. They prefer the least possible amount of activity when it's hot. Under natural conditions when grazing at pasture, they graze in the early mornings and late evenings until dark or even after dark if it's been too hot to graze during the day. If cattle are confined, don't feed during the middle of the day when it's hot. Very early morning and late evening is much better.

Stockmen often feed in the morning, but they don't start early enough, as heat production from eating peaks midday. Cattle eat better if fed very early or very late. If you can't get out at the crack of dawn, shift most of the feeding to evening so that when cattle generate heat from digestion and increased metabolism, it's not during the hottest part of the day.

If you know a heat wave is coming, cut down the amount of feed to help lessen the digestive heat load. It's better to have them gain less (or milk less) for a few days than have them die of heat stress.

Some types of forage hinder the ability of cattle to handle heat. If plants contain ergot or endophyte fungus, cattle suffer more heat stress (see chapter 17). Fungus-infected fescue also produces many problems for cattle in hot climates. The grass contains compounds that interfere with dissipation of body heat, due to constriction of blood vessels in the skin. Cattle build up core temperature, which leads to greater heat stress. Endophyte-infected fescue is the most common forage that creates trouble, but other types of grasses infected with ergot or fungi can cause the same problems.

Emergency Cooling

Sometimes you must take action to save overheated cattle. Watch weather forecasts, and check temperature and humidity indexes to know when the combination of the two is approaching the alert stage, danger stage, or emergency stage, in which cattle may die. Even if air temperature is only in the upper 70s (25 to 26°C), if there is humidity of 70 percent or above, you may be in the alert stage, and if the temperature gets to 80 (26.7°C), it's more serious. When the index combination reaches 84 or higher for more than two days in a row, animals may be in trouble. If it gets into the danger or emergency stage, do something quickly to save your animals.

If humidity and temperature both reach a point where cattle cannot cool themselves, you may have to hose them with water. In some instances stockmen call the fire department to hose down cattle to try to cool them. You must get their core body temperature back down, and this may be the only feasible way to do it. Don't use really cold water, however, because this causes blood vessels in the skin to contract and shut down, and body temperature will rise even higher. Cool or lukewarm water allows the blood vessels to stay dilated, bringing more overheated blood to the surface for cooling.

It's often best to spray or sprinkle cattle in early morning before they get too hot. Use large water droplets; a mist doesn't penetrate the hair coat as well. Spray for 5 to 10 minutes at a time, once or twice an hour. Continuous spraying or misting may add to the humidity or create mud underfoot. Also, if you start spraying the animals constantly, you have to keep doing it until the hot weather stops. This artificial cooling limits their ability to adapt to the heat.

It's not always easy to know when to use evaporative cooling like sprays or wetting the ground. If you put too much water into the air when humidity is already high, cattle can't lose heat through evaporation. In the hot, arid West, however, you can use water; evaporation is the best route for cooling.

Keep in mind that when air temperature climbs during the day, humidity goes down, unless you've had rain. As the temperature drops at night, humidity goes up. Use evaporation (spray) during the day when it gets hot and humidity has dropped. But if you've had rain and humidity is high, this is often when cattle start dying, and spraying cattle only adds to the problem.

If humidity is not too high, you also can cool down cattle in pens by spraying their bedding areas with water. If they lie on hot ground, body heat can't get away from the body. Dry surfaces in a pen may radiate heat up to 140°F (160°C) on a sunny day. If there are mounds in feed pens for cattle to lie on, keeping the mounds cool and damp by spraying them with water can allow for cooling and evaporation from the mound surfaces. Wetting about 20 square feet (1.9 sq m) of pen surface for every animal will give all of them enough room to utilize the cooler ground.

Temperature-Humidity Index

Air °F	Relative Humidity (%)																					Air °F
	0	5	10	15	20	25	30	35	40	45	50	55	60	65	70	75	80	85	90	95	100	
125	107	114	122	130	140	151																125
120	105	110	116	122	130	139	148															120
115	103	106	110	115	121	127	135	143														115
114	102	105	109	113	119	125	132	140														114
113	102	104	108	112	117	123	129	137	145													113
112	101	104	107	111	115	121	127	134	142													112
111	101	103	106	109	114	119	125	131	139	147												111
110	100	102	105	108	112	117	122	129	136	143												110
109	100	101	104	107	110	115	120	126	133	140												109
108	99	101	103	105	109	113	118	124	130	137	144											108
107	99	100	102	104	107	111	116	121	127	134	141											107
106	98	99	101	103	106	109	114	119	124	130	137	145										106
105	97	98	100	102	104	108	112	116	122	127	134	141										105
104	97	97	99	100	103	106	110	114	119	124	131	137	145									104
103	96	97	98	99	102	104	108	112	116	122	127	134	141									103
102	96	96	97	98	100	103	106	110	114	119	124	130	137	144								102
101	95	95	96	97	99	101	104	108	112	116	121	127	133	140								101
100	94	94	95	96	98	100	102	106	109	114	118	124	130	136	143							100
99	93	93	94	95	96	98	101	104	107	111	116	121	126	132	139	146						99
98	92	92	93	94	95	97	99	102	105	109	113	117	123	128	134	141						98
97	92	92	92	93	94	95	97	100	103	106	110	115	119	125	130	136	143					97
96	91	91	91	92	93	94	96	98	101	104	108	112	116	121	126	132	138	145				96
95	89	90	90	91	92	93	94	97	99	102	105	109	113	118	123	128	134	140				95
94	88	89	89	90	90	92	93	95	97	100	103	106	110	114	119	124	129	135	141			94
93	88	88	89	89	89	90	92	93	95	98	101	104	107	111	116	120	125	131	136	142		93
92	87	87	88	88	88	89	90	92	94	96	99	101	105	108	112	116	121	126	131	137	143	92
91	86	87	87	87	87	88	89	91	92	94	97	99	102	105	109	113	117	122	127	132	137	91
90	85	85	86	86	86	87	88	89	91	93	95	97	100	103	106	110	113	118	122	127	132	90
85	81	82	82	82	82	82	83	84	84	85	87	88	89	91	93	95	97	99	102	104	107	85
80	77	78	78	78	79	79	79	80	80	80	81	81	82	82	83	84	84	85	86	86	87	80
Air °F	0	5	10	15	20	25	30	35	40	45	50	55	60	65	70	75	80	85	90	95	100	Air °F
	Relative Humidity (%)																					

The temperature-humidity index formula calculates an apparent temperature, which is how hot the heat/humidity combination makes it feel. High humidity makes heat more dangerous because it slows the evaporation of sweat and the body is unable to cool effectively.

Avoid Working Cattle in the Heat

Exertion is dangerous when cattle are hot; it raises their body temperature even more. If you must round them up, move them a long way to new pasture, sort them, or put them through the chute for vaccinations or other processing, do it in early morning when it's cooler. Even evening work can be hard on the herd.

After sunset, it may take cattle six hours or more to dissipate accumulated body heat.

Work activity, stress, and jostling can elevate body temperature as much as 0.5 to 3.5°F (0.4 to 2.3°C), and put cattle into the danger zone for critical temperature. Anything you can do to minimize stress will help (see chapter 1). Among other measures, gather cattle slowly, work them in smaller groups, give them less standing time when they are confined, and never make them run. Minimize bunching up in a corral; crowding limits air movement between them. Give them plenty of rest stops if they must go a long way to the corral or to a new pasture. Young calves may overheat quickly, as will older calves with a lot of body fat. If any animals in the group start slobbering or panting, slow down or let the herd rest.

Transport Stress Is Worse in Hot Weather

If hauling cattle, do it at night or early in the morning. Open all the vents in a trailer or remove slats from a truck for airflow. Never leave cattle standing in a truck or trailer. Heat builds up rapidly when the vehicle is not moving. In hot weather load cattle more loosely (using fewer animals to fill the truck) so they are not tightly packed. If using bedding in the truck or trailer for cushion or traction, use cooler options such as wet sand or wet shavings.

Radiant Heat Research

Studies at the University of Missouri used environmentally controlled chambers to measure cattle responses to varying degrees of heat and humidity and the relationship of those climate factors with the intake of water and feed. Different feeds were evaluated, to determine best choices for hot weather, as was the ability of the cattle to transition through climate changes.

Some of these tests used chambers in which solar radiation was duplicated to understand the sun's effects combined with air temperature and humidity — important because much of the heat buildup in the body comes from radiant heat (sunshine). Researchers can now measure radiant temperature with a black globe thermometer. During hot weather, this globe may reach as high as 120°F (48.9°C) and is representative of an animal's temperature out in the sun. If you touch an object that's been in the sun, it's much hotter than the air temperature. On an animal with dark skin, the temperature of the skin can get as high as any other dark object. This is a significant consideration for stockmen.

CATTLE-DRIVE TRAGEDY

CATTLE IN FLESHY CONDITION and fat calves are most prone to overheating during or following physical exertion. On a cattle drive in July 2005, our son and his wife were gathering and moving range cattle to their high pasture (traveling several miles and climbing 1,500 feet. They noticed one of their larger steer calves was panting with his mouth open and beginning to lie down frequently. They left him and his mama behind, but when they went back later to get the pair, the calf had died from heat stress.

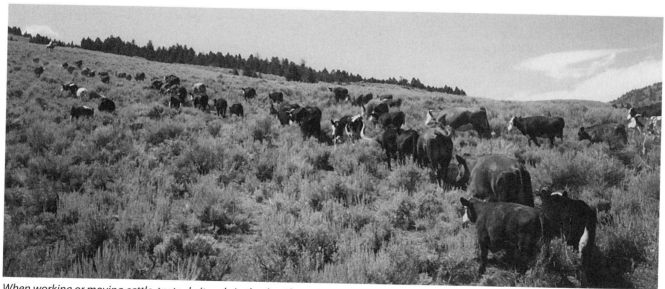

When working or moving cattle, try to do it early in the day. If weather gets hot, move them slowly, at their own speed, to avoid heat stress. These cows are traveling uphill on a hot day, to a new range pasture, following a rider and traveling at their own pace, rather than being herded or chased.

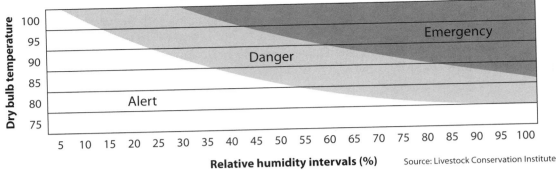

Livestock Weather Safety Index

Emergency

Danger

Alert

Dry bulb temperature: 100 95 90 85 80 75

Relative humidity intervals (%): 5 10 15 20 25 30 35 40 45 50 55 60 65 70 75 80 85 90 95 100

Source: Livestock Conservation Institute

As temperature and humidity climb, the danger for heat stress increases; if the combination approaches the emergency zone, steps must be taken immediately to cool the animals.

Studies have also been done using temperature transmitters that are swallowed by the cow and lodge in the gut for the life of the animal. The transmitter sends a signal every 5 to 10 minutes, giving the animal's body temperature. Rather than try to calculate air temperature, humidity, and wind speed, stockmen may one day be able to use these transmitters to monitor one animal in the herd to know whether or not heat stress is imminent.

The temperature/humidity index traditionally used by stockmen to figure out if cattle are at risk is not always an adequate indication for heat-stress danger as it does not figure in radiant heat, which can be a major factor. When the index was designed, it was based just on air temperature and humidity. Efforts are being made now to come up with another index that will incorporate radiant-heat load.

Scientists are also trying to understand how animals adapt to heat. Hot weather in early spring, for instance, can be harder on cattle than hot weather in midsummer, because they have not yet adjusted to the warmer weather. If springtime temperatures suddenly climb above 80°F (26.7°C), especially in the Midwest, where there may also be high humidity, this can be a problem for cattle, particularly if they have not yet shed their thick winter hair. They need time to adjust to heat. By August, they have adapted — the same high temperature is not as much of a problem for them as a sudden hot spell in May or June. Researchers at the University of Missouri found it takes cattle three to four days for their metabolism to drop to lower levels, thereby producing less body heat.

Cold-Weather Problems

Cattle often need extra care and feed during cold or wet weather to make sure they stay healthy and continue to milk well if they are lactating or grow well if they are young. Cold temperatures, wind, rain, and mud are all stressful to cattle. Feed intake, rate of feed passage through the digestive tract, and body metabolism all increase. The feed requirement of cattle may go up 10 to 15 percent. All of these changes contribute to an increase in heat production so the animal will be able to withstand winter temperatures without suffering cold stress. Management to prepare cattle for winter and minimize these stresses can save you money and reduce the incidence of sick animals.

Management for Pregnant Cows

Begin your winter management tasks with an assessment of body condition before cold weather begins. Plan to provide enough feed so cows maintain or regain moderate to good condition and can withstand the rigors of bad weather without losing weight. It helps if you have selected a type of cattle that performs well in your climate and maintains body condition on the feed your place provides without your having to purchase extra feed. If you manage pastures properly for your herd numbers (not overgrazing or running out of grass), cattle should not lose much weight during winter or lactation.

Start paying close attention to the body condition of cows at least three months before the start of your calving season, to have a chance to adjust the feed

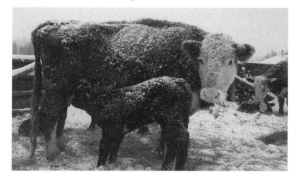
average body condition (score 5) or score 6 at calving and at the start of breeding season results in the highest pregnancy rates, but many factors can affect the reproductive success of a beef herd. Ideal body condition can vary with breed and cow type, season, and geographic location. As a general rule, cows in cold climates need more flesh covering than do cows in warm climates.

Newborn calves in cold weather are at greater risk for cold stress than their mothers because they don't yet have a functional rumen and don't produce as much body heat as older animals. They also don't have as much body fat for insulation. If you calve in cold weather, make sure calves get dry quickly and are able to get up and nurse. It also helps to have shelters so young calves can get out of the wind.

Many factors will influence the need and makeup of your winter feeding program, including climate, the type of cattle you raise, whether you utilize range or irrigated pasture, and crop types. It's usually more profitable to match cattle type to your feed sources than try to create a feeding program to fit cattle that can't do well in your particular environment.

Cows that get too thin during a cold or wet winter climate suffer more cold stress and must rob body-fat stores in order to keep warm. It becomes a vicious cycle; they can't keep warm so they rob more body fat and become even thinner. Calves born to thin cows may be compromised and more prone to disease during their first weeks of life. Calves may be born weak and unable to get up and nurse promptly enough to get the necessary colostrum in time. Thin

if necessary. You may need to increase the amount of hay, for instance, if cattle are losing weight due to cold weather.

Body Type

A three-year South Dakota study found that cows with higher body-condition scores return to heat sooner in the breeding season and are also more likely to become pregnant when bred. Thin cows (scoring 3 or less) have the poorest chance of getting pregnant. Several other studies have shown that

Not All Cows Are Created Equal

Many crossbred cows will milk well and breed back even if they are a little thin, due to hybrid vigor. This is especially true of composites and crosses between beef breeds and breeds traditionally used as dairy cows. These cows have enough internal fat for adequate reproduction and will keep cycling, whereas most purebred beef cows will not be fertile if they are thin.

A 10-year University of Alberta study examined the longevity and lifetime productivity of purebred beef cattle, beef crossbreds, and dairy-beef crosses under range conditions and found the dairy-beef crosses were the most productive group for breed-back, pregnancy rate, and longevity (ability to stay with the herd without presenting reasons for culling). Even though they gave the most milk, they also did better than traditional beef cattle under the same conditions (year-round natural grazing, except for 3 to 4 months of hay-feeding during winter). This type of crossbred cow is efficient and healthy at a lower body-condition score because she doesn't have to put as much flesh onto herself before she can come into heat.

cows may not produce adequate levels of antibodies in their colostrum; if they are underfed they may be short on protein — which is essential to production of good colostrum. Calf survivability is lowered in thin cows, as is the cows' ability to rebreed.

To help cows maintain health and body condition, keep vaccinations up to date, assess parasite populations, and deworm and delouse cattle if necessary (see chapter 7), so parasites won't rob them of nutrition when they need it most. Provide windbreaks and bedding during winter storms if you live in a cold climate, so cattle won't expend so much energy just to keep warm. Without bedding, energy requirements may increase by 12 to 15 percent just to offset the heat lost when cattle lie on cold ground.

Adjust Feed and Feeding Habits

How much hay or supplement a cow needs in winter depends on weather conditions; the age of the cow; her body condition; the quantity and quality of available pasture or crop residue; and whether she is still nursing her calf, is dry, is ready to calve again soon, or calved in the fall and needs extra nutrition to milk well and breed back again. Some herds do well in fall and winter on good native pastures without any other feed, especially if they are dry that time of year and not nursing calves, unless snow covers the grass or weather is bitterly cold. This situation is actually healthier for cattle than congregating them by feeding hay. When spread out on large pastures, they aren't exposed to as much fecal contamination, and their intestinal tracts don't get such a buildup of *E. coli* and *C. perfringens* that can be transmitted later to their calves (after calving).

Some kinds of dry-land bunch grasses in certain types of soil meet all the nutrient requirements of a dry cow except salt — as long as the grass isn't too dry. During a drought the grass may be short on protein and phosphorus. Salt should always be provided for cattle, since this is the mineral most lacking in forage (see chapter 16). Other kinds of pasture, especially "tame" or irrigated pastures or crop residues, lose some nutrient value once they dry up or freeze, and cattle will need supplemental feed (hay, silage, grain, or a protein supplement and mineral mix). Many regions are short on trace minerals, and you'll need to add copper, selenium, or other important elements to your salt-mineral mix.

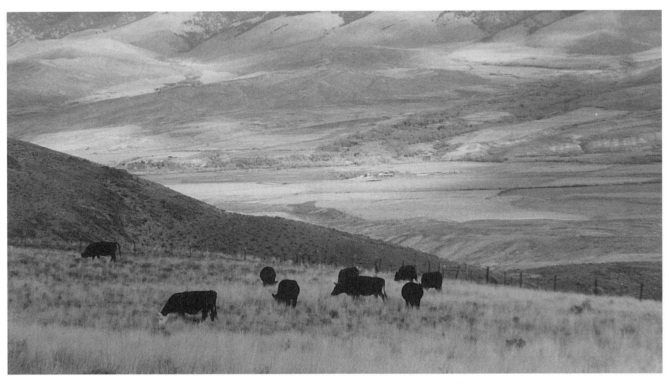

Some kinds of dry-land bunch grasses meet all the nutrient requirements of a dry cow except salt. These native grasses are adequate fall and winter feed unless the snow gets too deep.

Feed According to Need

In most herds cattle should be sorted into different groups for winter feeding and fed accordingly — or put in different pastures. Save your best pasture for weaned calves, yearlings, pregnant heifers, and 2-year-olds that just weaned off their first calves. The 2-year-old's winter is a critical time. Young cows are still growing while nursing their first calves, are pregnant again, and may go into winter a little thin. They need to catch up in body condition so they'll be able to give birth to healthy calves and rebreed. Mature, dry cows can get by on lesser-quality pasture or hay. If cattle are in separate groups, you can feed young or thin ones for growth and weight gain without overfeeding the rest of the herd. Feeding all the cattle extra rations or using up your best pasture too soon with the whole herd can be costly, especially since the older, bossier cows tend to eat more than their share of any hay or supplement.

Cows that calve early while weather is still cold and pastures have not yet begun to grow need more food than what winter pasture can provide. Dry grass does not contain enough protein and other nutrients for lactation. After calving, a beef cow's energy requirements increase 17 to 50 percent, depending on how much milk she's producing. A dairy cow's requirements will be even higher.

Inadequate feed for a beef herd during early lactation can reduce the weaning weights of calves by 20 to 50 pounds (9 to 22.7 kg), and reduce conception rates of cows as much as 25 percent when they start to rebreed. This is why it's often best to calve at the end of the winter (when green grass is starting) if you can, so you won't have to feed a lot of harvested or purchased feed.

In some situations, however, ranchers don't have much choice in calving season, as in areas of the West, where many ranchers must use public range for summer pasture. Most of them calve and breed cows early in the season so cows can all be calved (and maybe even already bred) before they go to summer range. Calving and breeding on the range is a counterproductive management situation because it's harder to keep track of cattle on huge range areas and harder for bulls to find all the cows in heat. Most ranchers calve early, in order to have

a uniform calf crop and fewer open cows. Thus they must feed more hay at the end of the winter when their cows are calving. There are always trade-offs in the cattle business; there is no "best" management that fits every situation.

If you must calve during cold weather at the end of winter, take special care to make sure cows have adequate nutrition. Don't overdo it, however, especially on protein, or cows may actually produce too much milk and create health issues for their young calves (such as enterotoxemia, see chapter 4). How much feed a cow needs during early lactation depends mainly on how much she's milking and on how cold or wet it is. If a cow is shortchanged on feed during cold or wet weather and can't supply her needs for lactation and body warmth, she'll lose weight and will have trouble rebreeding on schedule.

Closely monitor the body condition of cattle as they go into winter and through the winter, to know if their pasture is adequate or if you are feeding enough. Then if cows start to lose weight before calving, you'll be aware of it in time to correct the situation by feeding hay to supplement dwindling or snow-covered pastures or by increasing the hay ration if weather turns colder.

Fall Feed

Stockmen often underestimate the importance of adequate nutrition in the fall to make sure cows don't lose weight before winter. According to one veterinarian, probably 70 percent of the open cows in Montana are the result of inadequate nutritional intake in the fall, rather than improper spring nutrition. This plays a large role in their ability to properly feed their calves and breed back after calving.

Cows always need adequate, balanced feed in autumn, which may merely mean adding a trace-mineral supplement to native pasture, a little good hay or a protein supplement if the feed is too dry, or adequate hay if the feed is depleted or snowed under. If the cow is deficient in protein or phosphorus, she won't rebreed on time after calving.

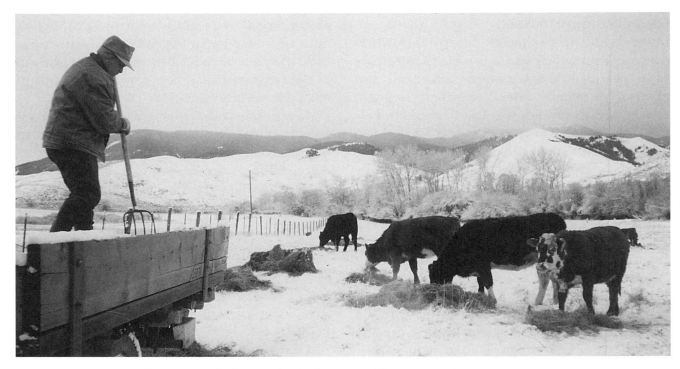

Sort cattle into groups and feed accordingly. These yearling heifers are in a different pasture for winter than the mature dry cows; the heifers need better-quality hay because they are still growing.

Food Choices

If weather is cold and windy, cows need to eat more, just to keep warm. If they stand around or huddle behind windbreaks instead of grazing, they can't eat enough to maintain body heat. Long, cold winter nights are part of the challenge of getting cattle to eat enough. Days (and grazing time) are short, so extra feed may be needed to make sure cattle eat enough to maintain condition and keep warm. They'll often eat hay during the night if it's too cold to graze.

Even if pasture is available, they may not start grazing till midday, when temperatures are warmest, and lose weight because they don't eat enough total feed during the day. This problem can be resolved by feeding some hay or supplement early in the day to get them going, and then they'll start grazing.

Cattle need to eat more roughage (forage) in cold weather to obtain calories for heat energy. If they don't eat enough fibrous feed — feed that not only provides nutrition but also furnishes them with the extra heat created by the fermentation process — pounds melt off them as they rob body fat to create the energy needed for warmth. More total pounds of roughage in the diet — all the pasture they can eat, or some extra grass hay, or even some good-quality straw — can keep them warm, as long as they have enough protein for the rumen microbes to digest it, since digestion and breakdown of cellulose create heat energy.

In cold weather, high-quality alfalfa hay by itself is not the best feed. Even though it supplies plenty of protein, calcium, vitamin A, and other important nutrients, it does not have enough fiber to produce heat energy during cold weather. Cattle on a diet of high-quality alfalfa may lose weight in winter. Alfalfa alone is not adequate for cattle when it's really cold; they gobble it up and stand around shivering. If a cow is cold, she should be given all the roughage she will clean up. You don't dare feed that much high-quality alfalfa, or she may bloat. She'll do better with a lower-quality alfalfa (containing more fiber and fewer leaves) or a mix of alfalfa and grass hay, with the amount of grass hay increased the colder it gets. High-quality alfalfa and good-quality straw (to supply the needed fiber for heat energy) often make a good mix.

Cold-Weather Adjustments

Cattle that have a chance to acclimate gradually to winter develop a thick hair coat and put on body fat if feed sources are adequate. Hair and fat both serve as good insulation against the cold. If you live in a region that has cold winters, select a type of cattle that has a naturally good hair coat and that fattens easily. They'll handle cold much better than the breeds that were developed for hot climates.

If you live in a cold climate and buy cattle from a warmer area, bring them home before cold weather starts so they have time to grow a good hair coat. With short summer hair, the typical beef cow may chill when temperatures drop toward 40°F (4.4°C), whereas with a heavy winter coat she can stay comfortable at temperatures well below 0°F (−17.8°C) if there's no wind. She also adjusts by increasing her metabolic rate, to boost heat production, which also increases her appetite.

Feed Digestability

If temperatures drop below the animal's comfort zone, not only is there an increase in maintenance requirements, but digestibility is also reduced, further increasing the feed needs. Research has shown there's a decline of 1 percent in feed digestibility for each 2°F (1.1°C) of temperature drop, but cattle adapted to cold weather have more efficient digestion at cold temperatures than unadapted cattle; they are more resistant to the depressing effects of cold on digestion.

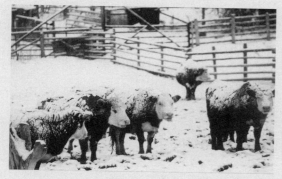

Cattle that have a chance to acclimate gradually to winter grow a thick hair coat and put on a layer of body fat if feed sources are adequate. Winter hair and fat serve as insulation against the cold.

Eating more will provide her with more "fuel" to keep warm. But if she gets too cold, heat loss and cold stress reduce her appetite and efficiency of feed conversion, since body metabolism is adversely affected if body temperature drops. Mammals must maintain a fairly constant body temperature to keep up the metabolic processes that enable the body to function.

Critical Temperature

If a cow has a good winter coat, she does fine until temperatures go lower than about 20 to 30°F (−6.7 to −1.1°C). Below that, she must compensate for heat loss by increasing her energy intake; she must increase heat production to maintain body temperature. Healthy cows in average body condition and acclimated to cold weather have a lower *critical temperature* point of about 20°F (−6.7°C). This is the point at which maintenance requirements increase: the animal must increase her rate of heat production, and you must feed her more. Lower critical temperature is defined as the lower limit of the comfort zone. This is also the temperature at which the rate of performance (growth or milk production) begins to decline, as temperatures become colder.

Daily Requirements

An 1,100-pound (499 kg) pregnant cow needs 11.2 pounds (5 kg) of TDN (total digestible nutrients) per day when temperatures are above freezing. If temperature drops 20°F (11.1°C) below her lower critical temperature, she needs 20 percent more TDN (2.2 more pounds (1 kg) of digestible nutrients). To supply that, you can feed her 5 pounds (2.3 kg) of hay containing 50 percent TDN. Your county agent or a

CRITICAL TEMPERATURES

Dry summer hair: 39°F (3.9°C)

Wet summer coat: 59°F (15°C)

Dry winter coat: 32°F (0°C)

Dry heavy winter coat: 18°F (−7.8°C)

If an animal is wet, this has the same effect as reducing the temperature by 20°F (11.1°C). With wet hair, she will chill at a higher temperature, or will need more feed to generate enough body heat to keep her warm.

cattle nutritionist can help you figure out the nutrient quality of your hay. In cold weather, a safe way to make sure cattle don't lose weight is to give them as much good straw or low-quality grass hay as they can eat and an adequate protein source (such as some good alfalfa hay or a protein supplement) to make sure they have enough protein to "feed" the rumen bacteria that process the roughage.

Wind or moisture makes the effective temperature (what's felt by the body) lower than the temperature stated on a thermometer. Always figure in the *wind chill* when arriving at the number of degrees below a cow's critical temperature point (see Wind Chill chart, page 74). For example, a 10-mile-per-hour (16 km per hour) wind at 20°F (–6.7°C) has the same effect on the body as a temperature of 9°F (–12.8°C) with no wind. A 25-mile-per-hour (40.2 km per hour) wind has the same net effect as lowering the temperature by 27°F (15°C). If temperature drops to 0°F (–17.8°C) (or the equivalent, figuring in the wind chill), the energy requirement of a cow increases by something between 20 and 30 percent — about 1 percent for each 1°F (0.5°C) of coldness below her critical temperature.

Cattle can't eat enough extra feed to compensate for heat loss at minus 50°F (–45.6°C) with a wind chill. In these conditions they need windbreaks to reduce their body-heat loss during winter storms. During severely cold weather, cattle also need bedding to insulate them from frozen ground and help conserve their body heat.

Cattle of British breeds and crosses, with normal winter hair coats, need about one-third more feed when exposed to a wind chill that brings the effective temperature down to 0°F (–17.8°C). Critical temperature for any individual will vary according to age, size, hair-coat thickness, moisture conditions, amount of body fat (that acts as insulation), length of time exposed to adverse weather conditions, and amount of wind. Feedlot steers, for example, with extra fat and access to windbreaks, are usually less affected by cold weather than are grazing cows.

Cold stress is also less severe if a storm is brief, compared with the chill and stress of continuous bad weather. Temperatures, wind-chill charts, and any measures of cold stress are based on 24-hour average temperatures. If cattle have windbreak protection so they can periodically seek shelter (using it when weather is bad or when they are resting after eating), their exposure to cold stress is intermittent rather than continuous, and thus the severity of wind chill is greatly reduced.

WIND-CHILL INDEX FOR CATTLE

Wind Speed	Temperature (Fahrenheit)																	
	–20	**–16**	**–12**	**–8**	**–4**	**0**	**4**	**8**	**12**	**16**	**20**	**24**	**28**	**32**	**36**	**40**	**44**	**48**
0	–20	–16	–12	–8	–4	0	4	8	12	16	20	24	28	32	36	40	44	48
2	–23	–19	–15	–11	–7	–3	1	5	9	13	17	21	25	29	33	37	41	45
4	–25	–21	–17	–13	–9	–5	–1	3	7	11	15	19	23	27	31	35	39	43
6	–28	–24	–20	–16	–12	–8	–4	0	4	8	12	16	20	24	28	32	36	40
8	–30	–26	–22	–18	–14	–10	–6	–2	2	6	10	14	18	22	26	30	34	38
10	–31	–27	–23	–19	–15	–11	–7	–3	1	5	9	13	17	21	25	29	33	37
12	–33	–29	–25	–21	–17	–13	–9	–5	–1	3	7	11	15	19	23	27	31	35
14	–35	–31	–27	–23	–19	–15	–11	–7	–3	1	5	9	13	17	21	25	29	33
16	–37	–33	–29	–25	–21	–17	–13	–9	–5	–1	3	7	11	15	19	23	27	31
18	–38	–34	–30	–26	–22	–18	–14	–10	–6	–2	2	6	10	14	18	22	26	30
20	–41	–37	–33	–29	–25	–21	–17	–13	–9	–5	–1	3	7	11	15	19	23	27
22	–43	–39	–35	–31	–27	–23	–19	–15	–11	–7	–3	1	5	9	13	17	21	25
24	–46	–42	–38	–34	–30	–26	–22	–18	–14	–10	–6	–2	2	6	10	14	18	22
26	–49	–45	–41	–37	–33	–29	–25	–21	–17	–13	–9	–5	–1	3	7	11	15	19
28	–52	–48	–44	–40	–36	–32	–28	–24	–20	–16	–12	–8	–4	0	4	8	12	16

To use the wind chill chart, determine the temperature in Fahrenheit and the wind velocity in miles per hour. The point at which these two intersect is the effective temperature. Cows stay comfortable until the combination of temperature and wind speed results in a wind chill index below the lower critical temperature (LCT), the temperature at which the cow needs additional energy to stay warm (LCT for dry hair coat is 30°F; LCT for wet hair coat is 50°F).

In dry conditions, increase TDN by 1% per degree below the LCT. In wet conditions, increase TDN by 2% per degree below the LCT. For example, a cow with a dry hair coat at 0° will require 30% more TDN than the same cow at 30°. If the cow is wet, at 30° she will need 40% more TDN than a cow with a dry hair coat at the same temperature.

Windbreaks

Natural windbreaks of trees or brush make good protection. Boards on fences can reduce wind-chill effects by up to 70 percent in pens or pastures without natural windbreaks. If you live in a climate with snow, however, remember that wind tends to curl up over a solid barrier and deposit snow drifts on the downwind side. A windbreak fence with a little open space between the boards can help prevent this, while still giving some wind protection to cattle standing or lying behind it.

Lower critical temperature with a dry hair coat is 20 to 30°F (–6.7 to –1.1°C) (depending on the individual and how well acclimated she is to cold), but with wet hair it will be 50 to 59°F (10 to 15°C). A rough rule of thumb to compensate for cold is to increase the amount of feed (energy source) by 1 percent for each 2°F (1.1°C) of cold stress. For thin cows with poor hair coats or any cows in wet conditions, figure a 1 percent increase for each degree of temperature (0.5°C) drop. A cow with a dry hair coat at 0°F (–17.8°C) will need about 30 percent more TDN than the same cow at 30°F (–1°C). Because wet hair loses its insulating quality, a wet cow will need 40 percent more TDN at 30 degrees than a cow with a dry hair coat at the same temperature.

With severe wind chill and wet conditions, it is impractical or impossible to feed enough additional energy to provide the calories cattle need to keep warm, especially if you try to use grain as the additional energy source. That much grain would cause digestive disorders (see chapter 8). It's better to provide windbreaks to offset wind chill and have cattle in adequate body condition (enough energy stored as fat) for these critical times.

When It's Wet

A wet storm is always harder on cattle than dry cold. Wet hair can't keep out cold; the cow will chill sooner. When dry, the hair is fluffy and traps body heat in tiny air spaces between the hairs, creating a blanket of insulation between the cow's body and cold air. Hair sheds water for a while because natural hair oils make the hair coat somewhat waterproof, but when completely wet, it lies flatter; its insulating quality is lost, and the cow becomes easily chilled. Cattle suffer a lot more cold stress in wet weather than in dry cold. They can be quite comfortable at 10 below zero F (–23.3°C) on a still, dry, sunny day, and quite miserable at 35°F (1.7°C) in a storm with rain and wind.

All too often stockmen overlook the effects of wet weather because the temperature isn't really low. Yet a cow's nutrient requirements may be greatly increased, since she has more trouble keeping warm. Try soaking your shirt in water and see how poorly it insulates you from the wind or cold temperatures. To make matters worse, while cold, dry weather stimulates the appetite, rain may create a temporary reduction of feed intake by as much as 30 to 100 percent. Having to stand or lie in mud during and after a rain will further decrease feed consumption. As the depth of mud increases or the temperature drops, feed intake is decreased even more. Cattle that have lost weight or are losing weight are very susceptible to cold- or wet-weather stress and are more apt to become sick, so keep close track of the body condition of your cattle during winter.

Mud

Moisture and mud always increase the effects of cold stress. If cattle have to stand or lie in mud (drawing heat from the body), this may increase their feed requirements. Cold mud has a greater effect on energy loss than frozen ground does. The adverse effects are greatest when there's no dry place for cattle, especially lactating cows and calves, to lie down.

It's also hard on growing animals. A study at South Dakota State University showed cattle living with 4 to 8 inches (10.2 to 20.3 cm) of mud and no access to dry or solid ground reduced their feed intake by 8 to 15 percent and reduced their daily weight gain by 14 percent. If mud is 12 to 24 inches (30.5 to 61 cm) deep, feed intake drops by 25 to 30 percent, and daily weight gain drops 25 percent.

Resolve this problem in pens by using concrete next to feed bunks so cattle don't stand in mud to eat and by creating mounds of higher ground where cattle can lie. Keep bedding areas and feeding areas cleaned off so they stay dry and don't get built up with mud and manure. It's always better if cattle can be out on large pastures with well-sodded or frozen ground, never having to contend with mud, but if they must be in a corral, you need a plan for reducing the effects.

If calving areas are muddy, a good solution is to have lots of bedding on higher, better-drained ground, so cows and young calves never have to lie in mud. In pastures where there are young calves, calf houses with floors to keep calves up out of mud and melting snow runoff will provide a dry place for them to sleep.

Water Needs

It's just as important to pay attention to water sources in cold weather, as it is when it's hot and humid. Cattle need adequate ice-free water. If they don't drink enough, they won't eat enough and will lose weight. In some instances they may become dehydrated and impacted. If contents of the smaller stomachs become too dried out, feed won't move through, and the digestive tract will become blocked, which will eventually kill the cow (see chapter 8). Signs that cattle are not drinking enough are loss of appetite; weight loss; lack of gut fill (looking "empty"); and firm, dry manure.

Moderate-size pregnant cows need about six gallons (22.7 L) of water daily in cool weather and twice that much when lactating after calving. The temperature of drinking water should be at least 40°F (4.4°C) or higher, if possible, in cold weather. If water is colder than that, cows won't drink enough. Extremely cold water may cause temporary paralysis of the digestive tract and loss of appetite, even though the cow needs a higher energy intake to maintain body temperature to warm the ice cold water in the gut. Sometimes a few dollars spent on warming the drinking water for cattle in cold weather, can save a lot of money on feed and health costs. Tank insulation and heating elements will help assure that the herd has enough to drink in cold weather.

Snow as a Water Source

Cattle can utilize snow for water intake in regions that get adequate winter snowfall and if snow stays powdery and not crusted. They must be able to sweep it up with their tongues.

People used to think that cows eating snow during cold weather required more energy to warm it to body temperature and therefore needed more feed, but research trials (with some cattle using snow and some using water) showed no difference in feed intake or weight gains. Cattle using snow just eat slower. They graze or eat hay for a while, then lick snow, eat some more, then lick more snow. They consume small amounts of snow through the day, whereas animals drink water only once or twice a day in cold weather. The intermittent eating of forage and snow seems to minimize thermal stress, and heat created by digestion is enough to warm the liquid to body temperature. It was also thought that cows deprived of adequate water (having to eat snow) would be at risk for impaction, but this is not true. Impaction is mainly a problem when cows must utilize coarse dry forage with low protein levels (see chapter 8) or do not have enough snow or water for adequate moisture.

Eating snow is a learned behavior, however. Cattle quickly learn by watching other cows, but those with no role models may go thirsty for a while before trying it. If snow is readily available and cattle learn to use it, they do well on winter pastures without water as long as snow is adequate but not so deep that it covers the forage.

A FROSTY DRINK

FOR MORE THAN 40 YEARS we've used a 320-acre (129.5 hectare) mountain pasture in late fall and early winter for our *dry* cows. We installed several water troughs to collect spring water. These work nicely unless weather gets severely cold and the troughs freeze over. We'd hike up there every day during a cold spell to break the thick ice, and cows would gang around the troughs to drink after we chopped it out. But we soon noticed there were a few individuals that never seemed interested in coming to water. We'd see them licking snow and worry that they weren't getting enough water.

After a time, we realized these cows were staying in good body condition and were not suffering from a water shortage. They had simply learned how to eat snow in cold weather and seemed to prefer periodic snow licking to tanking up on ice-cold water.

PART TWO
Common Diseases

CHAPTER FOUR

Bacterial Diseases

BACTERIA CAUSE MANY CATTLE DISEASES and infections. These one-celled microorganisms exist in large numbers in the natural environment and some have adapted to living in animals. Some, like those that live in the digestive tract and help with digestion of food, are "good guys." *Herbivorous* animals depend on these microbes to ferment and break down fibrous portions of plants, causing a chemical reaction that produces energy. Unlike humans, cattle can digest forage plants because they have these helpful bacteria living in the rumen. Some bacteria are pathogenic, however, and cause disease or infection if they get into the body.

This chapter examines some of the most common cattle diseases caused by bacteria. Other bacterial diseases and infections, such as pneumonia, mastitis, foot rot, pinkeye, wooden tongue, and lump jaw, will be covered in later chapters that focus on the body systems they affect.

Brucellosis

Often called Bang's disease after Dr. Bernhard Bang, a Danish veterinarian who first isolated the causative organism in 1897, brucellosis is the most common cause of abortion in cattle around the world, except where it has been controlled or eradicated by vaccination. Brucellosis affected as many as 25 percent of the cattle in the United States before the advent of control programs and vaccination.

Humans can get brucellosis *(undulant fever)*, and one of the main reasons for the development of *pasteurization* of milk was to kill brucella bacteria. Because human health was threatened, a rigorous program to eliminate this disease in cattle was begun as soon as a vaccine was created. Vaccination against this disease is not 100 percent effective, however, so a test-and-slaughter program was also used. Herd testing, slaughter of all infected animals, and vaccination of all healthy heifers eventually eradicated brucellosis in most parts of the United States.

Transmission

Cattle, hogs, goats, bison, and elk are *hosts* for brucellosis. As long as wildlife carry it, it can never be fully eradicated. Cases cropped up in a few cattle

What Are Pathogens?

Pathogens include certain types of bacteria; protozoa (one-celled animals); yeasts; viruses, which are smaller than bacteria and without a cellular structure; and fungi, a family that is multicellular and includes molds. Once a pathogen gains entrance to the body, it begins to multiply and may create disease if the body's immune defenses cannot combat the pathogen and halt the multiplication process.

herds in Texas, Wyoming, Montana, and Idaho in recent years. Bison and elk in Yellowstone Park carry brucellosis, for instance, and pose a threat to livestock whenever they come out of the park and mingle with cattle or contaminate pastures, livestock bed grounds, and feeding areas.

Today purchasing infected cattle poses the greatest risk of exposure to your herd. At calving, the disease is spread to susceptible (unvaccinated) cows via aborted fetuses, fetal membranes, and vaginal discharge from infected females. Most cows that abort become carriers and continue to shed bacteria for two to four weeks afterward, contaminating pastures and pens. The bacteria enter cattle via the digestive tract, move into the bloodstream, and infect the uterus and fetus of a pregnant cow. Other animals that sniff and lick contaminated areas or discharges become infected, and infected cows may also excrete bacteria in their milk, thereby infecting their nursing calves. Bulls can also become infected by ingesting the bacteria, but rarely transmit the disease unless the testicles become infected, and then they spread bacteria via semen.

Symptoms and Effects

The disease mainly affects sexually mature animals, causing abortion in the last trimester of pregnancy and a subsequent period of infertility for the cow, retained placenta, and unthriftiness. Bacteria take up residence in the udder and lymph glands and invade the uterus. Bacteria attack fetal membranes that supply blood to the fetus, eventually killing it and causing abortion or resulting in a weak calf. A few calves are born normal but may retain the infection throughout their lives, possibly spreading the disease at their first calving. Infected bulls may develop arthritis or inflammation of the testicles and subsequent infertility.

Prevention

Any cattle suspected of having the disease or any new additions to a herd that have no evidence of calfhood vaccination (a small metal tag and a tattoo bearing what's called a Bang's shield in the ear) can be tested. The veterinarian reads the tattoo when making a decision whether to test that cow or not. You can't depend on the metal ear tag alone, because these are often lost.

If you work with cattle that might be infected, take the following precautions to prevent spread of brucellosis to other animals and to humans:

- Use sterile gloves for all reproductive work.

- Don't keep horses with cattle; horses may carry the infection. Keep dogs out of livestock areas. They may spread the disease by chewing on or dragging an aborted fetus or placenta.

- If a cow aborts or calves prematurely, consult your vet, and wear gloves when handling the animals. Use plastic garbage cans or tubs to pick up an aborted calf and placenta; don't drag it through a pen.

- Scrub well after handling fetal material, and don't touch your eyes, nose, or mouth after touching a premature calf or aborted fetus.

- The area where the abortion occurred should be thoroughly disinfected and any remaining fetal or placental tissues burned or buried.

- Samples of aborted fetuses and placental material should be sent to a diagnostic lab for diagnosis by your vet to test for brucellosis.

- The aborting cow should be isolated from other cattle until you know the results.

- Keep any cow that retains her placenta (or any suspect cow with discharge from the *vulva*) separate from others for three to four weeks after she calves.

Brucellosis can be avoided if you buy females only from a herd that is known to be free of disease or that had calfhood vaccinations. If you have doubts, keep a purchased animal separate from others until she can be tested. If you live in a state that requires vaccination, vaccinate all heifer calves within the proper

UNDULANT FEVER

In humans, brucellosis is called undulant fever, an ailment with recurring symptoms of fatigue, fever, and chills. Chronic cases may produce arthritis, emotional disturbances, optic problems, and nervous system disorders. Humans can get brucellosis from direct contact with infected animals and by drinking infected milk or eating infected imported dairy products.

age limit. Most states are free of brucellosis, but since a few are not, some states won't allow any cows or heifers to come into the state unless they've been vaccinated. In a few states all heifer calves must be vaccinated when they are between 2 and 10 months. Consult your vet for state vaccination and cattle-movement regulations. These sometimes change if a state loses its Bang's-free status.

Leptospirosis

One of the most common causes of infectious abortion in U.S. cattle today (now that brucellosis is nearly eradicated) is leptospirosis, which is caused by spiral-shaped bacteria *(spirochetes)* that affect many kinds of animals, including humans. It is often present in wildlife populations, including rats and mice. The *leptospires* can survive in surface water, stagnant ponds, streams, or moist soil for long periods at mild temperatures. Leptospirosis is a common cause of infertility, delayed breeding, and abortions or birth of premature and weak calves.

Transmission

Lepto bacteria are spread by sick or carrier animal discharge (especially urine) that contaminates feed and water. Some animals, particularly with certain strains of lepto, appear to be healthy, yet harbor the bacteria in their kidneys and reproductive tract, shedding them in urine or reproductive fluids. Bacteria may enter a susceptible cow via nose, mouth, or eyes by contact with contaminated feed, water, or urine or through breaks in the skin on feet and legs when walking through contaminated water. Urine or contaminated water splashing into the eyes of susceptible animals can spread the disease, as can breeding. Calves infected before birth may shed bacteria. Once the leptospires enter an animal, they multiply in the liver and migrate through the bloodstream to the kidneys; they damage the red blood cells, liver, and kidneys.

Symptoms

The *incubation period* is three to seven days or longer after contact with lepto bacteria. There are more than 100 *serotypes* of leptospira — 40 of which can cause illness — but fewer than 10 that have been recognized in the United States. The disease in cattle may be mild or severe, depending on the type encountered. Symptoms last three to five days.

The disease may be acute, with loss of appetite, high fever, anemia, labored breathing, *jaundice* (yellow tinge on the whites of the eyes, gums, or other mucous membranes), and changes in the milk if lactating (sudden drop in volume, with milk becoming thick, yellow and sometimes blood-tinged). *Subacute* cases are mild, with intermittent fever. Subclinical (nonapparent) cases show very little sign of illness other than abortion and infertility.

Most adult cattle show no sign of sickness, but about 30 percent may have one or more symptoms of acute illness. In about 5 percent of cases the animal may die, due to *septicemia, anemia,* or malfunction of the liver and kidneys. Young cattle are often more severely affected than adults. After the animal recovers from the acute period of illness, the leptospires localize in the kidneys, and the animal continues to shed bacteria in urine for several months, serving as a source of infection for other animals. With some types of lepto, the cow may become a carrier and shed bacteria for several months or even for life.

Lepto infection may cause a pregnant cow to abort, usually one to three weeks after recovering from the acute stage of the disease. Even if she did not appear to be sick, she may abort. Sometimes an infected cow will give birth to a live, weak calf that dies a few days later. Abortion outbreaks from lepto are most common in the last trimester of gestation, but a cow may abort at any stage of gestation.

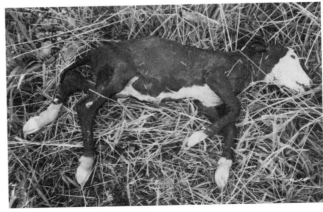

If a cow aborts, try to determine the cause. This is an aborted late-gestation fetus, which is common with lepto infections.

Diagnosis is not always easy in an individual animal because symptoms can vary so much, but the presence of lepto in a herd can usually be detected by taking blood samples from about 10 percent of the animals (or 10 animals in a small herd). Whenever there's a higher-than-normal number of abortions, lepto is a possible cause. With one type of lepto, however *(L. hardjo-bovis)*, its presence cannot be detected with a blood sample. *Titers* are inconclusive. The only way you can tell if an animal has *L. hardjo-bovis* is with a urine culture.

Treatment is most effective early in the course of acute disease, before it causes serious or irreversible damage to the liver and kidneys. Treatment in later stages of *chronic* infections can be helpful, however, to reduce shedding of bacteria and shorten the carrier stage. Consult your veterinarian regarding choice of antibiotic and duration of treatment.

Prevention

Recovered animals are generally immune to the type of lepto they encountered but still susceptible to infection from other types. There is a vaccine available against five of the most common kinds of lepto that affect cattle *(Leptospira pomona, L. grippotyphosa, L. hardjo, L. canicola, L. icterohaemorrhagiae)*, giving immunity for about six months. *L. hardjo* is a type found in Europe but not in the United States.

Another serotype, *L. hardjo-bovis,* is not covered in the five-way vaccine, but there is a specific vaccine that can be given to prevent it. Unlike the other types of lepto, hardjo-bovis seems to infect the animal for longer periods or even for life, residing in the kidneys and reproductive tract in cattle that may not show outward signs of disease. They continually shed bacteria and serve as a source of infection in the herd. This strain of lepto can also be passed from dam to calf in utero before the calf is born. For protection against all types of lepto, calves should be vaccinated at about four to six months of age, and cows should be vaccinated twice a year.

Lepto can be introduced to a herd by purchasing an infected cow, by pigs or wildlife mingling with cattle, or by rodent urine contaminating feed or water. Even if your cows never come into contact with other cattle, they can get lepto from dogs or mice or from wild animals such as raccoons, skunks, foxes, deer, elk, antelope, and other carrier animals urinating on a feed ground or into a water source. Deer feeding with cattle or in haystacks can be a big factor in spreading both lepto and IBR. Thus, the best protection against lepto is semiannual vaccination. It also helps to limit rodent and wildlife access to cattle feed and eliminate cattle's access to surface water used by other livestock. Draining or fencing off swampy areas that might harbor leptospires is another good preventive measure. Infected or recovered bulls should not be used for breeding until they have been treated to reduce shedding of leptospires.

Campylobacteriosis (Vibriosis)

Campylobacteriosis is a disease caused by the bacterium *Campylobacter foetus,* spread from cow to cow by the bull through breeding. This sexually transmitted disease is a common cause of infertility and "open" (nonpregnant) cows, unless the cows are vaccinated against it or care is taken to make sure no infected animals enter the herd. It can be introduced with a single breeding of an infected cow or bull.

Symptoms

Vibrio-infected bulls show no signs, even though, once infected, the bacteria usually live in tissue surfaces of the penis and prepuce for the life of the bull. During breeding, bacteria are passed from the bull into the vagina of the cow, causing an infection in her reproductive tract that may persist for several weeks or months. The disease can also be passed to cows via *artificial insemination (AI).* Infection in the cow may not interfere with conception, but it usually kills the *embryo.*

The cow loses the pregnancy early and returns to heat 40 to 60 days after breeding. She usually shows no other signs of disease. Her inability to become pregnant again may last from 2 to 6 months as her body fights off the infection. After that, most cows build immunity and can carry a pregnancy. In some instances, however, a cow may remain infertile or may conceive again and abort later. A few cows never clear the infection, even though they may eventually have a live calf. These silent carriers serve as a source of infection the next year, infecting any bull that breeds them. If inflammation in the uterus is severe, the cow may be permanently infertile, but most cows recover in about 5 months or less.

Diagnosis

Other sexually transmitted diseases can cause early pregnancy loss (including *trichomoniasis,* see chapter 6), so proper diagnosis is important when trying to eliminate a herd problem. The first sign of trouble is a high number of cows or heifers coming back into heat after being bred. Later signs include a large number of open cows at the end of breeding season or a very extended calving season the next year, with many calves arriving late.

Lab tests may be required for accurate diagnosis and to look for bacteria in cultures of mucus samples collected from infected females, from the *sheath* of an infected bull, or from tissues from an aborted fetus. Your vet can take samples to send for culturing and may also want to test the bulls for trichomoniasis at the same time.

Treatment

Antibiotic treatment of an infected cow may be successful if given in early stages, but often this disease is not detected early enough. Treatment in later stages may not be as effective. Recovery can be hastened by infusing the uterus with penicillin and use of *prostaglandins* (hormone drugs) to help the uterus flush itself.

Infected bulls can be treated, but ask your vet about the proper antibiotic and dosage, since this is an extra-label or off-label use (see chapter 2) of the antibiotic and requires a prescription. Work with your vet to arrive at the proper diagnosis and to plan treatment if vibrio is causing herd infertility.

Prevention

Vaccination of cows and heifers that might come in contact with an infected bull can usually prevent vibrio if carried out at the proper time to stimulate strong immunity by the time of breeding. Timing is very important, since the immunity produced is not long-lasting. You want to make sure immunity is at its peak during breeding season. If vaccination is too close to breeding, the animal may not have time to build immunity. If given too far ahead of breeding, immunity may be waning, and cows will not be protected.

Most stockmen vaccinate about a month before breeding. Bulls can be vaccinated at a higher dosage than cows to prevent the carrier state, but this is an extra-label use of vaccine and should be discussed with your vet.

There are several vaccines available, so be sure to ask your vet what would be best in your situation, and follow label recommendations for timing, especially if the vaccine requires two doses the first year.

Anthrax

This disease is one of the oldest killers of humans and livestock and was mentioned in some of the earliest recorded history, several thousand years ago. Anthrax, also known as splenic fever, charbon, milzbrand, and woolsorter's disease (in humans) is caused by *Bacillus anthracis* and occurs sporadically in the United States and Canada when conditions are right. This acutely contagious and deadly disease affects most mammals. Cases of anthrax in livestock must be reported to the state veterinarian or animal industry board.

The bacteria produce spores that can survive in contaminated soil indefinitely. Grazing animals may be exposed when drought and dust, flooding, or wind free up spores. *Alkaline* soils, high humidity, and high temperatures create perfect conditions for spore formation. Infections occur when the spores enter the body via breaks in the skin or by inhalation or ingestion (the most common route). If animals graze abrasive forage, spores may penetrate the lining of the mouth.

Cattle must pick up a *threshold number* of spores to develop infection; one or two spores will not cause disease. Thus, anthrax is likely to occur in areas where there are many spores, such as where animals have earlier died of this disease. Once the spores enter the body, they come out of their dormant state and begin to reproduce, multiplying rapidly and releasing toxins into the bloodstream. The toxins attack many body tissues, including the brain, and the animal soon dies. Before he dies he may shed bacteria via manure or other secretions, and when these bacteria come into contact with air, they form spores and complete the life cycle. The biggest source of spores, however, is the open carcass of a diseased animal exposing bacteria to the air.

Anthrax is generally not spread from live animal to live animal but is typically transmitted via spores that formed in the carcasses of animals that died of the disease. Other animals licking or sniffing a carcass may pick up spores. If the carcass is never opened, the bacteria die, especially in summer's hot weather. But any bloody discharge or opening of the carcass (via predators or postmortem examination) enables the bacteria to form spores when they are exposed to oxygen.

The spores are hardy and resistant to heat, cold, drying, and disinfectants; they may survive for years in soil and water, contaminating the surrounding area for a long time. They can be transported to other areas by flooding, dust particles carried by wind or birds, or farmers when they work the land where animal carcasses are buried. Drought may force livestock to graze closer to the ground, where they pick up spores from bits of soil. Flooding and erosion bring buried spores to the surface and concentrate them in puddles after evaporation.

When conditions are conducive, anthrax can kill many animals in a short time. This disease usually appears in warm, dry summer months, especially in regions where grass becomes short and conditions are dusty. A common sign of anthrax is black, tarry discharge from body openings in a dead carcass. Carcasses should be handled carefully, with a face mask and gloves, to reduce the risk of human exposure.

Symptoms

The acute form of anthrax kills quickly, sometimes within 1 or 2 hours of an animal's showing symptoms. The incubation period can range from 1 to 14 days (most commonly 3 to 7 days). First signs of illness are fever, lethargy, lack of appetite, bloody diarrhea, blood in the urine, and moderate to severe

Ancient Ghosts

Anthrax outbreaks are often a surprise because the original instance of disease may predate the memories of anyone who currently lives on the land. Animals that died of anthrax long ago can be a source of new outbreaks when weather conditions free up old, dormant spores and cause disease decades later.

In west-central Alberta, Canada, for instance, carcasses of bison that died of anthrax in earlier times were preserved for years in boggy, peat-moss soils. An outbreak in 1999 was attributed to spores that survived in the bone marrow of the skeletons in these peat bogs that became accessible to cattle during a drought, when wet areas had dried out enough to graze. Because of the drought, the grass was short, and the cattle grazed close to the ground, ingesting the anthrax spores. In those conditions, cattle were also drinking from small ponds in the peat bogs, and those sinkholes were probably full of anthrax spores.

bloat. There may be swelling around the neck, throat, and top of the shoulders. If the animal is still on his feet, he may be staggering or trembling. Usually the disease is so acute, however, that you just find the animal dead. A few cases become chronic, but the animal dies of it eventually. After death, the carcass decomposes quickly because it is so full of bacteria that were coursing through the bloodstream.

Once an animal in the herd dies, subsequent cases often occur, since cattle are curious and sniff around the carcass, thereby picking up lethal doses of spores. These secondary cases develop high fever and *toxemia* (toxins in the blood) and often die swiftly before presenting the other symptoms (such as bloody diarrhea) seen in the first cases. Toxins in the blood attack the brain.

If you find a dead animal, one of the clues that it could be anthrax is excessive bleeding from body orifices and lack of clotting. Toxins released by the multiplying bacteria inhibit blood clotting. Other signs are rapid bloating of the carcass, lack of rigor mortis, and swift decomposition.

Treatment and Prevention

If you find them early enough, treat diseased animals with massive doses of penicillin or tetracyclines to halt the infection. By the time symptoms are seen, however, it is often too late.

If anthrax is even remotely suspected, *do not* perform a postmortem examination, because tissues exposed to the air will stimulate spore production. Report the death to your state veterinarian so samples can be taken for testing. Diagnosis can be made by the vet via a blood sample taken from an ear, if done within 12 hours of death. The ear can be sent to a laboratory in a sealed bag. Once samples are taken for testing, the carcass should be limed (especially any body orifices that may be oozing fluid) and wrapped in a tarp to contain all fluids until a diagnosis is made. If the test results are positive for anthrax, the wrapped carcass, as well as the soil where the animal died, must be treated with the utmost caution, and disposed of properly.

There is a vaccine available. Anthrax was one of the first livestock diseases for which a vaccine was developed, in the late nineteenth century. An improved vaccine has been in use for several decades. For best protection, cattle should be vaccinated 2 to 4 weeks before going out on risky pastures; this should give them 6 to 12 months of immunity. In outbreak situations all herdmates should be vaccinated after infected animals are destroyed, and a booster is recommended 2 to 3 weeks after that first vaccination. Cattle should be vaccinated if they are grazing in areas historically known to have cases of anthrax. The vaccine has a long withdrawal period; vaccinated animals should not be sent to slaughter for at least 60 days after vaccination. Consult your veterinarian for proper use of the vaccine.

Carcass Disposal

Control of anthrax depends mainly on proper carcass disposal. All carcasses and any soil, bedding, or feed that may have been contaminated by the dying animal should be burned or buried at least 10 feet (3 m) below the ground surface with an ample supply of lime added to reduce the chances of environmental contamination. If the carcass must be moved, all soil contaminated by the carcass should be burned and limed. Once the carcass and soil around it is burned, spread lime over the top of the burned debris afterward. Be very careful when handling carcasses or contaminated debris. Wear disposable gloves and a mask, if possible, then burn them, and wash your hands and equipment thoroughly.

Because this disease can be contracted by humans and must be reported, your state vet can advise you on proper handling procedures and answer any questions you may have.

Clostridial Diseases

There are a number of very serious cattle diseases caused by a group of bacteria called *Clostridia*. These bacteria have the ability to form a protective shell-like spore form when exposed to adverse conditions such as drying. The spores can remain alive but dormant indefinitely. Some live in the soil for many years and infect animals later when ingested with feed. They can also exist within bodies of animals in a *latent* state without causing disease, then suddenly grow when conditions become favorable.

Clostridia can produce deadly toxins that may kill the animal if they get into the bloodstream. Toxins of different types of *Clostridia* vary in their effects and the way they gain entrance to the bloodstream. They grow in the absence of oxygen and, unless the animal is previously vaccinated, they release toxins faster than the body can mount a defense, killing the animal suddenly.

Many of these bacteria are found in the intestinal contents of normal animals and humans as part of gut flora. They also exist in soil that contains old manure. They cause disease in certain circumstances, as when dietary or management changes produce an environment more favorable for swift multiplication. Because most of these bacteria are ever-present in the environment, the only way to protect cattle is by vaccination. There is an eight-way combination vaccine to protect against most clostridial diseases — including blackleg, redwater, *malignant edema, black disease, enterotoxemia* — and a separate vaccine for tetanus. All of the clostridial diseases can be deadly, but they are also unique in that they can be effectively prevented by vaccine.

Blackleg

Blackleg is an acute and highly fatal disease mainly affecting cattle under 2 years old; it is caused by *Clostridium chavoei,* a spore-forming bacterium capable of living in soil for long periods. Spores enter the body via the digestive tract, where they pass through the gut wall into the bloodstream and end up in muscles and other tissues. They may live in the gut, spleen, and liver without causing problems and can lie dormant in muscles for a long time until conditions are right for swift multiplication.

The bacteria start to grow and produce deadly toxins whenever there is bruising or injury to the muscles or any other condition that reduces the oxygen level in the tissues. Muscle trauma associated with exertion, transport, herding, and handling may also trigger multiplication of these bacteria. In an unvaccinated herd, cattle of all ages are susceptible, but this disease often crops up in the fastest-growing calves. The usual cause is ingestion of contaminated feed or soil.

Symptoms

Blackleg comes on suddenly. A stockman may find a few animals dead without having seen signs of illness. The first signs are depression and lameness; the animal is very dull. The infection causes inflammation of the muscles, resulting in lameness, swelling of the upper part of the affected leg, severe toxemia, and death. The animal has a high fever, up to 106°F, but by the time symptoms are obvious, the temperature may have dropped to normal or subnormal.

Swelling, caused by gas bubbles in the muscle tissue, can often be felt under the skin, which crackles upon being touched, especially on hips and shoulders. The swollen leg is hot and painful, but soon becomes cold and painless as swelling enlarges and blood supply to the area diminishes. Skin is discolored and becomes dry and cracked. The animal usually dies within 12 to 36 hours, often so quickly that you just find him dead without knowing he was sick. In some cattle, swelling occurs only in the heart and *diaphragm,* with no outward evidence. In most cases, however, postmortem examination reveals black, *necrotic* (dead) tissue in infected areas of the larger muscles (and sometimes tongue and jaw), containing pockets of gas bubbles.

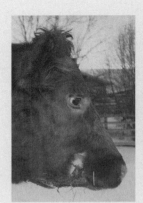 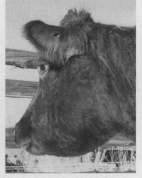

Treatment and Prevention

Unless begun very early, at the first sign of symptoms, treatment is generally of little value. Large doses of penicillin may save the animal at that stage. In the face of an outbreak, it may help to vaccinate the herd and administer penicillin at the same time. The penicillin will halt proliferation of bacteria in exposed animals and give them time to develop immunity from the vaccine.

Many cattle died of blackleg before the advent of vaccination; this was the first cattle vaccine developed. Today the only blackleg vaccine available is a combination vaccine that includes protection against other clostridial diseases.

Calves are generally vaccinated at 2 to 4 months of age, with a booster at weaning time. A two-dose regimen is needed, which generally gives lifelong immunity against blackleg. Calves vaccinated at less than 4 months of age should be revaccinated at 5 to 6 months or at weaning, since early vaccination may not give lifelong immunity. Some of the other clostridial diseases (such as redwater and black disease) can be a threat at any time during the life of the animal, so the combination vaccine is often given annually or even more often if redwater is a problem in the region.

Expect a Local Reaction with Clostridial Vaccines

Clostridial vaccines are given subcutaneously (beneath the skin), preferably on the neck. These vaccines are notorious for creating local reactions, with heat and swelling. When given in the neck, the result may be a temporarily stiff neck and a reluctance to move the shoulder forward. The vaccine sometimes causes permanent lumps under the skin.

If a permanent blemish is a concern with show cattle, an alternative injection site just behind and under the elbow can be used. Swelling in this area may make the animal sore and lame for a few days, but a permanent knot under the skin will not be so readily noticed.

Malignant Edema

This disease affects cattle of all ages and is caused by *Clostridium septicum*, found in human and domestic animal *feces* and in the soil where livestock population numbers are high. The bacteria gain entrance to the body via deep wounds, any contaminated surgical sites that are not adequately disinfected, or vaginal or uterine injuries after a difficult calving.

You will observe dullness, loss of appetite, swelling around the wound and lower parts of the body, high fever (106 or higher), and death within 24 to 48 hours when a cow suffers from this disease. There may be a wet, doughy swelling around the wound or the break in the tissues where the bacteria have gained entrance. This swelling may gravitate toward lower parts of the body. Postmortem examination will reveal dark, foul-smelling, necrotic areas under the skin, often extending into the muscle.

Massive doses of penicillin can sometimes save an affected animal if given early in the course of the illness. Malignant edema can be prevented only by vaccination — usually a combination vaccine that protects against most clostridial diseases.

Black Disease

Black disease is caused by *C. novyi* and is seen more often in feedlot cattle than in cow-calf herds. The bacteria reside in the soil, are extremely resistant to heat or freezing, and may live indefinitely. Spores gain entrance into the body via wounds or possibly may be ingested. They take up residence throughout the body in the muscles. Anything that damages cells and reduces oxygen in tissues near the spores can enable them to reproduce and produce toxins.

Symptoms are similar to those of malignant edema, but most often the affected animal is found dead because this infection is so swiftly fatal. There is generally no time for treatment, so no treatment is recommended. Prevention requires two doses of vaccine.

Sudden Death (SORD)

C. sordellii is another clostridial bacterium that is so highly fatal that symptoms are rarely seen; the animal is typically found dead. This is generally a disease of feedlot cattle. The route of transmission is unknown but is thought to be ingested. Like blackleg, these bacteria can reside in muscle tissue and may remain harmless until triggered into growth and toxin production by an event that lowers the oxygen content of the tissue. The toxin is more deadly than that produced by blackleg or malignant edema. Cattle of all ages are susceptible, but calves and young adults are most often affected. Protection is by vaccination.

Redwater (Bacillary Hemoglobinuria)

This disease is caused by *C. hemolyticum* and occurs primarily in the Rocky Mountain regions of the American West and some areas along the Gulf Coast. The bacteria are durable, and their spores can survive in the environment for many years. The disease often occurs in marshy areas where there are snails that serve as an intermediate host to liver flukes (see chapter 7). Liver damage from flukes enables the bacteria to proliferate in liver tissue, producing powerful toxins. The disease is less commonly seen in cattle pastured where there is no access to marshes or surface water.

Bacteria are spread by feed contaminated with feces and by contaminated surface water or soil. After being ingested, they localize in the liver and remain dormant there and suddenly begin rapid multiplication if the liver is damaged. Damage may be due to flukes, abscesses, chemicals, plant toxins, or bacterial or viral infections.

Symptoms

The first signs of infection are sudden loss of appetite, a drop in milk production, the sudden halting of rumen and bowel movements, shallow and labored breathing, and a reluctance to move. Toxins from multiplying bacteria destroy red blood cells. The breakdown of red cells releases hemoglobin pigment, which ends up in the urine; hence the term "redwater" disease. The animal is dull, with a high fever of 103 to 106°F, bloody diarrhea, dark red foamy urine, blood- or bile-stained feces, and anemia.

The sick animal may collapse and die before you know she is ill. Pregnant cows may be sick for only 10 or 12 hours before they abort or die, but nonpregnant cows, steers, or bulls may live for 3 to 4 days. Postmortem examination shows red-stained urine in the bladder, pale tissues, thin watery blood, and usually a large necrotic area in the liver.

Treatment and Prevention

Treatment for redwater is often of no use because the animal is found dead. If the disease is observed in the early stages, large doses of penicillin given every 12 hours may help, along with immediate antitoxin treatment. IV fluid should be given and the animal protected from bad weather.

Control of liver flukes can help reduce the incidence of redwater. In years past, a bacterin was available to prevent redwater and was given to susceptible cattle every six months, but it is no longer made. Cattle can be protected with an eight-way clostridial vaccine that now contains *C. hemolyticum* and various other clostridial antigens. Vaccinate every six months for protection and even more often in low-lying regions with marshy pastures and constant exposure to flukes.

EXPERIENCE WITH CLOSTRIDIAL DISEASE

MY FIRST ENCOUNTER with clostridial disease was in 1958 on my father's ranch, when we found two cows dead on our upper pasture. Our vet did postmortem examinations and determined that redwater — a disease we'd never heard of until then — was the cause. The vet had seen several other cases in our valley that year. The theory was that cattle from other regions had brought this disease with them. There was a vaccine available, so we vaccinated all our cattle and have been vaccinating them every six months ever since.

The only other loss we've had to clostridial disease was in 1978, when we had a young cow with a calving problem. Her calf had a bony ridge on his forehead and would not fit through the pelvis. Our new vet, who had just moved here, performed a C-section without antibiotics, despite the fact that he used clippers and surgical instruments that were not disinfected between uses. By the next day the cow was very sick. We started her on antibiotics, but it was too late. After she died we cut her open and found the tissue around the incision black and dead. The vet came back out and diagnosed it as malignant edema.

Enterotoxemia Caused by C. Perfringens

Enterotoxemia is a term that simply means toxic infection of the intestines, but stockmen commonly use it to refer to infection by certain clostridial bacteria. There are five types of *C. perfringens* (A, B, C, D, and E), classified by the type of toxins they produce. These organisms are found worldwide in the lower intestinal tract of humans and most mammals, but cause disease, such as toxic intestinal infections in calves and food poisoning in humans, only under certain circumstances.

C. perfringens type C causes acute and fatal intestinal infection in calves unless they've been vaccinated. Types C and D primarily cause enterotoxemia, with signs ranging from acute abdominal pain and diarrhea to *convulsions*, blindness, *coma*, and swift death. Since these bacteria are normal inhabitants in the digestive tract, a specific set of circumstances must exist in order for the calf to be affected. Type C bacteria must have an abundant supply of carbohydrates before they can multiply rapidly and produce toxins.

In order to develop enterotoxemia, the calf must experience the following three conditions:

1. Type C strain must be present in the intestinal tract

2. The bacteria must have an abundance of nutrients, especially carbohydrates (as supplied by milk)

3. There must be a slowdown or stoppage of intestinal-tract movement, allowing toxins to accumulate and be absorbed by the gut

If a calf ingests a large amount of feed, as when loading up on milk after a period of not eating, it can bring about the intestinal slowdown. The large volume takes more time to digest, creating a slowdown in gut contents.

Symptoms

Signs of disease include severe abdominal pain that comes on suddenly; the calf kicks at his belly or throws himself on the ground. He is dull and may be slightly bloated, with abdominal distension due to gas in the intestines and *abomasum* rather than the rumen. If not treated with antitoxin immediately, he goes into shock (and may present with convulsions and paddling of the feet) and soon dies, often within 12 hours or less.

If the calf lives more than a few hours, he may develop diarrhea with blood in the feces. The postmortem exam will show a red-purple section of small intestine and thick blood-tinged fluid in the gut. A prompt postmortem (and tissue samples sent to a lab within six hours of death) can give a definitive diagnosis. Some years ago the samples had to be frozen immediately to preserve the toxins in the tissues so they could be inoculated into mice, but now a *polymerase chain reaction (PCR) test* can be done to detect the toxins.

Type D generally affects older calves, and toxins can escape from the gut into the bloodstream without causing significant gut damage. These calves don't show the massive bloody intestinal *lesions* at postmortem. This toxin is acutely lethal, and the calves die very quickly once it gets into the bloodstream. Type D is triggered to multiply and produce toxins by the intake of feeds such as grain that are high in soluble carbohydrates or by a sudden change in diet, as from hay to grain or when the ration in a feedlot is changed.

Treatment and Prevention

It is often too late for treatment by the time you find the calf, but if a young calf is found before he goes into shock and coma, antitoxin (type C) may reverse the condition. If he's found early, a large dose of *castor oil* and neomycin sulfate solution given orally (or an oral dose of penicillin) may combat the infection and stimulate the gut to start moving again and move the offending material on through. Castor oil can bind to the toxins and render them harmless. Activated charcoal may also help absorb toxins.

Some herds experience problems in calves less than a week old; the best prevention calls for vaccinating the cows a few weeks ahead of calving so they'll have a high level of antibodies against *C. perfringens* type C. If the calf ingests plenty of colostrum right after birth, he will be protected. Other herds experience problems in older calves (1 to 4 months of age) after the temporary immunity from colostrum is gone, since temporary immunity lasts only

Type A Attacks the Gut

In recent years type A has become prevalent as a cause of gastrointestinal disease in both adult and young animals. In calves it causes abomasum ulcers and intestinal bleeding and in some instances is now showing up more commonly than types C and D, possibly because vaccination has kept types C and D at bay. Calves have a sudden onset of abdominal distension, with pain, bloat, depression, refusal to eat, and sudden death.

4 to 6 weeks. In these herds, vaccinating calves soon after birth will give protection. Most vaccines contain both C and D toxoid.

Hemorrhagic Bowel Syndrome

In mature cattle *C. perfringens* type A is thought to be associated with *hemorrhagic bowel syndrome (HBS)*. No single cause has been identified, but these bacteria are commonly found in the gastrointestinal tracts of affected animals. HBS begins with a sudden and sometimes massive hemorrhage in the small intestine, which can result in blood clots that obstruct the intestine. Because the hemorrhage is sudden, affected cattle are often found dead without any warning signs.

Most clostridial vaccines do not contain protection against *C. perfringens* type A, but there is a type A toxoid available. If you suspect that you might have this problem, work with your veterinarian for diagnosis and help with prevention. Often, correcting nutritional and environmental factors that might promote overgrowth of clostridial bacteria or impair immunity can prevent HBS.

Tetanus

Although cattle are less susceptible to tetanus (caused by *C. tetani*) than most mammals, it sometimes occurs in cattle when bacteria enter the body via a wound, when surgery is done without the appropriate disinfectant, or through the moist umbilical stump of a newborn calf. These bacteria live in the intestines of many animals and are present in soil where animals have lived or where manure has been used as fertilizer.

The bacteria remain in the area where they enter the body and can remain dormant until conditions are right. They multiply best in an airless environment, such as deep puncture wounds with damaged tissue and not much blood or oxygen circulation at the site.

Symptoms

Powerful toxins are released when the bacteria multiply, attack nerve tissue, and eventually affect the brain and spinal cord. The animal develops muscle spasms (obvious when trying to react to sudden sounds or touch). In early stages the main sign of tetanus is incoordination, with ears up and tail held stiffly elevated. About 60 percent of affected cattle die.

Treatment and Prevention

Treatment consists of tranquilizing the animal and giving penicillin to halt bacterial multiplication and production of toxins. Tetanus antitoxin is sometimes given in large doses. Supportive treatment (force-feeding by *stomach tube* or giving IV fluids) must be given until the animal is able to eat and drink again. This may take as long as 1 to 4 weeks.

To prevent tetanus, make sure the environment is free of sharp objects (such as nails sticking out of boards or poles or old metal parts on abandoned machinery) that might create puncture wounds and by using very clean techniques and antibiotics for any necessary surgery. In geographic regions where the risk is great, some veterinarians give tetanus antitoxin at the time of surgical procedures and may also recommend vaccination in some instances.

Botulism

Botulism is caused by *C. botulinum* and occurs in cattle only rarely but can be devastating. Toxins produced by these bacteria are some of the most potent known. The bacteria form spores that can live in soil a long time, being resistant to heat, boiling water, light, drying, and radiation. These spores are common in the environment but need warmth, alkaline conditions, and low or no oxygen to germinate. After they germinate they release neurotoxins. The bacteria can be found in the decomposing bodies of animals, especially in an airless environment, as when small animals like rabbits, mice, or snakes are baled in hay. The powerful toxins released by germinating spores build up in the decomposing animal and leak out into surrounding feed. On occasion the disease may also be transmitted via contamination of open wounds with the bacterial spores.

Botulism can also occur when cattle eat spoiled silage — whenever the pH of the silage rises above 4.6 or when large round bales are baled green and put into silage bags for fermentation and then get tears or punctures in the bags that allow air to enter and cause improper fermentation. It can also occur in some situations in baled alfalfa or alfalfa cubes.

Symptoms

When cattle eat contaminated feed or become infected in another way, they become weak and develop paralysis (are unable to get up), followed by death in 1 to 3 days. It takes only one bite of bad feed to cause severe illness, with muscles becoming weak and paralyzed. Once the respiratory muscles are affected, the animal can't breathe.

One way to tell if she is suffering from botulism is to pull on her tongue, extending it out of her mouth. A normal cow will immediately pull her tongue back, but a cow with botulism usually has trouble retracting it back into her mouth. If you try this, however, use a protective glove so no saliva will touch your hand, because this symptom may also be typical of rabies (see chapter 3).

Treatment and Prevention

There is no effective treatment for botulism. There is a vaccine for horses, but since the disease is uncommon in cattle, there is no vaccine for cattle.

E. Coli

Escherichia coli is a bacterium that occurs commonly in the environment and in the digestive tract of animals and humans. There are many different strains, some of which are nonpathogenic and some that cause disease, especially in young animals. Because these bacteria are common in manure, young calves born in crowded conditions are susceptible. They may pick up the organisms soon after birth if born in a dirty pen or a pasture contaminated with manure or if they nurse a dirty udder or lie in manure and then lick themselves.

There are basically two forms of disease in calves possibly caused by different strains of *E. coli*. The *enteric* form involves the digestive tract, damaging the intestinal lining and causing acute diarrhea. This

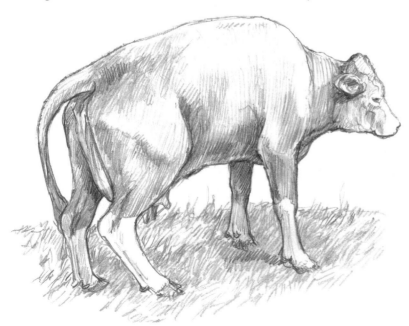

Toxins from Clostridium botulinum *infection cause incoordination and then paralysis of the hind legs.*

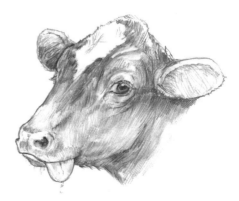

Botulism often results in tongue paralysis and an inability to eat or drink. The cow can't retract the tongue back into the mouth.

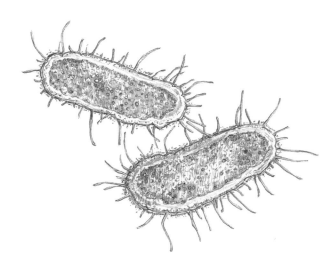

E. coli *bacteria that cause calfhood diarrhea have fingerlike projections called* pili. *These projections attach the bacterium to the intestinal wall and secrete harmful toxins.*

most commonly occurs in calves less than 3 days old. Since a young calf dehydrates quickly, severe diarrhea may be fatal unless treated swiftly with frequent administration of fluid and *electrolytes*. In other instances, bacteria proliferate in the gut and damage the intestinal wall, enabling bacteria and their toxins to move through it and into the bloodstream, thereby producing septicemia, which can also kill the calf quickly.

Symptoms

The enteric form of this infection usually appears in the first week of life. The calf has a moderate fever, but the first sign noticed is foul-smelling diarrhea. He quits nursing and may also have abdominal pain. He dehydrates quickly due to fluid loss from watery diarrhea. Without treatment, the calf soon becomes weak and usually goes into a coma and dies within 2 to 5 days. Most calves are affected within 12 to 48 hours of birth.

In calves that develop septicemia, the disease may be so acute that the animal dies before there's much sign of diarrhea, or he may stagger and become extremely weak after a short bout of diarrhea. The infection circulating through the bloodstream attacks various organs of the body, and unless the disease is quickly reversed with proper treatment, the calf goes into shock and dies.

Treatment

Treatment is usually successful if begun early, before the calf is dehydrated, weak, or in shock. Consult your vet regarding an appropriate oral antibiotic. Immediately administer oral fluids containing electrolyte salts if the calf is still on his feet, able to absorb fluids via the digestive tract. Fluid should be given every four to six hours, depending on the age of the calf and the seriousness of the diarrhea. If he is too weak to stand or his legs are cold, this means blood circulation to his extremities is already shutting down and his gut is also too compromised to absorb fluids. If he is this weak, or in shock, he needs intravenous electrolyte fluids (see chapter 2).

Prevention

The best preventive measures include providing clean areas for calving; having clean, uncrowded pastures for cows with young calves; and making sure every calf receives an adequate amount of colostrum within the first hour of life. Older animals have developed resistance to *E. coli;* the cow will have protective antibodies in her colostrum (see chapter 1) that she will pass to her calf if he nurses soon after he's born.

Some types of *E. coli* infection that affect calves early in life can be prevented by vaccinating the cow ahead of calving, so that her antibody levels are high. This will help, however, only if the calf gets a full nursing of colostrum soon after birth. There are commercial antibody products that can be given orally to newborn calves, but they protect against only a few strains of *E. coli* and must be given immediately after birth to be effective.

Navel Ill and Joint Ill

Navel ill and *joint ill* are common terms for septicemia, a bacterial infection in young animals that circulates through the bloodstream to all parts of the body. The umbilical stump (navel cord opening) is often the portal of entry, and the infection may settle in the joints, causing septic arthritis. Some of the common bacteria that cause navel ill include *E. coli, Proteus, Staphylococcus, Actinomyces pyogenes,* and others that are often present in the environment.

Bacteria may also enter the bloodstream of the newborn via other routes, such as the digestive tract (see *E. coli,* above). Bacteria or their toxins may compromise the intestinal lining and slip through into the bloodstream to cause serious, quickly fatal disease. These bloodstream invaders may also cause infection in various sites in the body, such as a navel abscess or enlarged, damaged joints.

Symptoms

Navel infection may be localized, as with an abscess at the navel; spread through the body as septicemia affecting multiple organs; or settle in joints to cause painful arthritis (joint ill).

▸ **Local infection** results in inflammation and swelling that may be confined to the navel or spread upward into the abdomen. The navel is enlarged and painful. The calf may or may not be sick.

▸ **If infection is circulating through the body,** the calf may be very ill, off feed, with fever. Without immediate and extensive treatment he will go into shock and die, and even with treatment may end up with arthritic joints.

▸ **If the infection settles in the joints** it causes swelling and lameness. The calf may or may not be acutely ill. Joint infections may result in permanent crippling, however.

Treatment

A number of antibiotics can be used to treat early cases of navel ill. If infection is confined to the navel area, draining and flushing the abscess usually results in healing, though in some instances your veterinarian must surgically remove all infected umbilical tissue.

If the calf is ill with septicemia, your vet can recommend an appropriate antibiotic and give advice on dosage, frequency, and route of administration. Blood serum taken before the calf is treated can be cultured to find out which pathogen is involved and which antibiotic would be most effective against it. But growing a *culture* may take several days and the calf can't wait that long for treatment. The vet will usually recommend a *broad-spectrum antibiotic,* and it's used until results of the culture are available. It may take several weeks to completely halt

the infection, and treatment should not be discontinued until the calf is completely back to normal. Supportive treatment, such as force-fed fluids and nutrients if the calf isn't nursing, may be necessary until the calf feels better again.

PIPSY'S BIG JOINTS

ONE OF OUR SON'S CALVES developed septicemia after a navel infection, and even though diligent treatment saved her life, she ended up with permanent swelling and enlargement in all of her leg joints — especially her knees and hocks. Amazingly, after she got over being sick, she eventually got over being lame.

Because of her big joints, she could not be sold with the other calves that fall, and our son kept her. She's now an eight-year-old cow with big knees, raising a calf every year, and still doing fine.

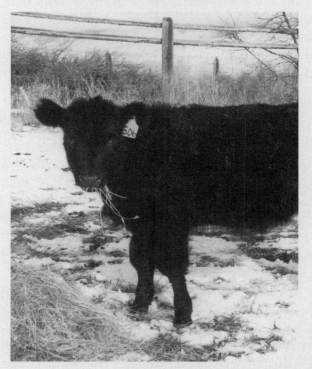

Pipsy as a weanling, with enlarged knees and hocks, due to joint infection acquired as a newborn calf.

Prevention

The best prevention is sanitary conditions at birth, to avoid bacterial contamination of the moist navel stump. Calves born on clean, grassy pasture rarely develop navel ill, whereas calves born in a corral or barnyard or anywhere else previously used by livestock may be at risk, since the soil is contaminated by manure, body discharge, and other foreign material. Birth in a clean barn stall bedded with fresh straw is safer than a birth in a dirty stall or on the ground. Dip the navel stump in tincture of iodine as soon as the cord breaks to prevent infection.

Tips for Navel Stump Dipping and Care

Immediate disinfection of the navel stump with iodine is crucial. If the calf has already flopped around on the ground and in manure for a while, dirtying his navel stump in his efforts to get up, you may be too late to prevent contamination. You may still be able to prevent navel ill, however, if you diligently dip the navel several times during the first 24 hours of life until the stump is completely dry. Make sure the stump is completely immersed and saturated. Swabbing the navel stump is not enough to kill all bacteria that may have entered the tissues; dipping is more effective. To do this:

▸ Dip the navel stump in a small widemouthed jar containing at least ½ inch (1.3 cm) of tincture of iodine.

▸ Hold the jar up tightly against the abdomen, sloshing it around.

▸ Be careful not to spill iodine on the calf when dipping the stump; iodine is quite caustic and can burn skin or eyes.

▸ Make sure the navel stump dries up completely during the first 24 hours; as long as it remains moist, it presents an open doorway for bacteria.

▸ It may take repeated dipping to dry up the stump, especially for a bull calf. A heifer may have a dry, shriveled navel stump within 12 hours after just one application of iodine, but a bull calf may keep the stump moist longer if he urinates while lying down.

▸ If the stump is moist with urine, it may take several more dips to hasten drying and sealing off.

▸ Several disinfectants are recommended for preventing navel ill, though they are not as effective as iodine. Some vets suggest that the navel stump can be dipped in *chlorhexidine (Nolvasan),* for instance, but 7 percent solution iodine has the advantage of being astringent, which helps the cord dry faster (weaker solutions won't help dry the navel cord). Iodine is also surer protection; Nolvasan is inactivated if it comes into contact with organic material such as manure or straw. If the navel is already dirty by the time you dip it, Nolvasan won't be very effective. And if you use the same dip for another calf, the solution has become contaminated and has lost its potency.

Along with dipping the navel stump, make sure the newborn calf nurses his dam within an hour of birth and gets adequate colostrum. The maternal antibodies in colostrum (see chapter 1) can help protect him against some of the infections he may encounter soon after birth, including pathogens that cause navel ill and septicemia. Calves born in a clean environment, whose cords are diligently disinfected, and who receive adequate colostrum, rarely develop navel or joint ill.

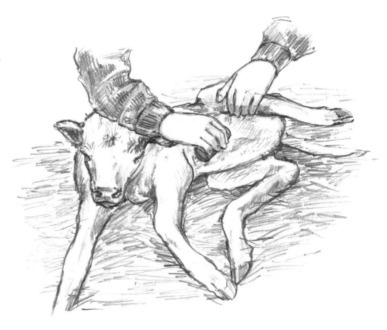

Dipping the navel stump of a newborn calf in iodine immediately after birth is the best prevention for navel ill and joint ill, along with making sure the calf is born in a clean place.

Salmonella

There are more than 2,200 known types of salmonella bacteria, but only five are thought to cause disease in U.S cattle, and only two are common — *Salmonella typhimurium* and *S. dublin*. *Salmonellosis* generally causes diarrhea but sometimes affects other body systems instead. These bacteria are ingested and spread from one animal to another via feces or feces-contaminated feed. *S. typhimurium* is highly fatal to calves, but if they recover, they will not be carriers. Cattle outbreaks and deaths from this type of salmonella are therefore sporadic, as when infected rodents spread the disease. By contrast, *S. dublin* can be a long-term problem on a farm or ranch because it tends to persist in some cattle even though they do not show signs of disease.

Susceptibility can be influenced by the stress of hauling, bad weather, malnutrition, and calving, among other things. Young calves may be most at risk for severe outbreaks and high death loss. *S. typhimurium* can also be transmitted to humans, so care must be taken when handling sick animals.

Salmonella bacteria are hardy, surviving in dried manure, dust, old barn bedding, and contaminated feed for many years, though sunlight and temperatures above 70°F (21°C) will kill them. Salmonella can survive in soil, manure, and drinking water for up to nine months. Bonemeal and fishmeal sometimes fed to cattle can be contaminated if the source animal carried salmonella, and grain may be contaminated with infected bird or rodent droppings. Salmonella almost always enters via the mouth, from contaminated feed or environment.

Symptoms

Symptoms include fever, severe diarrhea with a putrid smell, abdominal pain, and sometimes blood or mucus in the feces. Occasionally the disease progresses to pneumonia or joint infection due to septicemia; if bacteria are circulating through the bloodstream, the infection may settle in the lungs, joints, or other areas of the body.

Early symptoms with *S. dublin* are not as readily apparent, and a symptom-free animal may carry this strain. Infection with *S. dublin* may begin with an upper respiratory problem or generalized weakness accompanied by fever as high as 107°F (41.7°C). This strain often infects lungs, liver, kidneys, brain, and joints when calves are 2 to 3 months old. Diarrhea may not be seen or may occur just in the later stages of the illness. Many calves infected with *S. dublin* die or grow poorly if they survive. *S. dublin* can cause severe illness in humans who drink infected, unpasteurized milk.

Calves that pick up only a few bacteria during the first day of life and receive adequate colostrum may not show signs of sickness but may still spread the disease. Later, if they are stressed by bad weather or other illnesses or conditions, they may become sick. The stress of weaning may bring on symptoms and contaminate the weaning area.

Treatment

Treatment for salmonellosis should always be done under veterinary supervision. The vet will culture the organism to determine the cause (because diarrhea may be due to other types of pathogens) and then recommend the drugs that will be most effective. Systemic antibiotics injected into the muscle, under the skin, or into a vein can be very helpful if given early in the course of the disease, but they will not cure carrier animals. Your vet may prescribe anti-inflammatory drugs to reduce fever.

Treatment also involves intensive supportive care, such as prolonged use of oral electrolyte solutions or intravenous fluids if the calf's gut is too damaged to absorb fluid. Treating a calf with respiratory symptoms for pneumonia may not be effective.

Prevention

Decreasing stress and minimizing contamination of feed and the environment are crucial for preventing outbreaks. Even one carrier cow can rapidly spread the disease through a dairy operation or a confined calving situation. Infected cows shed bacteria in feces, urine, and milk when they are stressed, most commonly during calving. Severity of the disease is often related to how many bacteria are taken in due to crowding and unsanitary conditions or the degree of contamination in feed.

Stress levels also affect the severity of infection. Stresses such as feed and water deprivation, bad weather, shipping, recent calving, change in diet, overexertion, surgery, the presence of another disease, among others, may cause a carrier or sub-clinical animal to show signs of salmonella or make a healthy animal more vulnerable to infection.

Protection for calves depends on reducing stress and making sure each calf receives an adequate amount of colostrum immediately after birth. Careful use of antibiotics can also help. Overuse of oral antibiotics when treating diseases may kill the normal bacteria in the gut that ordinarily compete with pathogens like salmonella, allowing them to multiply more rapidly and cause disease.

Tuberculosis (TB)

Several species of *mycobacterium* called *tubercle bacillus* cause tuberculosis, a disease infecting all warm-blooded animals. *Mycobacterium bovis* causes bovine tuberculosis and can also infect deer, and occasionally humans. It primarily affects the respiratory system, but it may be several years before signs become evident. Cattle typically remain in good condition even after the bacteria become established in the lungs, where they attack the *lymph nodes* and create lesions in the lungs. If calves drink milk from infected dams, the bacteria can also cause lesions in the calves' intestinal tracts.

Early symptoms are rarely recognized, since the disease advances very slowly. Symptoms may include lethargy and persistent coughing and weight loss in later stages. Since these symptoms are seen in many kinds of infection, the possibility of TB is often overlooked, especially in early stages.

If an animal is found to have TB, the animal is sent to slaughter rather than treated, since the United States is trying to eradicate this disease. TB has been eradicated in most areas of the United States but re-emerged in Texas and California via infected cattle from Mexico, and in Michigan via infected deer. California and Texas regained their disease-free status in 2007 after intensive testing, quarantine, and eradication programs, but Michigan's efforts are still ongoing. Federal veterinarians work closely with state veterinarians to make sure that any producers with infected herds round up their cattle for testing.

Johne's Disease (Paratuberculosis)

Johne's disease is caused by a bacterium called *Mycobacterium paratuberculosis,* which is similar to the one that causes tuberculosis in humans. It affects ruminants (such as cattle, sheep, goats, deer, and

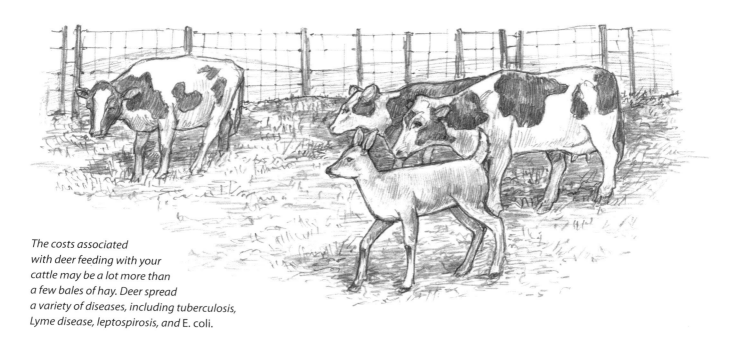

The costs associated with deer feeding with your cattle may be a lot more than a few bales of hay. Deer spread a variety of diseases, including tuberculosis, Lyme disease, leptospirosis, and E. coli.

bison), but signs of disease don't show up for several years; the bacteria grow in body cells of the host and multiply very slowly after the animal becomes infected. It may take 2 to 10 years for symptoms to develop, though the animal is continually shedding bacteria into the environment via manure. The incubation period averages 3 to 4 years, but it sometimes takes as long as 12 years before obvious symptoms are seen. Diarrhea, emaciation, and loss of productivity are the result of gradual, irreversible destruction of function in the intestine. An infected animal can infect many other animals long before he appears sick. Most cases are noticed in animals 2 to 6 years old. First thought to be a problem only in dairy cows, Johne's is now prevalent in beef herds also.

The disease was first described by Heinrich Albert Johne (pronounced Yo-knee) in 1895; the bacterium was discovered in 1911. This organism is hardy and may survive on pasture or moist ground for more than a year. Animals are usually infected as calves. Healthy-looking infected animals may shed bacteria, though those with diarrhea are the worst shedders, passing billions of bacteria in manure. Usually about 95 percent of infected animals in a herd are not yet showing symptoms; the ones that do are just the tip of the iceberg.

There are four stages of this disease:

- **Stage 1** is not detectable. Infection progresses slowly and may take months or years to reach stage 2, in which the animal becomes a shedder of bacteria, unbeknownst to the stockman.

- **Stage 2** cattle are usually more than 2 years old and appear healthy but are shedding enough bacteria to be detected by fecal culture even though blood tests may not pick it up yet. Animals in stage 2 are a hidden threat to herd health unless fecal samples are being checked.

- **Stage 3** is clinical disease; the animals suffer from diarrhea and weight loss. These signs usually don't show up until after 2 years of age, but in some instances may appear as early as 12 to 14 months. Usually the younger the animal is when he develops symptoms the higher the likelihood of a high infection rate within the herd and the greater the level of contamination.

- **Stage 4** animals become more emaciated and very weak, and die.

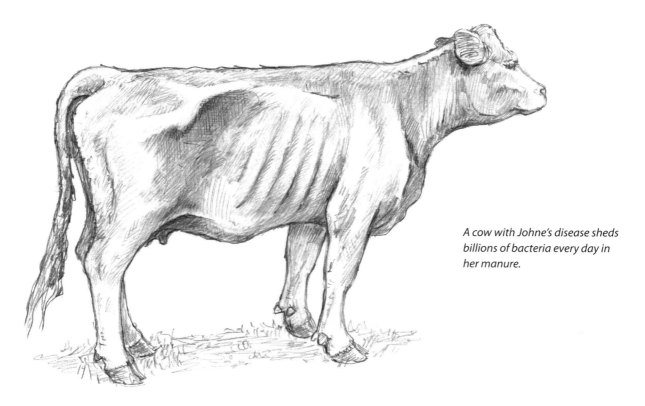

A cow with Johne's disease sheds billions of bacteria every day in her manure.

Transmission

Cattle ingest these bacteria when they take in contaminated feed or water or nurse a dirty udder. They can also be infected via breeding. The bacteria can pass between all ruminant animals; cattle may pick up Johne's disease from infected deer, sheep, and goats. Young calves are at highest risk of picking up bacteria from manure and may be infected before birth if the dam has Johne's disease. About 30 percent of calves from infected cows are born infected. The calf picks up bacteria before or soon after birth but seems healthy until signs appear several years later. During the latter part of that time he seems healthy, but he is actually shedding bacteria and infecting more calves.

Calves can also be infected by their mother's colostrum or that of another infected cow, so even in a clean environment a calf can get Johne's disease. Beef calves fed colostrum from dairy cows are at risk. Some cases of Johne's have been traced to embryo transplant calves with Holstein recipients; the calves get the disease in utero from the surrogate mother. Johne's has been introduced to several herds by the practice of buying dairy calves to be raised by beef cows that lose their calves. Purchased or leased cattle can also infect a herd.

Once the bacteria enter the digestive tract, they infiltrate and reproduce in the lining and adjacent lymph nodes of the lower part of the small intestine, cecum, and colon. The resulting chronic inflammation triggered by the animal's immune response in an attempt to get rid of these pathogens results in a thickened, leathery inner lining of the bowel, hindering absorption of fluid and nutrients from the digestive tract.

The bacteria can also multiply in the uterus, mammary glands, and testicles of infected animals. Bulls can pass the disease to cows they breed. Infected cows may shed large numbers of bacteria in milk; their calves ingest bacteria from both milk and feces from the dam. Some animals spontaneously recover after infection, while others become lifelong carriers and shedders. A small percentage of this group develops symptoms. In cows, the onset of visible signs often follows stress from their first or second calving. In bulls, the onset often occurs during the stress of breeding season.

Symptoms

At first the bacteria affect just the lower small intestine, causing gradual thickening of the lining and impeding absorption of fluid and nutrients, hence the diarrhea and weight loss. Low protein levels result in edema under the jaw and belly. Temperature, general demeanor, and appetite remain normal, but the animal keeps losing weight, and hair color may fade. Eventually the bacteria spread from the gut to other parts of the body, circulating through blood and lymph systems. Johne's should be suspected if a mature animal with chronic weight loss and diarrhea fails to respond to treatment for other ailments.

This disease can enter your herd quietly; by the time you realize you have a problem, it may have spread through the entire herd. You might buy an infected animal that looks healthy, and a year or so later it develops diarrhea. Most people don't connect the two events, because they never realize that the animal was infected at the time of purchase.

Treatment

There is no effective treatment; the disease is not responsive to antibiotics and is always fatal. When the animal enters stage 4 he becomes more emaciated and dies. In stage 4 the diarrhea is a watery, bubbly "pea soup" with very little odor. The animal becomes weak and often develops *bottle jaw* — edema and swelling between the lower jawbones. This fluid-filled bulge under the jaw can also be a sign of parasites or liver damage, however, and not only Johne's disease. Diarrhea and weight loss can also be due to parasites, BVD, liver failure, salmonellosis, and other diseases, so it's not always easy to know what you are dealing with. If an animal is diagnosed with Johne's disease, he should be sent to slaughter before the final stages (the meat is safe for human consumption). If an animal dies, the disease can be confirmed with postmortem examination, by checking the lymph nodes and the intestine.

Sometimes the stage 3 appearance of symptoms is brought on by stress, such as calving. Infected cows may have severe diarrhea following the stress of calving, resulting in fecal contamination of teats and udder, which then infects the newborn calf. Animals that break with diarrhea when stressed may seem to recover temporarily but relapse the next time they're stressed. The severity of signs may change with the seasons and feed. Diarrhea and weight loss are easily misdiagnosed as a parasite problem (see chapter 7). For a while, an infected animal may respond favorably to treatment for internal parasites (if infested with parasites), but "recovery" is brief, and the animal soon goes downhill again.

Even though many animals get culled before they actually show diarrhea, Johne's disease may eventually affect many animals in the herd, since shed bacteria can survive in water for up to a year and in manure and soil for more than a year. The disease gradually mushrooms; within 15 to 20 years of its entering a herd, a number of young cows could be dying of Johne's at 3 to 4 years of age.

In confined herds like dairy or feedlot operations, the combination of constant fecal contamination and stress of confinement results in widespread infection. Infected animals are usually culled due to poor productivity before they show signs of disease. The economic impact of poor production and high rate of turnover in the herd can be enormous.

Prevention

It's not easy to get rid of Johne's in a herd, but it can be done. Even though it's hard to diagnose definitively before death (a *biopsy* of intestine or lymph nodes at postmortem can confirm the diagnosis), tests in live animals can be useful. Fecal cultures may show bacteria but are often impractical in most initial diagnostic cases because the culture grows so slowly (6 weeks to 4 months), and *false negatives* are common.

Blood tests are better, but even if all your cattle test negative, you can't be over 85 percent sure that your herd does not have Johne's. By testing, you can generally identify and get rid of shedders, however. If a cow turns up positive, you can be fairly sure her calf is infected also, and both should be culled. If Johne's has been diagnosed in any of your cattle, every animal over 2 years old should be tested annually. Any animals identified with the disease should be sent to slaughter. Eliminating all cattle that test positive will cut down the source of contamination, and if you practice good sanitation (see box on previous page) the disease will eventually wear out. Most vets recommend continuing to do fecal cultures on every cow until you get three consecutive negative tests for the whole herd.

Since no treatment exists, and common disinfectants are not effective, the best way to protect your herd is never to bring in cattle from unknown origins. Johne's is always a purchased disease, being introduced onto farms disguised as healthy-looking bulls, replacement females, an older cow, a dairy nurse cow, or even a gallon of colostrum bought from a dairy. Purchase your cattle from a reputable breeder who is willing to show the cattle's health records and give you names of other stockmen who have purchased his or her animals. It's best if you can maintain a closed herd, raising your own heifers and being very careful about where you buy bulls.

Listeriosis (Circling Disease)

Listeriosis is caused by *Listeria monocytogenes,* which is common in soil and sometimes in surface water. *Listeria* bacteria have been found in mammals, birds, fish, insects, and crustaceans and are often present in human and animal feces. They can survive for several years in some types of fecal material, for six months in cattle manure or dry straw, almost a year in damp soil, and more than two years in dry soil. Freezing won't kill them. Since these bacteria are present in many environments, there's no definitive conclusion about why some cattle get listeriosis and others don't, but stressed cattle may be more susceptible.

Plants are sometimes contaminated and serve as a source of infection. Once bacteria are ingested, some animals remain infected, shedding pathogens in manure and milk. For the bacteria to multiply to dangerous levels, they need an environment low on oxygen. This can happen when silage is improperly fermented or hay is not baled under the best conditions. Tight bales or tightly packed silage are safest, since the bacteria need a little oxygen and a pH higher than 5.5 to multiply. Moldy silage is sometimes mistaken as having higher risk for listerosis, but *mold* requires more oxygen than *Listeria* does to multiply, so silage free from mold can still be dangerous.

When eating contaminated feed, animals may become infected via breaks in the lining of the gut or mouth, due to eating coarse feeds. The bacteria penetrate the lining and migrate along nerves in the facial area or in the bloodstream, traveling to the brain where they create tiny abscesses. Symptoms vary, depending on which brain functions are affected.

Symptoms

Infected animals with the brain form of listeriosis become dull and disoriented, indifferent to their surroundings. The head may be tilted to one side. They stop eating, have a fever, and usually wander away from the rest of the herd. In early stages they may wander into fence corners and push their heads against fences or other objects. When trying to walk, the animal may be uncoordinated and stumbling (always on the same side), moving in a tight circle, always in the same direction.

The tongue may protrude, with slobbering, drooling and difficulty swallowing, due to paralysis in the facial area. Some individuals can't close their eyes if the infection spreads to the *optic nerves.* When the animal can no longer get up, he will always lie on the same side, returning to that position even if you roll him over. Death is due to respiratory failure, usually one to two weeks after the appearance of symptoms.

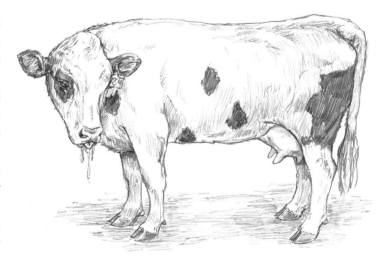

Cows with severe listeriosis often look dull, compulsively circle to the left (or sometimes to the right), and salivate excessively with the tongue protruding.

Treatment

If treated with broad-spectrum antibiotics such as penicillin or *chlortetracycline* in early stages, the animal generally recovers. The earlier this disease is diagnosed and treated, the better the response. Intravenous injections of chlortetracycline or administration of injectable *oxytetracycline* (such as LA-200) or *Nuflor* can save the animal if given soon enough and continued for an extended period. Consult your veterinarian. The sick animal should be isolated.

Prognosis is good if treatment is begun when the animal is still on his feet and in the circling, stumbling stage but not so good if the animal can't swallow. In those instances you must be diligent with daily administration of fluids and electrolytes. Prognosis is poor for cattle that are unable to get up.

Prevention

If one animal in a herd gets sick, this is a warning that others may become infected if they are eating the same feeds. Evaluate your feeding program to see what might be causing the problem. Silage is often the culprit, especially if its poorly packed. The risk is also increased if there's soil contamination in the silage, as happens when it's made from crops on mole-infested fields. Your veterinarian or county Extension agent can help you prevent future cases.

Silage is often to blame but is not the only risk factor, since cattle may pick up bacteria through contact with infected feces, urine, aborted fetuses, and uterine discharge. Healthy, minimally stressed, animals seem to be most resistant to infection.

Thromboembolic Meningoencephalitis (TEME)

This infectious cattle disease causes a wide variety of conditions, including respiratory disease, *laryngitis*, arthritis, foot rot, vaginal and uterine infection, eye and ear problems, mastitis, and, occasionally, abortion. The offending bacteria are a common resident in the respiratory tract of adult cattle — in some herds as many as 50 percent of cows carry antibodies against them — but most often cause disease in young animals. The bacteria survive for long periods in infected nasal discharge and on equipment contaminated with blood, and may be present in water troughs, feed bunks, or handling chutes.

When stress lowers immunity, bacteria present in the upper respiratory system quickly multiply and gain entrance to the bloodstream, causing septicemia. They damage the inner lining of blood vessels, creating clots that break loose and lodge in smaller arteries. The tissues where blood supply is blocked by infected clots are quickly invaded, resulting in abscesses and disease. In some instances this occurs in the brain and is highly fatal; death may occur as soon as 36 hours after the first symptoms appear.

This complex of diseases is caused by *gram-negative bacteria*, a *coccobacillus*, an oval-shaped bacterial cell called *Haemophilus somnus*. These bacteria thrive in an environment containing carbon dioxide, are commonly found in the respiratory tract, and probably enter with air breathed in by the animal. Respiratory disease caused by *H. somnus* will be covered in chapter 11.

Symptoms

Septicemia resulting from rapid proliferation of bacteria in the lungs causes high fever, rapid breathing, lethargy, and weakness. Clots lodging in the small arteries of the larynx, kidneys, feet, and brain create problems in those parts of the body. Young cattle in crowded, stressful conditions may develop a cough about 3 weeks after being penned together, then suddenly develop pneumonia that rapidly progresses to difficult breathing, high fever, and sometimes disorientation. Unless treated quickly, the animals with pneumonia may die within 12 hours.

Laryngitis and *diphtheria* may occur as an *epidemic* within a group of infected calves and is different from typical diphtheria (see chapter 11). Blood clots in the larynx cause severe swelling that shuts off airways. Affected calves have loud, difficult breathing as they force air through the constriction. Foot rot may also occur as an epidemic in a pen of calves; a high percentage may become lame within 48 hours. Blood clots in the feet create conditions ideal for bacteria that cause foot rot (see chapter 12).

H. somnus may invade the joints after an animal develops septicemia. Shoulders, *stifles*, hocks, and elbows are most commonly affected, and surrounding tendon sheaths may be distended. The joints are very swollen, but the animal is usually not as lame as when affected by other forms of joint infection.

Vaginal and uterine lining infection can cause infertility in females. The disease may cause a prolonged interval between calving and conception, since females may not become pregnant until after several heat cycles. This infection can occasionally cause abortion in late gestation. Bulls may also carry the bacteria in their penile sheaths.

The brain-infection condition generally affects cattle 1 to 3 years of age and is most common in feedlot cattle, especially weanlings and yearlings. Stress associated with weaning, shipping, handling, or breeding may lead to outbreaks. Often the first sign is a dead animal or a down animal unable to get up. If a clot in the brain is large, the animal may die suddenly of a massive stroke. More commonly, many small clots lodge throughout the brain, causing multiple symptoms depending on which part of the brain is most damaged. Common signs are one-sided circling or animals lying down with head turned around toward one side. If you find the animal before it dies, early signs include loss of appetite, fever of 105 to 107°F (40.6 to 41.7°C) (though the temperature often drops toward normal as the condition progresses), depression, lameness, lack of coordination, reluctance to move, stiffness, and knuckling of the *fetlock joints.*

The head is often held up with nose extended, or tilted, with rolling eyes. The affected animal may walk in circles or seem blind in one or both eyes. Once down he may have muscle tremors and make paddling movements with the legs. Death usually occurs within a few hours after the animal goes down. Examination of the brain (to find lesions created by clots) may be necessary for diagnosis, because symptoms may be confused with those of listeriosis.

Treatment

Treatment for TEME is most effective if begun in early stages, especially for brain lesions. The animal usually responds to high levels of antibiotics such as oxytetracycline, which should be administered intravenously to get high blood levels quickly. For brain infections, use an antibiotic that will cross the blood-brain barrier in high concentrations. Consult your vet, since a prescription is needed.

Early, aggressive treatment usually results in rapid recovery of acutely ill animals. Dramatic recovery of animals that were near death is typical of this infection. Repeat treatments are usually needed. Since it is difficult to identify the sick animals early, however, a 50 percent recovery rate is considered good. Animals with prolonged pneumonia may be slow to recover, but unlike cattle with *Pasteurella* pneumonia (see chapter 11), recovery is usually complete. In a herd outbreak of a group of weaned or feedlot animals, adding high levels of antibiotic to a feed ration can help reduce the incidence of TEME.

Prevention

TEME prevention is accomplished by vaccination. Calves should be vaccinated at about 4 months of age, with an annual booster for feedlot animals. Two vaccinations are required, with at least a three-week interval between doses. Vaccine is not effective during an outbreak; it must be given before exposure.

Other ways to help prevent infection include minimizing stress, dust, and overcrowding; carefully cleaning water troughs, feed bunks, handling facilities, and trucks and trailers used for hauling cattle; and not mixing groups of cattle. Since a high percentage of cattle are carriers of this pathogen, the less mingling of cattle and the fewer newcomers added to a group, the better. A good vaccination program to protect cattle against other respiratory diseases can help prevent secondary invasion of the lungs by an opportunistic *H. somnus* infection.

CHAPTER FIVE

Viral Diseases

THERE ARE MANY VIRAL INFECTIONS that affect cattle. Viruses are often spread from one animal to another by direct contact, contaminated feed and water, infected discharge from a sick animal, or coughing. Viruses are so small that they often slip through body tissues into an animal, passing through mucous membranes of nasal passages, the mouth and throat, the eyes, and other orifices.

Inside the new host, some viruses survive even after being engulfed by white blood cells and may travel through blood and lymph systems inside these cells to get to sites where they can multiply. Once a virus reaches its preferred location in the body, it multiplies in the tissues. Some viruses start multiplying in the bloodstream, creating *viremia*. This is the stage of the illness when the infected animal is most likely to shed the virus and infect others.

Infectious Bovine Rhinotracheitis (IBR)

Often called *"red nose"* because of the reddened mucous membranes, infectious bovine rhinotracheitis was first recognized as a disease in feedlot cattle during the early 1950s. This *herpes virus* is similar to the *Herpes simplex* virus that attacks humans. Today, IBR is recognized as a common infection of the upper respiratory tract. It is present in most cattle herds but causes illness mainly in animals with no previous exposure (hence, no immunity) or those

with poor immunity due to stress or other diseases. The virus exists in healthy carrier animals that have been exposed or were sick and recovered, and is shed during times of stress. When complicated by bacterial infection, IBR commonly causes pneumonia.

IBR also causes abortion; eye problems; infectious inflammation of vulva and vaginal tissues *(pustular vulvovaginitis); encephalitis* (inflammation of the brain); diarrhea in calves; and, occasionally, a fatal septicemia in young calves, marked by respiratory distress, *ulcers* in the stomach lining, and peritonitis. IBR is one of the most common viral infections of cattle in the United States. It is spread by direct contact, airborne particles, breeding, and sometimes from dam to calf *in utero,* or during birth as the calf passes through the dam's infected vagina. Because many cattle can carry the IBR virus and then shed it when stressed, it can spread rapidly when cattle are grouped for weaning or at a sale or feedlot. The incubation time is 4 to 6 days; infected animals are usually sick for 10 to 14 days.

Symptoms

IBR often causes upper respiratory disease with fever (104 to 107°F [40 to 41.7°C]); dullness; lack of appetite; nasal discharge (clear and watery at first, then sticky and yellow, hanging from the nose in long strands); reddened mucous membranes (inflamed, tender surface that crusts and peels off); nostril and muzzle tissue damage; ulcers in the nose, throat, and windpipe; coughing; rapid or difficult breathing; and sometimes secondary pneumonia (see chapter 11).

There may be watery discharge from the eyes that becomes sticky if eyelid inflammation develops. The windpipe is inflamed and may fill with mucous. All animals in a group may be infected and coughing. They usually recover in two weeks unless the disease becomes complicated by secondary infections due to weather or other types of stress.

Symptoms depend on the tissues infected, the animal's resistance, and the severity of the infection. IBR is a common cause of abortions because the infection destroys the *corpus luteum (CL)* on the ovary that produces *progesterone,* the hormone that protects the pregnancy. These abortions are often mistaken for lepto (see chapter 4). Abortions from IBR may occur at any time during gestation but are most common in the second half. In a herd outbreak, more than half the cows may abort, depending on the number of susceptible cows in advanced pregnancy. Cows may or may not show signs of respiratory disease; often the only evidence of IBR in adult cattle is abortions, which may occur any time from several days to six weeks after contracting the virus. Once the cow recovers from the abortion, she usually breeds back with no problems.

Some animals have *conjunctivitis* (inflammation of the membrane lining the inner eyelid and eyeball) with the respiratory form of IBR; others have eye inflammation with no other signs of illness. The animal has a wet face from excessive watering of the eyes; it becomes dirty when dust collects in the hair. The edges of the eye may be crusty from dried discharge. Watering and inflammation of the eyes may be mistaken for pinkeye (see chapter 9). Eye infection may occur when calves have some immunity to IBR but not enough to completely avoid the infection.

Calves with partial immunity have some circulating immunity and antibodies but are latently infected with IBR, which can become active again *(recrudescence).* IBR is a herpes virus; the disease can stay in a latent (dormant) stage in nerves at the base of the brain, the tonsils, and a few other places in the body. Then, when the animal is stressed or gets an injection of cortisone (such as *dexamethasone*), the infection will recrudesce and return to the oral cavity and/or create an eye infection. This viral dormancy and reactivation are characteristic of human herpes virus as well. Like cattle with IBR, humans have herpes "cold" sores that appear, heal, and then reappear a couple of months or so later if the person is under stress. Because the virus is contagious whenever it is activated, each time it reappears, affected animals may spread the virus to other cattle, such as pregnant cows — which may then abort.

Occasionally, the IBR virus causes vaginal inflammation in cows and inflammation of the prepuce and penis in bulls, with pustular lesions and discharge. An infected cow has a mild fever and white discharge from the vulva; she holds her tail out and switches it due to discomfort. A dairy cow has a temporary drop in milk production. Calves infected before birth may be aborted, *stillborn,* born prematurely, or sick or unable to nurse at birth. Some calves may develop encephalitis; brain lesions may be found postmortem.

Because several respiratory diseases have similar symptoms, diagnosis may depend on careful observation of lesions and on laboratory tests. When in doubt, call your vet.

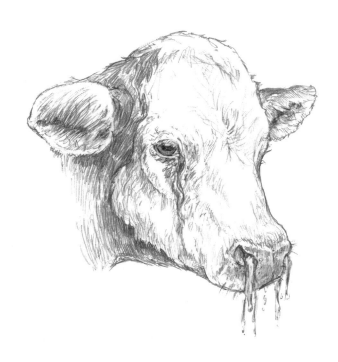

Infectious bovine rhinotracheitis (IBR) is characterized by nasal discharge, runny eyes, a cough, and labored breathing.

Treatment and Prevention

Treatment is of little value against viral infection, but if the animal has severe respiratory signs, antibiotics are usually given to help prevent or combat secondary bacterial pneumonia.

IBR can be prevented by vaccination. Modified live-virus (MLV) vaccines generally give longer protection than killed products (and protect with one dose, versus two doses for most killed products), but pregnant animals should not be given MLV vaccine because it can cause abortion. Abortions due to vaccination, if they are going to happen, usually occur 2 to 10 weeks after the injection. Killed vaccines or intranasal products (sprayed up the nostril) are safer for pregnant cows. Intranasal products immunize surfaces of the upper respiratory tract against future invading viruses and can produce antibody response within 3 days. They are helpful in the face of an outbreak because they provide quicker (if shorter) immunity than injected vaccines.

Calves nursing immune dams obtain temporary protection via antibodies in the colostrum, but this passive immunity interferes with development of active immunity from vaccination, so it is usually not worthwhile to vaccinate calves until they're several months old. If calves in a herd have problems with "summer pneumonia" (which is actually IBR), however, it can sometimes be halted by vaccinating calves at 1 or 2 months of age. Usually calves are vaccinated for IBR at about 6 months of age, or they are revaccinated at that time.

Intranasal vaccine can help to halt a herd epidemic but may not immediately stop IBR abortions because of fetuses that were infected before the vaccination. To avoid this problem, vaccinate cows each year when they're not pregnant — after calving and at least three weeks before rebreeding.

Calves should be vaccinated at weaning to start building immunity. If they are to be vaccinated while still nursing their dams (to start building immunity and protect them during weaning stress), use intranasal or killed vaccine. Otherwise, because the vaccine causes a mild form of the disease, the modified live virus may be transmitted from the calf to his dam by nose-to-nose contact, and the cow may abort. In herds where cows are always vaccinated with modified live-virus vaccine every spring before breeding,

they may still have enough immunity in the fall to be protected from the virus, and their calves can be given live vaccine without risk to the cows.

Parainfluenza 3 (PI3)

This respiratory disease can be relatively mild by itself but may cause severe problems when combined with bacterial infection. It is part of the respiratory disease complex called *shipping fever* (see chapter 11).

PI3 virus can damage the lining of air passages, enabling resident bacteria to invade the tissues. Cattle of all ages are susceptible. Transmission is through direct contact between animals and airborne droplets (from breathing and coughing) containing the virus. Affected animals shed the virus in nasal secretions for several weeks. Many IBR vaccines include PI3, to immunize cattle against both viruses at the same time.

Bovine Respiratory Syncytial Virus (BRSV)

Bovine respiratory syncytial virus is a major cause of respiratory infections (see chapter 11). It is most often a problem in weaning-age calves, feedlot animals, and young dairy stock. BRSV infection damages the cilia (tiny hairlike appendages lining the windpipe), enabling bacteria to bypass them and invade the lungs and causing air to be trapped in lung tissue.

Calves with BRSV are usually dull, with heads hanging down, runny noses and eyes, and raspy coughs. The cough may linger for weeks or months, especially following exertion, even after the animal seems otherwise recovered. In later stages of disease, the sick animal may have labored breathing or breathe with his mouth open. There's usually thick discharge from the nose and eyes and a harsh cough. In acute cases the animal may die within 48 hours of first symptoms. BRSV is often mistaken for other viral infections because symptoms are similar to those of IBR and PI3.

If your vet diagnoses this virus as a problem in your herd, there are vaccines available: killed vaccines (with two initial doses required, to start building immunity), and also modified live-virus vaccines.

Bovine Viral Diarrhea (BVD)

Bovine viral diarrhea virus causes abortion and birth defects and is an indirect cause of other types of illness due to adverse effects on the immune system. It's been estimated that 80 percent of cattle in the United States have been exposed to BVD and that 70 to 90 percent of infections go undetected, without visible symptoms. The first descriptions of BVD in North America (outbreaks of diarrhea, digestive tract ulcers, nasal discharge, abortion) were reported more than 60 years ago.

Two Biotypes, Two Genotypes

The BVD virus is an elusive villain because there are two biotypes that have different effects within body cells. These effects are called *cytopathic* (making obvious changes in cells and killing them) and noncytopathic (the virus does not destroy or change the shape of cells). The main difference is that the cytopathic virus infects cells in the lymph tissues of the gut, while the noncytopathic virus infects a wider range of body cells, including those in the respiratory tract, blood, and lymphoid tissue. The noncytopathic virus also persists longer in the animal.

There are also two basic genetic types (genotypes) of the virus and several different strains within each genetic type. Each type or strain may be either cytopathic or noncytopathic.

The two virus genotypes (Type I and Type II) can both be present in the same animal. They can also change their genetic composition during multiplication. This explains the great variation in disease symptoms and variations in how each animal's immune system handles the virus. Thus, there are several forms of the disease, ranging from *subclinical* infections (in which the animal shows no obvious signs) to a severe and highly fatal form called *mucosal disease.*

BVD can affect the digestive, respiratory, nervous, reproductive, and immune systems. It can cause abortion in cows, *mummification* of the fetus (it dies but remains in the uterus), stillborn full-term calves, or calves with birth defects or immune deficiencies and/or persistent infection with the virus. Noncytopathic BVD viruses cause more than

> ## Contrasting Acute and Persistent BVD
>
> The cytopathic biotype generally causes acute rather than chronic infection. The illness is temporary; it may be mild or severe, and the animal sheds the virus for up to 15 days after infection, then clears it from the body. These animals are not as big a threat to herd health as persistently infected animals because they do not shed the virus continually. They get sick, shed the virus, and then get over it.
>
> By contrast, persistently infected cattle are infected before birth, shed larger numbers of virus particles in body secretions, and continue to do so throughout their lives.

90 percent of BVD outbreaks and are always the cause when cattle are persistently infected.

The BVD virus can mutate or change, and because there are several strains, the infected animal may or may not be able to mount a protective immune response or be protected by vaccination. Because BVD can be so varied, some infections do not cause obvious disease, while others affect the animal's ability to fight off the infection. The disease's appearance in different systems (such as digestive, respiratory, or reproductive) and in different situations depends on the type of virus and the animal's immune status.

Mucosal Disease

The most serious form of BVD was first called mucosal disease because it damaged the mucous lining of the intestine. This is a highly fatal impairment of the small intestine in which the virus has a cytopathic effect: it changes and destroys cells. Mucosal disease occurs only in cattle infected before birth with a noncytopathic version of the virus, due to infection in the dam. These calves seem normal at birth but are persistently infected, with no immunity to the virus. If at some point they come into contact with a cytopathic type of the BVD virus, they cannot develop immunity, even if they've been vaccinated. This makes them vulnerable to severe effects of the cell-killing version of the virus if it's a strain

IN JUNE OF 1975, one of our yearling heifers, Lulubelle, started losing weight while on summer range. By July, she appeared to be ill, so we brought her home, treated her for pneumonia and hardware disease, and tried to get her to eat more. In spite of good nursing care, she died. That same summer a neighbor who ran cattle with us on the range had a cow he called "Old Diarrhea" that got progressively thinner on the range and died out there.

The next year we lost two more yearling heifers in similar circumstances; they died in spite of intensive treatment. That summer, Vaquina, a 4-year-old cow, started losing weight, so we brought her and her calf home from the range and had our veterinarian check her. We treated her with antibiotics and vitamins, but the vet suspected she had BVD, a disease we (and other ranchers in our valley) had never heard of at that time. He told us there was no effective treatment, so we weaned her calf to minimize his mama's stress and butchered her later that fall for hamburger since she was too thin for any other cuts of meat.

We learned that there was a vaccine available, and our vet got us started on a herd vaccination program for BVD. That fall we vaccinated our replacement heifers with modified live-virus vaccine after they were weaned and again the following February before being bred. Since then we've vaccinated all of our cows annually with modified live-virus vaccine a few weeks before breeding season, and we have had no more instances of BVD.

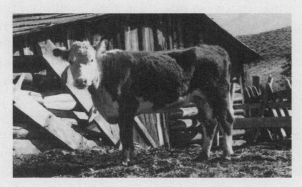

Our 4-year-old cow, Vaquina, became emaciated with BVD virus.

closely related to the persistently infecting virus — although not every combination of noncytopathic and cytopathic BVD virus in a persistently infected (PI) animal results in mucosal disease.

Cattle 6 months to 2 years old are the most likely to develop mucosal disease. Though only a small percentage of a herd may be affected, nearly all affected animals die. Of those who die, most are persistently infected with a strain of noncytopathic virus before birth and then exposed to an animal shedding a cytopathic BVD virus of the same strain.

Mucosal disease often causes profuse watery diarrhea that may contain blood and intestinal lining. Diarrhea usually develops 2 to 3 days after the animal starts to show weakness, fever, depression, and lack of appetite. There are often lesions in the mouth that may involve the lips and the tongue or the inside of the nostrils. Diarrhea results in emaciation and dehydration. Acute cases usually die in a few days or weeks. A few become chronic, and may survive for up to 18 months, becoming increasingly emaciated.

Diarrhea in chronic cases may be continuous or intermittent, and some animals develop chronic bloat. Lesions in the mouth and skin are slow to heal, and the animal may be lame. Treatment is not recommended because even if there's a slight chance of recovery, the animal will be infected for life; she should be sold for slaughter or humanely destroyed.

It's important to work with your vet for proper diagnosis to know whether it's worth trying to treat the sick animal or not. Diarrhea from acute and temporary BVD infection caused by a cytopathic biotype of the virus is usually mild and followed by rapid recovery. But mucosal disease (which may be acute or chronic) is the result of dual infection with both cytopathic and noncytopathic biotypes and generally causes death in persistently infected animals.

The Problem of Persistent Infections

If a cow is infected while pregnant, the virus easily crosses through the placenta. Even if the dam does not show signs of illness herself, her unborn calf may be infected. The outcome of fetal infection depends on the age of the fetus at the time it's infected. If infection occurs prior to 100 days of gestation, BVD infection may result in birth defects or the death of the fetus (through absorption, mummification, or abortion). The fetus may be aborted at the time of infection or up to several months later.

Calves infected during the third trimester (after 150 days) may be normal at birth, having developed immunity. They have a titer to BVD virus. Their immune systems were mature enough at the time of infection to create antibodies to protect themselves.

The biggest problem occurs when a noncytopathic BVD virus infects fetuses before they've developed a competent immune system (before 140 to 150 days of gestation). These calves may end up persistently infected with BVD because their immune systems do not recognize the virus as anything other than a normal part of their body and do not produce any immune response against it. The calf's body tolerates the virus and can never get rid of it. The virus continues to multiply, infect more cells, and be excreted from the animal. These calves may appear normal and healthy at birth, but they continue to shed BVD virus throughout their lives. These carriers of BVD are the biggest threat to herd health and the main source of transmission within and between farms or in a feedlot.

The PI (persistently infected) animal sheds high numbers of virus particles in nasal discharge, saliva, semen, milk, urine, and tears. Feces contain virus particles but in lesser numbers. Acute BVD infections, by contrast, are less likely to spread the virus. Acute infection causes illness and shedding of the virus for up to 15 days after infection. The typical shedding period is 7 to 10 days. Then the animal mounts an immune defense, clears the virus, and is no longer a source of infection.

If you keep a PI heifer, however, she sheds BVD virus for the rest of her life, and all her calves become infected during her pregnancies. This is one of the main ways BVD persists within a herd, and these PI cattle are always at risk for mucosal disease if they encounter a cytopathic form of the virus.

PATHS TO PERSISTENT INFECTION

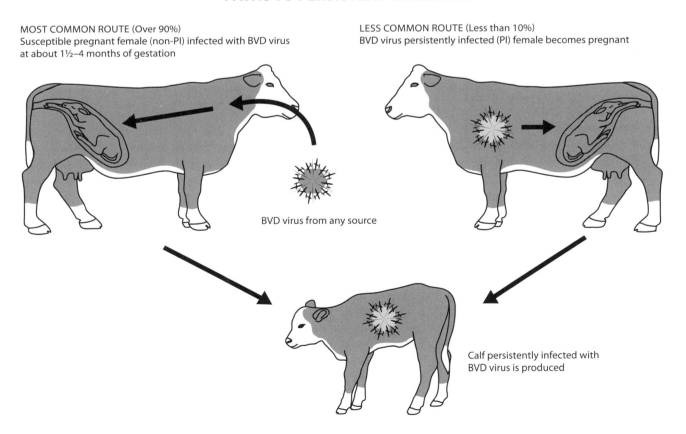

MOST COMMON ROUTE (Over 90%)
Susceptible pregnant female (non-PI) infected with BVD virus at about 1½–4 months of gestation

LESS COMMON ROUTE (Less than 10%)
BVD virus persistently infected (PI) female becomes pregnant

BVD virus from any source

Calf persistently infected with BVD virus is produced

PI cattle are also at risk for other diseases because the BVD virus in their bodies hinders the immune system. PI calves have a higher incidence of scours and pneumonia and a higher *mortality rate*. They may be unthrifty (fail to grow) and not gain weight well. PI heifers may not be selected by stockmen as replacements just because they don't grow as well as other calves.

Birth Defects

BVD infection at any stage of gestation may retard fetal growth, resulting in low birth weight and poor bone growth. Infection between 50 and 150 days (in the second trimester) may result in birth defects rather than fetal death. Lung development may be incomplete. Skeletal defects may include a short jaw or fused joints. Sometimes an infected calf will have no hair, less than the normal amount of hair, or curly hair.

When the fetus is between 100 and 150 days old, the nervous system is in the final stages of development. Defects of infected fetuses involving the nervous system include inadequate brain development (calves may have trouble standing up), water on the brain, and other brain problems. Congenital defects involving the eyes include cataracts, opaque cornea, inflammation of the optic nerve, atrophy or abnormality of the retina, and varying degrees of blindness in the newborn calf.

BVD Diagnosis and Testing

To determine if your herd has a BVD problem or is at risk for problems, look at current pregnancy rates and death loss and whether you've added new animals that might have brought BVD to your farm. Testing can be done to find and remove any PI animals before the next breeding season so that no females will be exposed during breeding and pregnancy. That way, you will eliminate the risk of having any PI calves born in your herd.

PI animals are created before birth, when the dam encounters BVD between 40 and 125 days of gestation. Once a calf is PI, it will always be infected. If a calf is not PI at birth, it can never become PI (once an animal has tested negative for BVD, it never needs to be tested again for PI status). The key to eliminating PI animals is to protect your cows from BVD during pregnancy, so no fetuses become exposed.

Cattle can be tested; if BVD virus is present, it can often be isolated from a blood sample or from tissues of an aborted fetus or an infected weak or unthrifty calf. You might test a cow because she aborted or gave birth to a weak or abnormal calf. To screen the herd, most testing programs focus first on finding any PI calves in the new calf crop before the next breeding season; an infected calf can spread the virus to a pregnant cow. If a calf is found to be PI, his dam can be checked, too.

Take an Ear-Notch Sample for Testing

A small skin sample can be checked for the presence of BVD. Since PI cattle have high levels of virus in their bodies, it can be readily detected. Your vet can collect the ear notches if you wish, but they are easy to collect if you follow the steps on the next page.

1. Fully restrain the animal that is to be tested.

2. Using a medium-sized pig-ear notcher or large-diameter hole punch, take a ¼-inch (0.6 cm) to ½-inch (1.2 cm) square piece, about the size of a pencil eraser, from the lower edge or the outermost tip of the ear. Rinse the ear-notch tool in disinfectant after notching, and rinse again in clean water before taking a notch from the next animal. If notching many animals, alternate the use of 2 ear-notchers, leaving one in the disinfectant while you use the other.

3. Place the sample in a labeled container — a sandwich bag or, as is the preference of some labs, in a labeled blood vial.

4. Samples must be kept cool but don't need to be frozen while awaiting testing.

5. Send the samples to a diagnostic lab by express or overnight mail with a cool pack inserted in the package.

Any animal that tests positive should be checked again in four weeks to see if he had an acute infection or is persistently infected. The virus level will be dropping by the second test if the animal had an acute infection, but the virus level will remain high if the animal is PI. Cull all PI animals.

In the first year of testing, all calves, heifers, and bulls (and any cow that may have lost a calf) should be tested before breeding season. If tissue samples are

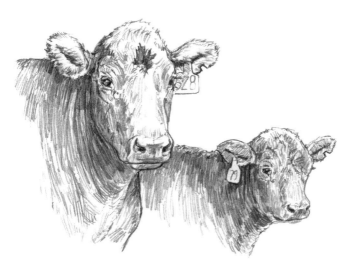

One type of BVD test uses an ear-notch skin sample to detect the disease.

Preventing Introduction of BVD to Herd

Any cattle coming to your farm or added to your herd (even home-raised heifers) should be tested to see if they are PI and isolated from the breeding herd until test results are received. Then you'll know if you can safely add them or should cull them. One of the main ways BVD is introduced or perpetuated on farms is through the introduction of new animals. Don't bring in extra calves to graft on cows that lost their calves, or purchase bulls, cows, heifers, or pairs without testing them. Introducing new animals always carries a risk of transmitting BVD to susceptible animals. PI cattle can be hard to recognize because they rarely show visible signs, yet they continually infect other animals.

Any cow or heifer that conceived a calf somewhere else (bred on the range or communal pasture or purchased as a bred animal) should be isolated until her calf is born and tested. Purchased pregnant animals can be PI negative themselves and still carry a PI fetus infected during pregnancy; the dam may have recovered from the infection that affected her fetus and will test negative. But once her calf is born, he can expose your cattle to BVD.

Avoid communal pastures or fenceline contact with other cattle, especially during the time of year when your cows are in early to mid-pregnancy. Make sure your cows and heifers are adequately vaccinated to provide a high level of protection in case they become exposed to BVD during pregnancy.

taken from suckling calves before cows are rebred, you can then test the dam of any calf that tests positive (if a calf tests negative, the dam is ok). All PI calves and their dams can be removed from the herd before they come in contact with any pregnant animals, thus eliminating risk of passing the virus to a fetus. If you can keep BVD from reaching a fetus, there will be no more PI calves produced. In subsequent years, only the young calves in a herd and any newly purchased animals need to be tested. An individual only needs to be tested once; if he's PI-negative he will never become PI.

In addition to testing live animals, it pays to perform necropsies on any stillborn calves, aborted fetuses, and calves that die of scours, pneumonia, or any other cause. If a calf is PI, this means the dam was infected. The best way to eliminate BVD is to check all animals in the herd at the beginning of an eradication program, cull any shown to be PI, and then keep the herd on a good vaccination program. No new animals should be added unless they are free of BVD.

Vaccination for BVD

There are several killed and modified live-virus vaccines containing various strains and concentrations of BVD virus. Health programs utilizing vaccination of the cow herd are aimed at preventing infection of the fetus, but this goal is more difficult to achieve than just protecting an animal against acute BVD infection. Calfhood vaccination (if properly boostered to stimulate adequate immunity, then boostered annually with modified live vaccine) will usually protect the animal himself from BVD unless he was born persistently infected.

It's harder to obtain 100 percent protection for the fetus if the dam is exposed to BVD. The cow may have enough immunity from previous vaccination (or earlier exposure to the disease) so she won't get sick, but the virus can still occasionally infect the fetus. If a cow is exposed to the BVD virus in early pregnancy, the damage is done. Annual fall vaccination of pregnant cows with killed vaccine will not correct the problem that's already occurred. The best protection against BVD is to eliminate all sources of infection within a herd, keep up a regular vaccination program using modified live-virus vaccine ahead of breeding or an oil-based killed-virus vaccine (so cows have the strongest possible protection in early pregnancy), and never let cattle become exposed to infected animals.

In a herd that has already experienced BVD, starting a vaccination program may not show immediate results unless you also test for and eliminate PI cows. They can't produce an immune response to vaccination and will continue to carry the virus. Without testing, it may take three years of vaccinating and culling (removing cows that are late breeders or produce unthrifty calves) to rid a herd of BVD.

> ## Vaccination Boosts Overall Herd Health
>
> An added benefit to vaccination and keeping a herd free of BVD, with no PI calves produced, is stronger immunity to other diseases, since BVD hinders an animal's ability to mount immune defenses. If an animal is PI, she cannot develop immunity. PI calves usually die from something before they grow up. If you test your cattle and find any PI animals, most veterinarians recommend that they be destroyed.

Live or Killed Vaccine?

A modified live-virus (MLV) vaccine contains the virus itself, but it has been altered so it won't cause disease. It retains some of its original characteristics, however, so the animal's body will recognize it and mount a strong immune defense, just as it would if confronted with the actual disease. Because of this, the MLV produces a stronger and longer-lasting immunity than aluminum hydroxide–based killed vaccine. The oil-based killed vaccines stimulate excellent results, however, and produce better vaccine titers than either the modified live or other killed vaccines. They are slower to be absorbed, safer than the MLV vaccine, and give an animal time to mount a strong immunity.

In many herds, an annual booster (after the initial series of shots in a young animal) with MLV vaccine is enough to keep cows protected. Because MLV vaccine is so potent, however, there's a risk that giving it to a pregnant cow may infect her fetus, unless you are vaccinating her during the last trimester. You have to be sure of the cow's stage of pregnancy to be safe with this vaccine, and do it only on the advice of your vet because this is off-label use (see chapter 2). There's no reason to use it in pregnant cows now, however, since today there are better killed-virus vaccines (oil based) that are just as effective.

There's also the risk that a vaccinated calf that's still nursing his dam (as when vaccinated preweaning) might pass the virus to the cow and infect her fetus. Label directions state that MLV vaccines should be given only to nonpregnant animals and to calves not nursing their dams. MLV vaccines are commonly given to young animals and once a year to the cow herd after calving and before rebreeding — preferably 3 weeks or longer before breeding, to ensure full immunity before pregnancy begins. MLV vaccine given at the time of breeding or soon after (to cows with no prior immunity) may result in embryo death. And there is an occasional cow vaccinated with modified live-virus vaccine before breeding that carries the virus in her ovarian tissue for 60 to 90 days, hindering her ability to become pregnant.

By contrast, a killed vaccine will not reproduce itself in body tissues. There's no chance for it to cause disease in pregnant cows or calves that are nursing pregnant dams. But it doesn't give protection that's as strong or as long lasting unless it's oil based. Most vets recommend giving it twice a year to cows, and calfhood vaccinations also require more boosters. Killed vaccines require two doses at least two weeks apart to confer immunity.

Some ranchers and veterinarians feel the most protection can be obtained by giving MLV vaccines to cows after calving (before rebreeding) and using a killed vaccine in the fall on pregnant cows as a booster. This gives more immunity through winter and better levels of antibodies in colostrum at the next calving.

Calfhood Vaccination for IBR and BVD

Many stockmen vaccinate calves preweaning to develop immunity before calves are stressed and more vulnerable to disease. Killed vaccine is generally used preweaning so dams are not at risk, even though the IBR portion of the vaccine doesn't give calves as much or as long-lasting protection as the BVD portion and must be boostered. While working with their vets on a total herd health program, some stockmen have found that if the herd has strong immunity with annual vaccinations kept up to date there's little risk of cows developing a reaction to calves' vaccinations. These ranchers, on the advice of their veterinarian (because it's not recommended on the label), use MLV vaccine in preweaning programs for calves and have no need for an additional booster.

If cows were vaccinated with MLV vaccine the previous spring before breeding, it's usually safe to vaccinate their calves with MLV vaccine before weaning. If the immune status of the herd is in question, however, MLV vaccine should not be given to calves until after weaning. Discuss this with your vet.

The combination IBR-BVD vaccines generally give calves good protection against BVD but may be inadequate to protect against IBR. There are still latent carriers, and neither the modified live-virus nor killed products can solve that problem.

The best protection against BVD for young heifers or bulls going into the herd is three vaccinations (preferably MLV vaccines or oil-based killed products) before breeding age. The first injection can be given at 1 to 2 months of age before the dam is bred again, the second at weaning age, and another just before the animal's first breeding season. This gives a heifer the strongest protection against becoming infected in early pregnancy. After that, annual MLV vaccination prebreeding is usually adequate for the rest of her life.

BVD Can Cause Other Disease Outbreaks

Since BVD suppresses the immune system, infected cattle have a higher incidence of sickness. Pregnant cows may abort from lepto, IBR, and other diseases simply because they couldn't develop immunity. A herd health program may not be effective because cattle with BVD don't respond to vaccination. Even if you vaccinate against common diseases, BVD cattle may still get those diseases. You may think the vaccine was bad, but in reality the animal was unable to respond.

If you have problems with calf scours and respiratory disease, BVD may be part of the problem. In one study BVD was the virus most often found in the lungs of older calves with pneumonia, often in conjunction with *Pasteurella*. The BVD virus is associated with outbreaks of respiratory disease and can impair the ability of calves to fight lung infections caused by IBR. Many vaccines combine IBR and BVD to give protection against both.

A 1992 study showed that use of killed IBR-BVD vaccine given at 1 to 3 months of age resulted in a strong immunity to BVD when boostered just before weaning. The first dose of a killed vaccine gives little protection, but boostering with an oil-based vaccine 30 days later stimulates the calf to build immunity. Some stockmen and vets who adopted this program began using MLV vaccine, instead of killed vaccine, for young calves whose dams were not yet pregnant (vaccinating calves at the same time that the cows were being vaccinated prebreeding) and found an added benefit. They discovered that calves developed immunity after only one dose and had less calfhood illness from all causes (including scours, pinkeye, diphtheria, pneumonia, and ruptured stomachs from abomasal ulcers).

If calves are not vaccinated until after bulls have been put with the cows, killed vaccine is safer, but water-based or aluminum hydroxide adjuvants (immune-system stimulants) won't give calves protection until they receive a booster at or before weaning. (Some protection is achieved with one shot, using an oil-based killed product.) Even if you use MLV vaccine in young calves, a booster at weaning time is essential, since the immunity gained by the young calf may last only a few months.

Bluetongue

Bluetongue is spread by bloodsucking insects — most often, a specific type of gnat called *Culicoides variipennis*. In climates with cold winters, cattle are the main *reservoir* for the virus during months when insects are not active. Gnats become infected while feeding on infected cattle, then transfer the disease to other cattle or sheep as they fly from animal to animal to suck blood. Bluetongue can also be transmitted through infected semen and spread by bloodsucking lice or certain types of soft tick. There may be mechanical spread of the disease, with the virus merely "riding" on biting flies and hypodermic needles used on multiple animals. There are at least 25 strains of the virus, but only 6 have been identified in the United States. Bluetongue is usually seen from mid-summer until first frost, but in areas with mild winters, where gnats are active year-round, the disease can appear at any time.

A blood sample taken from a newborn calf before he nurses can determine if the calf was affected in utero. Many countries, including Canada, require a negative blood test for bluetongue before allowing an animal to enter the country, and some require a quarantine period in conjunction with the test to be sure an animal isn't developing the disease. Some countries won't allow animals to enter from regions or countries where bluetongue has been diagnosed, even if the animal has a negative test, since a few animals that carry the virus may still test negative.

Bluetongue is more serious in sheep than in cattle, and there is controversy regarding the extent of its effects on cattle. Some researchers feel it's relatively common, while others feel it's rarely a problem. There are three ways bluetongue can affect cattle: it can interfere with reproduction, cause birth defects, and infect them for life.

Reproductive effects include abortion, infertility, mummification of the fetus, and birth of a full-term dead calf.

Congenital defects occur if the virus damages but doesn't kill the fetus. The fetus is most vulnerable to these effects if the virus is encountered at 60 to 140 days of gestation, resulting in weak or *dummy calves* (calves that are lethargic and "retarded" at birth) or calves with deformed legs and feet, blindness, white eyes, an *overshot* lower jaw (protruding farther than the upper jaw), or a persistent gum covering over the front teeth.

Persistently infected cattle were previously infected with one strain of the virus (which can occur before birth when the fetus is past 140 days gestation) but show no evidence of disease until reinfected with the same or another strain. The resulting illness may be moderately to extremely serious.

Symptoms
Ulcers may appear in the mouth, nose, *trachea,* esophagus, or rumen. The animal may be lame with muscle stiffness, laminitis, hoof cracks, or coronary band inflammation. Capillaries are affected, resulting in a loss of blood supply to tissues; the hoof horn may *slough off.* Skin inflammation, hair loss, sloughing skin, oozing crusts on skin or muzzle, or ulcers on udder or teats may occur. The sick

animal may have fast, shallow respiration, excessive salivation (drooling long, stringy strands), and a swollen, protruding tongue that is bluish from lack of oxygen in the tissues. Fever may be as high as 106°F (41.1°C).

Treatment and Prevention

Good nursing care that includes shelter and good feed, if the animal will eat, and washing affected areas with a mild disinfectant solution recommended by your vet may provide some relief from discomfort, but there is no effective treatment to halt the virus.

There is a vaccine available for sheep but not for cattle. Some of the difficulties in creating a safe vaccine may be overcome in the future with the use of DNA vaccines, in which a segment of viral DNA is inserted into something else, such as a bacterial plasmid, to stimulate immunity to the virus.

Draining stagnant ponds and standing water, use of insecticides, and periodic spraying of animals are all techniques for managing disease-carrying gnats. Some ranchers house cattle in the early morning and evening, when gnats are most active.

Never use the same hypodermic needle on multiple animals in regions where bluetongue exists, and be sure to thoroughly clean and disinfect equipment between animals when castrating, dehorning, or tagging to avoid blood contact.

Bovine Leukemia

This disease is also called bovine *lymphosarcoma* and *bovine leukosis* and can be a viral-induced form of cancer (see chapter 19). Infection may occur before birth or via colostrum if the dam is infected, but it usually doesn't show up in young calves. The disease generally does not become apparent until months or years later. In affected animals it is eventually fatal. Some family lines seem more susceptible, and the disease is more common in dairy cattle than beef breeds. The white blood cell count may show evidence of disease before an animal shows symptoms. A high white count with many immature cells is typical of leukemia.

Once infected, the animal produces an antibody response and has antibodies present in the blood for

> **HUMAN INFLUENCE**
>
> Bovine leukemia can be transferred from one animal to another by infected blood. It also can be spread by human handling when surgical instruments, hypodermic needles, or dehorning tools are not disinfected between animals.

the rest of his life, showing that he has been exposed. Not all exposed animals develop persistent *lymphocytosis* (an excess number of lymphocytes in the blood) or lymphosarcoma (cancer).

Symptoms

Lumps under the skin are an indication of enlarged lymph nodes caused by this disease. Internal swollen nodes can't be seen, but in the chest or abdomen they may interfere with lung or digestive function and mimic other diseases. Enlarged nodes may be discovered by accident during exploratory surgery or by rectal palpation. Symptoms vary depending on which body system is affected by the nodes. Often, the only sign is unexplained weight loss or a decline in milk production. Occasionally, young calves are affected and have various enlarged lymph nodes, infiltration of the bone marrow by certain types of white blood cells, and anemia.

Prevention

There's no treatment for bovine leukemia, but a blood test can reveal antibodies, showing the animal encountered the virus at some point. Survey tests have shown that about 20 percent of dairy cows in the United States (and fewer beef cattle) have been exposed, but prevalence of the actual disease occurs in less than 1 percent. With blood testing, some European countries tried to eliminate the disease with test-and-slaughter programs, but prevention in individual herds is difficult. An animal with obvious signs should be culled. Blood tests and blood counts can identify animals that might be in early stages; this provides a tool for culling and for checking prospective replacement animals.

Because the disease can be passed from one animal to another via infected blood, it may be spread by biting flies that feed on multiple animals. Control of horseflies may reduce the incidence of transmission. Surgical instruments, dehorners, ear-tattoo pliers, castrating tools, and hypodermic needles may spread the virus from one animal to another. All tools should be disinfected between animals. Studies have shown that infection can be reduced from 80 percent to 4 percent in dairy heifers being dehorned just by altering dehorning methods. The virus can also be transmitted by rectal examination of cattle, especially in dairy herds if the same obstetrical sleeve is used when palpating multiple cows. Changing sleeves between animals or using a blood test rather than palpation to check for pregnancy may limit the spread of this disease.

Rabies

Rabies is a viral infection of the central nervous system and is always fatal in livestock. It occurs in all warm-blooded animals, including humans and cattle, and is transmitted by the bites of infected animals or by contact with their saliva on broken skin or mucous membranes. In a rabid animal the virus may be present in saliva before symptoms appear; the animal may be infective for up to five days before signs of rabies become evident.

Cattle are not a common source of infection for other animals. They rarely bite even if they have rabies, but can still transmit the disease to humans. If you examine the mouth of a sick cow or calf and get saliva in a break in your skin, the virus can gain entrance to your body. Anyone who handles the sick animal is at risk, whether or not the animal bites. Wear protective clothing and gloves when handling a suspect animal. Use household bleach to disinfect any equipment or instruments that come in contact with the animal's saliva.

Rabies virus is fairly fragile. It dies in dry saliva within a few hours and is easily killed by disinfectants. But if it enters the body through a wound or break in the skin, it starts attacking the nerves. Unlike other viruses that travel through blood, the rabies virus starts multiplying at the site of the bite or broken skin and begins traveling along nerve networks, eventually reaching the brain. It reaches the salivary glands via cranial nerves and is transmitted to other victims via the saliva.

Symptoms

The incubation period (the period between when the victim is bitten and when disease signs appear) is variable, depending on the location of the bite, the amount of the virus in the saliva, how long it takes the virus to reach the brain and spinal cord, and the susceptibility (immune status) of the bitten animal. A cow bitten on a hind leg may not show symptoms as quickly as a cow bitten on the nose, for instance. But once signs appear, the disease is always fatal.

The incubation period for cattle is between 3 and 15 weeks. When the virus enters the spinal cord and brain, it creates encephalitis (brain inflammation) or *meningitis* (inflammation of the protective membrane around the brain) and destroys nerve cells. One of the first and most common signs is difficulty swallowing. Other signs include fever, blindness, depression, abdominal pain, seizures, and behavior changes. The cow may try to eat, taking food into her mouth, but can't chew or swallow it. She may try to drink but can't. Because she's unable to swallow, saliva may drool from the mouth.

Inability to swallow is often misdiagnosed as choking; every year humans are exposed to rabies as the animal's owner or vet examines the mouth and throat or tries to reach down the throat to find

---

Stages of Rabies

Rabies has three phases of progression, but you may observe only one or two.

- **Stage one** lasts one to three days: the animal has a change in behavior. An aggressive animal may become friendly, and a wild one may lose his fear of humans.

- **Stage two** brings on the excitability often referred to as "furious" rabies. The animal is easily agitated and bites at anything that comes near, and the muscles that control swallowing are paralyzed.

- **Stage three**, the final phase, involves loss of muscle control, eventual coma, and death.

a suspected obstruction. Diagnosis of rabies is one of the most difficult yet important duties of a vet because there is the possibility of human exposure, especially with cattle, since rabies is usually the last thing you expect. You may spend time and effort working with the sick animal. Symptoms of rabies also can be mistaken for an injury to the head, poisoning, or other conditions that affect the nervous system.

In cattle, rabies may show a variety of symptoms, lumped into two categories — *dumb rabies* and *furious rabies* — with some cases falling in between.

▶ **In the dumb rabies (paralytic) form,** the *brain stem* is affected. The animal is lethargic and depressed and may look dazed, hang her head, and drool. Temperature, pulse, and respiration are normal. There's no sign of pain or shock. Mucous membranes are normal. The animal is usually uncoordinated, with hind legs knuckling under at the fetlock joints and hindquarters sagging and swaying if she tries to walk. She becomes less and less coordinated and eventually is paralyzed and unable to get up.

▶ **In the furious rabies form,** the *cerebrum* (the front part of the brain) is affected, and the animal becomes aggressive, tense and alert, and more sensitive and attracted to movement and sound. She may pace around, run wildly, or charge at anything that moves. This acute change in personality may be the first apparent symptom.

There's no set pattern in the development of symptoms. Gradual hindquarter paralysis in dumb rabies may be followed by excitement and convulsions. Death is usually caused by respiratory paralysis; muscles needed for breathing no longer function. Not all animals with rabies have esophageal paralysis, however. Some continue to eat, and may try to eat strange things like wood or rocks. Pulse, temperature, and respiration may be normal and then rise as the animal becomes more frenzied. Muscle tremors, staggering, and uncontrolled violent actions are characteristic of rabies. Some cases run a course of 6 to 7 days while in others the animal dies within 36 to 48 hours. In the final stages the animal becomes paralyzed and goes into convulsions.

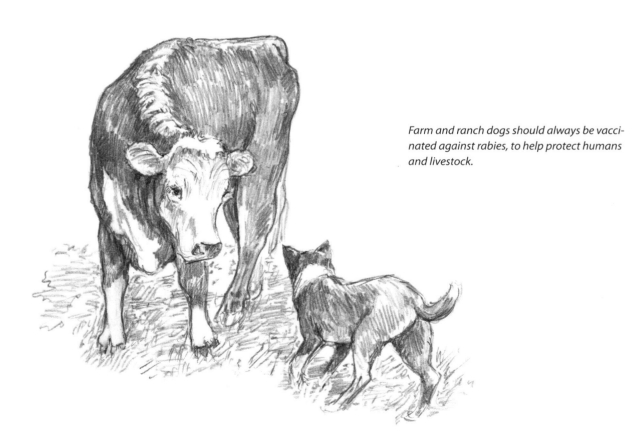

Farm and ranch dogs should always be vaccinated against rabies, to help protect humans and livestock.

Diagnosis

Rabid cattle don't always have aggressive behavior or excessive salivation. Furious rabies occurs in about 50 percent of cases involving dogs, raccoons, and foxes; 75 percent of cat and skunk cases; and 66 percent of horses cases — but only 25 percent of cattle. A cow sick with rabies is more apt to be dull and have muscle tremors, lack of coordination, and paralysis of the hindquarters.

If you see an animal acting abnormally, keep the possibility of rabies in the back of your mind. Know your cattle. If any are out of character or there's something different that you can't quite put a finger on, be suspicious. Remember: Uncommon presentations of common diseases are more common than common presentations of uncommon diseases. Rabies in cattle can have many faces. The fact that rabies can be mistaken for other problems is what makes it so dangerous; the veterinarian or stockman may not suspect it soon enough to prevent human exposure.

Rabies can be tentatively diagnosed by examining the animal and his history of symptoms, but positive diagnosis can be made only by tests on the brain after the animal dies, to confirm the presence of the virus. It is not detectable in blood, saliva, or urine — only in brain tissue. If a cow is suspected of having rabies, she should be euthanized and the brain removed by a vet and submitted to a diagnostic lab. Make sure the brain is not damaged. If the animal must be shot, don't shoot her in the head.

Prevention

There's no treatment. Once symptoms begin it's always fatal. Because of the long incubation period, humans and animals can be vaccinated after exposure. If vaccination is started soon enough, the body builds immunity in time to prevent fatal brain inflammation. Humans are treated with multiple injections of vaccine over a 28-day period. But with animals you rarely know when they're exposed. It's safer to give them annual vaccinations in areas where rabies is a problem. Cats and dogs should always be vaccinated, since they pose the most risk to humans. Horses and cattle can also be vaccinated, with an annual booster. Vaccine is usually adequate protection, but any animal bitten by a rabid animal should receive a booster shot immediately and be quarantined for 90 days. An unvaccinated animal is more at risk. Postexposure vaccination is routine in humans, but public health officials often recommend immediate euthanasia (killing the animal and destroying the carcass) or slaughter of animals.

You may not know if a cow has been exposed to rabies. The bite of a raccoon, fox, skunk, squirrel, or bat is often small and unnoticed. It heals, leaving no clue until the cow starts showing symptoms. Cattle are curious if a small animal staggers through the pasture, barnyard, or barn. They usually try to smell it and may be bitten on the nose. Even if they don't approach the rabid animal, it may attack and bite them since rabid animals have no fear during the aggressive phase of the disease.

Incidence of rabies in wildlife increases and decreases in cycles, with a corresponding increase of the disease in domestic animals due to bites by rabid wild animals. Your cattle are at risk if you live in a region where rabies occurs in wildlife. Consult your vet about vaccination. There are several types of rabies vaccine, but not all are safe for cattle.

Viral Diarrhea in Calves

Two groups of viruses, rotavirus and coronavirus, cause diarrhea in young calves. Rotavirus affects calves less than a week old (sometimes as young as 1 to 3 days) while coronavirus affects calves more than a week old. Most of the serious cases are in calves that have concurrent bacterial infections, creating severe and life-threatening diarrhea. These viruses by themselves are not nearly as dangerous as the combination. Spread of the virus is via contamination, as when a newborn calf nurses a dirty udder; the virus is present in feces of carrier cows.

Treatment and Prevention

There's no effective treatment for viral scours except supportive therapy: reducing stress and keeping the calf well hydrated with fluids administered either orally or by IV if the gut is compromised by infection and dehydration. Antibiotics are usually given, however, to combat secondary bacterial infection, as it's the combination of viral and bacterial infection that generally kills a calf.

The best way to prevent viral scours is by maintaining a clean environment for calving cows and newborn calves. If your herd does not already have these diseases, don't bring in new animals that might harbor them. If your herd has problems with viral scours, vaccinate cows several weeks ahead of calving so that their colostrum contains high levels of antibodies. To gain the protection, the calf must nurse the colostrum immediately after birth before he ingests pathogens. It's important to make sure that the calving area and the cow's udders are very clean and the calf is up and nursing within an hour of birth.

There is also an oral vaccine that can be given to calves if cows were not vaccinated ahead of time, but it must be given to calves immediately after birth, before they encounter viruses in their environment. Consult your veterinarian for advice on vaccine products and how best to protect calves in your particular situation.

For a broad examination of the topic of viral diarrhea in calves, refer to *Essential Guide to Calving* (Storey 2008), the companion volume to this book.

How Rotavirus and Coronavirus Do Their Damage

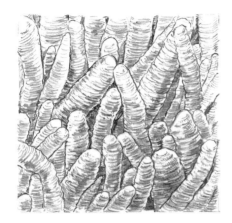

A. Normal villi (threadlike projections covering the surface of the intestinal lining) absorb fluid and nutrients.

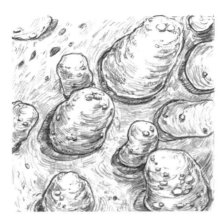

B. Damaged, denuded villi infected by rotavirus result in diarrhea.

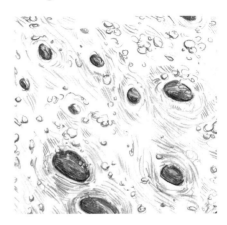

C. Coronavirus infection completely destroys the villi.

CHAPTER SIX

Protozoal Diseases

PROTOZOA ARE ONE-CELLED ANIMALS. There are many kinds, and most are harmless, but there are several cattle diseases caused by pathogenic varieties. Texas cattle fever, caused by protozoa in the bloodstream and spread to cattle by ticks, was a serious problem in the Southeastern United States before an extensive eradication program began in 1906 to rid the region of the tick that transmits the disease. Although another one-celled invader, trichomoniasis, is a sexually transmitted reproductive disease caused by protozoa in the reproductive tract, most bovine protozoal diseases are transmitted via the fecal-oral route. The troublesome organism is shed in feces of infected or carrier animals and picked up by a susceptible animal ingesting contaminated feed or water.

Two common diseases, coccidiosis and *cryptosporidiosis,* occur most often in calves, causing severe diarrhea. Some protozoal diseases require two hosts to complete their life cycles and reproduce, such as a canine and a grazer in a predator-prey relationship. *Neosporosis* and *sarcocystosis* are examples of organisms that require a two-host life cycle.

Coccidiosis

There are many types of coccidia protozoa. Some affect birds, and some affect various mammals. All cattle are infected to some degree by *coccidia* that live in their intestines, and the protozoal infection occurs in almost every herd, often without any signs. There are at least 15 kinds that live in cattle, but only 2 are pathogenic. These may give calves severe diarrhea (coccidiosis) any time in the period between 3 weeks and 1 year of age. Immunity developed against one type of coccidia does not protect against another, so a calf can suffer from more than one bout.

By the time calves reach 6 months of age, most have been exposed and harbor coccidia in their intestines, though only 2 to 5 percent of calves show actual signs of disease. Constant low-level exposure enables a calf to build immunity, but calves with little or no immunity that are exposed to high levels of coccidia or are stressed will break with diarrhea. Adult cattle have immunity and are rarely affected by coccidia unless they become so stressed the immune system is hindered. Even though adults don't usually get sick, they continue to pass a few parasite eggs *(oocysts)* in manure, serving as a continual source of infection for calves.

STRESS INHIBITS THE IMMUNE SYSTEM

Drought, cold or wet weather, weaning, and transport inhibit the immune system and allow protozoa to divide more rapidly and move through more life cycles before a calf can begin to resist the parasite. This allows for more damage to the gut lining, which subsequently takes longer to heal.

Most calves haven't gained enough immunity to fight effects of the protozoa if they ingest a high concentration, as is sometimes the case when environmental conditions are right for picking up large numbers of oocysts. If calves lie in manure and then lick themselves, or nurse a dirty udder, or eat hay contaminated with manure, they are at risk.

Coccidiosis causes diarrhea, weight loss, and lowered resistance to other diseases. It can sometimes be fatal in young calves or weanlings with no immunity. In baby calves, damaged intestinal tissues are susceptible to bacterial and viral infections. There is often more than one pathogen involved when they have diarrhea, which can make it much worse.

The parasite is found in all healthy cattle, causing illness only when animals are stressed or have overwhelming numbers of protozoa. Growth rate through 2 years of age can be affected, even if cattle are not showing symptoms. Visible illness may occur only when cattle are confined in small areas, allowing the small number of oocysts passed in manure to build to infective levels.

In an outbreak, most animals in a group become infected, but only a few show signs of disease. In a serious outbreak, however, up to 80 percent may be sick, and the mortality rate can be as high as 10 to 15 percent unless calves are all treated in early stages. In the calves that don't show symptoms, subclinical infection may slow their growth until their intestines are fully healed.

Serious outbreaks often occur when warm weather brings to life the dormant oocysts in old manure around feeding areas where cattle are congregated or when calves are put into contaminated weaning pens. Many outbreaks occur during the first 30 days after calves are placed in weaning areas or feed yards, especially if wet conditions stimulate development of oocysts shed in manure.

Coccidia enter a susceptible animal with contaminated feed or water or when grazing a wet, contaminated pasture or licking a hair coat covered with manure. The protozoa destroy the gut lining while releasing millions of oocysts, which pass out with manure to further contaminate feed, water, and bedding and begin the cycle again.

COCCIDIA LIFE CYCLE (21–28 DAYS)

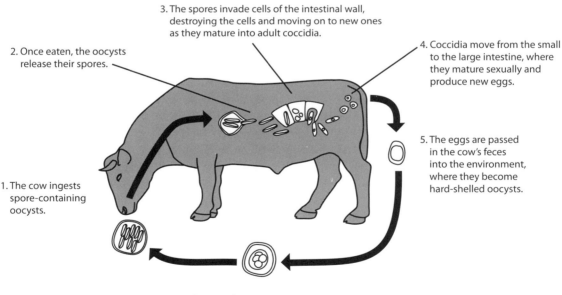

3. The spores invade cells of the intestinal wall, destroying the cells and moving on to new ones as they mature into adult coccidia.

2. Once eaten, the oocysts release their spores.

4. Coccidia move from the small to the large intestine, where they mature sexually and produce new eggs.

5. The eggs are passed in the cow's feces into the environment, where they become hard-shelled oocysts.

1. The cow ingests spore-containing oocysts.

6. The coccidia oocysts survive in feces, pasture, and feed.

Incubation

Incubation for coccidiosis begins when the calf ingests oocysts and lasts until he breaks with diarrhea — approximately 16 days or longer. While coccidia are still in the small intestine, the calf looks normal. On about day 16, protozoa move into the large intestine, where they produce male and female cells to create and fertilize more oocysts. When these develop and mature, they rupture through the intestinal cell lining. By day 18 or 19 the calf has diarrhea, and there may be blood in the feces. By day 21 there are oocysts passing out with the manure.

Protozoal Living Conditions

These protozoa build up wherever cattle are congregated: in corrals, feeding grounds, calving areas, or an intensive pasture-rotation system. Oocysts can survive on the ground from one year to the next. They just need warmth, moisture, and oxygen to become infective. Infection is common when cattle are fed on the ground, with fecal contamination of feed. Outbreaks can occur when cattle gather at water sources, hay feeding areas, and mineral boxes.

Oocysts passed in manure need moisture and mild temperatures (53 to 90°F [11.7 to 32.2°C]) to *sporulate* (reproduce). Heat and dryness impede them. They can survive freezing (down to 18°F [–7.8°C]) for a couple of months, but temperatures below minus 22°F (–30°C) usually kill them. Oocysts can sporulate in the winter on the hair of cattle dirty with manure even if it's too cold for sporulation on the ground. When cattle lick themselves or each other, they ingest protozoa.

Large numbers of sporulated oocysts must be ingested, however, before signs of coccidiosis appear. This can happen with continual reinfection and buildup of contamination in the environment, as when calves are confined or crowded or there are a lot of cattle on irrigated pasture. Calves brought into weaning pens from large pastures may carry only a few oocysts, which build up to large numbers in the small area, especially if conditions are moist.

Some farms have problems in young calves if cattle are in the same fields, pastures, or pens at calving time each year and when weather is wet there. Other farms have problems in older calves or at weaning or in groups of replacement heifers during winter.

Sometimes a late-born calf doesn't encounter many coccidia and builds no immunity, so that in the fall, when exposed to contaminated conditions, he gets coccidiosis. Early calves that picked up a few oocysts in the spring may not have developed diarrhea but still serve as a source for the later calves (who have less immunity) at weaning or on winter pasture if they are gathered together.

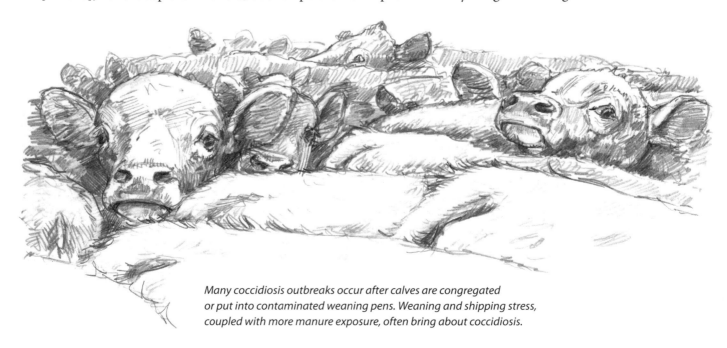

Many coccidiosis outbreaks occur after calves are congregated or put into contaminated weaning pens. Weaning and shipping stress, coupled with more manure exposure, often bring about coccidiosis.

Coccidia Are Prolific!

In the gut, an oocyst hatches into eight sporozoites. Each of these invades a cell in the intestinal lining, destroying the cell as it forms a packet of new oocysts that then ruptures to release more than 100,000 new oocysts. Theoretically each oocyst can eventually develop into 28 million new organisms. Ingestion of about 125 sporulated oocysts could cause destruction of more than 12 billion cells as they hatch and multiply, interfering with digestion and absorption of food and causing bloody diarrhea.

To understand what a calf faces, imagine the microscopic oocyst as the size of a BB. At this size, multiplication from one oocyst in a 28-day reproductive cycle in a calf's intestine would produce enough new oocysts to fill the back of a pickup truck. If all of those riding in the pickup reproduced, in one more month they would cover 160 acres of land — 250 feet deep! This massive proliferation rate enables coccidia to exist anywhere there's cattle manure in pens and pastures.

A cow passes about 50 million oocysts each summer, some of which may be ingested by calves. Light infection causes no signs of disease, and the calf builds immunity. Moderate infection causes diarrhea; then the calf starts building immunity. Ingesting a large number of oocysts results in serious infection that may kill a calf unless you give him intensive care.

Symptoms

Coccidiosis causes diarrhea, bloody feces, anemia, and emaciation. The rupture of cells in the intestinal lining during swift multiplication of protozoa results in diarrhea. Fever may occur in early stages, but the sign first noticed is the sudden onset of severe diarrhea — foul-smelling, watery, brown feces containing blood or mucus. Blood may be dark and tarry or fresh and red. The calf's rear end, hind legs, and tail are covered with sticky, mucous-streaked feces that become matted around the tail head. If the calf has had coccidiosis for long, he may have dull, rough hair and appear sluggish and unthrifty or potbellied. After the coccidia stop multiplying and the intestinal lining heals, manure firms up, but this may take a while if he is constantly being reinfected.

WATCH FOR STRAINING

Straining to pass a bowel movement is a common sign of coccidiosis. The damaged large intestine and rectum are irritated, and the calf continues to strain after passing watery feces or without passing anything. In severe cases, constant straining results in prolapse of the rectum.

If there's only one life cycle, the disease runs its course soon. But often a calf is reinfected because he's in a contaminated environment. There are generations of protozoa at various stages of life cycle within the gut, until the process has gone on long enough for his immune system to build resistance. A long course of diarrhea may also mean that he has had a concurrent bacterial or viral infection or extensive gut damage that takes a long time to heal.

If the calf has lost a lot of blood, he is weak and staggering, with pale mucous membranes. Most calves go off feed for a while or eat poorly. A baby calf stops nursing his mother. A weanling only picks at his feed. Some calves take a long time to recover, and their growth is stunted because the intestine can't absorb fluid and nutrients. Without good care and supportive treatment, a calf becomes susceptible to other diseases such as pneumonia.

In mild cases there may be diarrhea and poor weight gain but no blood in the manure. Subclinical cases may have poor growth but no diarrhea. Most subclinical cases last just a short time; the digestive tract is irritated, interfering with food absorption for two or three weeks. Then the calf builds immunity and throws off the infection but continues to shed a few oocysts in manure for the rest of his life.

Some cases of acute coccidiosis affect the brain, and the animal shows signs of nervous system damage (muscle tremors, problems in coordination, convulsions) and has a high risk of mortality in spite of treatment. Affected calves may die within 24 hours after the onset of bloody diarrhea and nervous signs, or they may linger for several days in a coma before dying.

Diagnosis

Coccidiosis is not always easy to diagnose even if your vet looks at a fecal sample with a microscope to check for oocysts. Finding oocysts in feces does not always mean the calf has coccidiosis; many normal calves shed a few oocysts, and there are several kinds of coccidia that are not pathogenic. Oocysts may not show up in a fecal sample if you check the manure before the sick calf starts shedding them. If you check the calf's manure again in a few days, there may be some.

A fecal sample must be analyzed in light of an animal's history and symptoms. A single sample from one calf is not always an accurate diagnostic tool. It's more revealing to take samples from several calves in the group. Diagnosis is made more difficult by the fact that there's often more than one pathogen involved. A young calf may have cryptosporidiosis (see page 124) and also be passing a few coccidia, leading to misdiagnosis as coccidiosis.

Preventive Management

There's no vaccine against coccidia, and disinfectants won't kill them. Control depends on cleanliness, avoidance of stress and crowding, and use of a good *coccidiostat* (a drug that suppresses multiplication of the protozoa) in situations where calves are exposed to more than a minimal level of infection.

Cleanliness

Young calves are susceptible because they have not yet developed immunity. Calves or weanlings may develop coccidiosis if hay is fed in the same area all winter or cattle are grouped around big bale feeders. The best way to control coccidiosis is to limit the spread of coccidia in manure by keeping group sizes small, feeding in new, clean areas, and using clean bedding in wet weather so cattle don't get manure on their hair or udders.

If cattle are spread out on pasture and ground-feeding areas and bale feeders are continually moved, oocysts in manure are widely scattered over a larger area, and calves won't pick up enough to cause massive infection. They encounter the protozoa and begin to build immunity but don't ingest enough oocysts to develop disease. Cows are passing small numbers of oocysts, but a young animal with diarrhea will spread thousands. It's better to prevent coccidiosis than to treat it after calves get sick.

Protozoan-Suppressing Drugs

If calves start getting coccidiosis, isolate the sick and move the others to a clean area. If you can't move the herd to clean ground during wet weather, protect calves with a drug such as *Deccox (decoquinate),* or *Corid (amprolium)* that inhibits coccidia. Mix it in the feed (if calves are fed grain) or in the water. If weaned calves drink from a water trough in a corral, for instance, Corid can be added to the water.

Young calves using a calf creep can be fed Deccox in their feed mix. If they're eating 3 to 4 ounces (88.7 to 118.3 mL) of feed daily (and getting their full dose of Deccox) at 3 weeks old, this will prevent coccidiosis until you can move them to clean pasture or spread them out and away from the contamination. Deccox in feed works as a preventive in young calves if you start them on it before they get sick.

Sick calves won't eat enough of the daily dosage to hinder coccidia. Deccox can be used in salt, but the most reliable source of the medicine for young calves is in feed.

Calves stay healthier at weaning if treated for coccidiosis along with their usual vaccinations just prior to the stress of weaning. Studies have proven that calves treated with a coccidiostatic drug before weaning experience less sickness (especially respiratory problems) and suffer fewer deaths. The calves remain healthier, grow better, and have a chance to develop a stronger immune response to vaccinations. Some stockmen who've had problems with coccidiosis in weaned calves use a coccidiostatic drug for a few weeks before weaning, giving the drug in creep feed, and this halts the problem. Like so many illnesses, outbreaks of coccidiosis are stress-related; calves tend to become ill when they are weaned or experience bad weather.

Several feed additives can prevent coccidiosis, but all animals in the group must eat the recommended amount. It's also important to feed the proper amount for age and weight of the animal. Some drugs can be toxic if overfed, and none is effective if underfed. Individuals that don't consume enough should be separated from the group and treated individually.

Treatment

Many stockmen harbor misconceptions about treating coccidiosis. Symptoms subside when the multiplication stage is past, and many treatments are credited with curing it without taking this into account. Drugs commonly used for treatment have little effect on late stages of coccidia. Most drugs just have a depressant effect on early stages of the protozoa and keep them from multiplying.

Even though damage to the gut is already done by the time you see diarrhea, it's still worthwhile to treat the calf. Treatment may shorten the course of an otherwise long, debilitating illness. In most cases, this disease is an ongoing process because all the coccidia are not developed and multiplying at the same time. There may be a few coccidia in the environment; then, as more calves get sick and start shedding ingested oocysts, there are coccidia in each calf's gut in various stages of development.

Silent Robber

Most people don't use a coccidiostatic drug unless calves have symptoms they can see, yet all calves are affected to some degree by coccidia. A study in New Mexico used 1,300 calves in a feeding trial at weaning: half the calves got Deccox in their supplement (fed daily as cubes), and the other calves did not. They were in large grass pastures for 45 days after weaning before being shipped to a feedlot. Weather was ideal for weaning, with mild temperatures and no rain.

There was very little sickness in any of the calves, but at the end of the test when they were weighed, there was an 8-pound (3.6 kg) difference in average weight between the two groups. Feeding a coccidiostat was cost effective in a good year — when they didn't seem to have sickness problems — and even more beneficial in bad years.

Effects of coccidia in groups of weaned calves or yearlings are typically subclinical. A calf may have lower feed efficiency (less weight gained per pound of feed consumed), but you're not aware that there's a problem. Subclinical coccidiosis reduces growth rate and makes cattle more vulnerable to other diseases.

Some of the damage is already done, but you should still treat the calf because of the potential for secondary infection with other pathogens and also to limit the contamination the calf is putting into the environment.

Corid (amprolium), Deccox (decoquinate), monensin, or sulfa will usually halt new life cycles. If a calf has a secondary bacterial infection, sulfa will hinder that, too. Several drugs are effective if given early, before symptoms appear, but are less effective after the calf is already sick. In outbreaks, all the calves in the group should be treated even if they are not all sick. Those that are sick may also need supportive treatment to save them.

Rectal Prolapse

Once a calf has prolapsed his rectum due to constant straining, he will continue to do so, even if you put it back in. If the rectum is prolapsed, take the following steps to return the rectum to its proper position and stitch it in place:

1. Wash the prolapsed tissue with warm water and a mild disinfectant.
2. Apply an anesthetic ointment to the rectal tissue to reduce pain and straining.
3. Gently push the rectum back in.
4. Stitch across the rectal opening with two or three stitches of *umbilical tape* (thick cotton "thread"). Be sure to anchor the stitches in the skin around the rectum, leaving room for feces to pass.
5. Stitches can be removed later after he recovers.

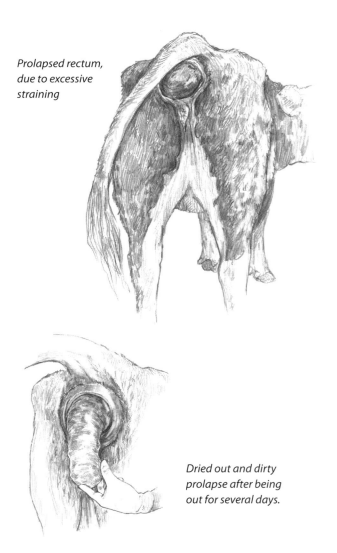

Prolapsed rectum, due to excessive straining

Dried out and dirty prolapse after being out for several days.

Anemia

If a calf has lost a lot of blood, he'll be anemic. Supportive treatment with fluids via stomach tube or IV may be needed to combat dehydration and prevent death. In a severe case you may have to continue feeding the calf via tube for a while if the animal doesn't want to eat. A young calf can be force-fed milk or milk replacer during this recovery period. An older calf with a functional rumen may do better with *propylene glycol* given by stomach tube. This can supply some quick energy and help keep the animal alive until he can eat again.

Cryptosporidiosis

A protozoan found almost everywhere causes cryptosporidiosis. Various types infect humans, sheep, deer, squirrels, and many other animals, but only one infects cattle (and can also infect humans). These protozoa survive in moisture and can live for 170 days in streams. They can live on wet, contaminated calving grounds, but drying and freezing will kill them.

Cryptosporidia multiply in the intestine, creating diarrhea. It's rare to find this organism in adults or calves older than 4 months, but many beef and dairy calves are infected during their first 4 months of age. In earlier years, this disease was a problem only in dairy cattle. It was estimated to affect up to 70 percent of dairy calves 1 to 3 weeks of age, with the rate of infection on some farms as high as 100 percent. The disease now appears in beef herds as well. Though it is often mild and *self-limiting* (the sick individual gets over it without treatment), "crypto" can be life threatening in any human or young animal with a compromised immune system.

In one study, 5 percent of cows tested were carriers. These organisms are common in the environment and water. The best defense is a healthy herd kept in good body condition and in a clean environment. Herd health is affected by nutrition, and whenever you are dealing with crypto, you also want to take a hard look at the trace-mineral status of the animals — especially that of selenium and copper, since these minerals are crucial to the immune system, seem to be an especially important factor in cattle's susceptibility to crypto, and are often lacking in some geographic areas.

IN SEPTEMBER 1971, I was riding the range, checking cattle, and found a sick calf deep in the bushes, out of the hot sun. The calf was wild but very weak. He tried to charge me when I got off my horse to look in the brush to see whose calf he was. The calf had been sick with coccidiosos a while; his rectum was prolapsed, dried out, and dirty. I rode home and called our neighbor to tell him about his calf.

A few days later I was riding in the same area again and saw the calf. I was surprised that the neighbor had not come to get the calf to treat it and also surprised that the calf was still alive. He was weaker by then and could not get up. More surprising was the fact there was *another* sick calf nearby, also belonging to the neighbor. The second calf hadn't been sick long; he was still alert and bright but was starting to prolapse his rectum from continually straining.

I rode home and called our neighbor again, who said he didn't have time to go get the calves and that if we wanted to try to save them, he'd split their value with us if they lived. Lynn and I hate to see an animal suffer and die, so we drove up there in our jeep and with the help of two other people loaded the big calves into the back of the jeep. It was a struggle because they each weighed about 500 pounds (226.8 kg). They were both so weak they simply lay in the jeep, unable to get up as we took them to town.

The only area vet was gone to England on vacation, but his receptionist helped us wash, replace, and stitch the calves' prolapsed rectums. We gave both calves injections of several types of medication and gave George (the calf that had been sick the longest and who was the most dehydrated) some IV fluid. We brought the calves home, put them in a shed (out of the hot sun), gave them more medication and oral fluids via stomach tube.

By 11 p.m., the "better" calf was dead, and George was trying to stand up and charge at us when we came to the shed door. He had a fighting spirit that may have kept him alive. But it was a long uphill battle to save him; he went down again and could not get up for several weeks. We fed him three times a day by stomach tube (fluid, milk, electrolytes, and extra protein) and gave him daily injections of vitamin B_{12} because he was so anemic. We also gave him probiotics to try to start proper digestion again.

Finally he was stronger and able to stand and eat hay, and in a few more weeks he recovered. But he never lost his wild, defiant attitude. He (and his buddy that died) taught us that an animal's will to live (or lack of it) is one of the most important factors in whether or not you can successfully treat and save him. The other calf, who was in much better shape than George, simply gave up. George never did.

Wildlife occasionally pass crypto to livestock. The disease can be deadly if young calves are challenged with another pathogen at the same time. Calves with severe, hard-to-treat diarrhea usually have more than one infection. Once you've had crypto on your farm, it is almost impossible to eradicate; each crop of calves may become infected.

The life cycle of cryptosporidiosis is different from that of coccidiosis (see page 121). In the latter, calves don't get diarrhea until they're at least 3 weeks old. By contrast, a calf can break with crypto diarrhea when as young as 4 days if he was born in contaminated conditions and ingests a large number of protozoa. After an oocyst is ingested, it attaches to the intestinal lining to sporulate and multiply, similarly to the multiplication stages of coccidia, but the incubation period is only 2 to 7 days. Thousands of new oocysts are then passed in feces for 3 to 12 days. Infection persists until the calf develops an immune response to eliminate the parasite.

When protozoa attach to the intestinal lining, white blood cells migrate to the site to fight the infection, creating intense inflammation. The only way the calf can get rid of the pathogen is to rid himself of the cell it's attached to, so the lining is shed. The raw gut can no longer absorb fluid and nutrients, so everything the calf eats or drinks shoots through, creating watery diarrhea. Peak diarrhea occurs 3 to 5 days after a calf ingests oocysts. The gut usually heals in a few days, but without intensive supportive treatment, the calf may die from dehydration before it heals. Calves younger than 3 weeks usually dehydrate more quickly and take longer to regenerate the damaged gut lining than does an older calf.

As with coccidiosis, after a calf gets over the infection, he has some resistance. If he encounters the protozoa again, he's less likely to get sick, but he may continue to shed a few oocysts. Adult cattle usually don't become ill with crypto, but they can serve as a source of infection for calves.

Symptoms

Calves with crypto usually have diarrhea, which persists for several days even if you treat them, since protozoa do not respond to antibiotics. Diarrhea is usually watery, pale, or green (sometimes yellow, cream-colored, or gray), but unlike that of coccidiosis it does not contain blood because the damage is not that deep. You may see mucous or shreds of tissue in feces. The calf may be dull and not nursing, may be dehydrated, and may show signs of abdominal pain. Persistent diarrhea may result in weight loss and emaciation. If complicated by concurrent infection with bacteria or viruses, the calf is usually much sicker; it may take diligent nursing care and frequent fluids to keep him alive long enough for the gut to heal.

Treatment and Prevention

There's no medication for crypto available, but supportive care that includes administering nutritional and hydrating fluids can often save the calf if started early. If the calf is not nursing, force-feed milk (or milk replacer) as well as extra fluids, or he may become weak. An injection of Banamine will help reduce inflammation and make the calf less miserable and more apt to keep nursing. IV fluids may be necessary for calves unable to absorb oral fluids.

Make sure that you never bring this bug to your place. Since it's a common problem in dairy calves, don't buy them to raise on bottles, nurse cows, or beef cows that lost their calves unless you are very sure that they are healthy and have not been exposed to crypto. Even if they look healthy, isolate them for five days to be sure they are not incubating the disease. Don't buy *any* dairy or beef cows from a herd or farm known to have crypto.

If this disease is already on your place, keep calving cows and young calves in a clean environment so calves won't be exposed to the disease early in life by ingesting contaminated feed or water or nursing

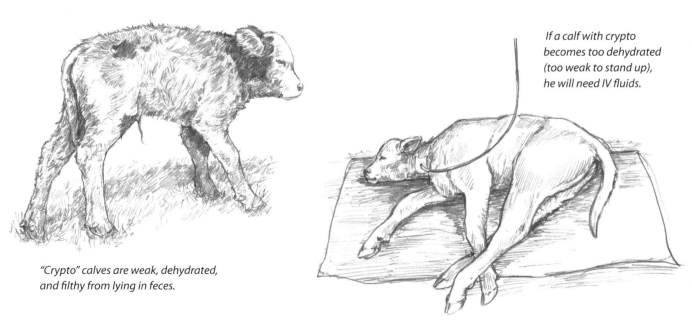

"Crypto" calves are weak, dehydrated, and filthy from lying in feces.

If a calf with crypto becomes too dehydrated (too weak to stand up), he will need IV fluids.

a dirty udder. Isolate any calf that develops diarrhea; take the cow and calf out of the herd to a "sick pen" and keep them separate for several days after he recovers so the calf won't spread protozoa and infect other calves. Be careful you don't inadvertently spread the disease. Change clothes and footwear or rinse your boots in disinfectant, wash your hands, and don't track feces from the sick pen to any other location on your land.

Sarcocystosis

The protozoan sarcosystis has a two-host life cycle in a predator-prey relationship. There are several types; one goes from canines to cattle, another from dogs to sheep, another from cats to pigs. Cattle can be infected with more than one type. The protozoa spend part of their life cycle in dogs or cats and are transmitted to ruminants via fecal matter contaminating livestock feed. When eating muscle tissue of a ruminant animal infected with the protozoa, the predator ingests an *encysted* (enclosed in a cyst in the muscle) parasite. Oocysts form in the cells of the canine intestine and *sporocysts* (cysts or sacs containing spores or reproductive cells) are passed in feces, which contaminate cattle feed (hay or pasture plants) directly or indirectly after drying and blowing about as dust.

After a cow eats contaminated feed, oocysts disperse through her body, causing lesions in all body tissues and organs but mainly in skeletal muscles. Cysts that form in the muscles stay there indefinitely and serve as a source of infection for predators that eat the carcass, perpetuating the life cycle of the protozoa. The most common result of this disease in cattle is the appearance of lesions in muscles found during meat inspection. The tiny, round, purplish red spots or blue purple patches (a condition called *sarcosporidiosis*) are caused by small hemorrhages.

Infection with these protozoa can hinder growth rate. A high level of infection from massive contamination of feed can cause fever, lack of appetite (symptoms sometimes mistaken for shipping fever), emaciation, nervousness, lameness, loss of tail switch, anemia, or abortion. Continual exposure to small numbers of sporocysts (as when grazing pasture with canine feces) can stimulate cattle to create

Colostrum for Health

Make sure every calf gets adequate colostrum soon after birth. Even though cows don't produce many antibodies against crypto, they produce some if they've been exposed to it, and this may give their calves a little protection. Healthy, stress-free calves with high levels of antibodies from colostrum won't develop other diseases that might put them at risk for a serious case of crypto.

immunity, but large doses of contamination may produce body lesions or outbreaks of illness. Muscle cysts can be a cause for meat condemnation.

Prevention

Minimize contamination of cattle feed by canine and feline feces. It's hard to keep dogs and livestock separate, but the farm dog can't spread infection if all meat fed to him is thoroughly cooked. Management of barn cats and farm dogs won't resolve the problem of wild predators (coyotes, foxes, bobcats) spreading the disease by defecating in a pasture, however.

Neosporosis

This disease causes abortions and premature birth in cattle and is similar to sarcocystosis in that it has a two-host life cycle between predator and prey. Neospora protozoa are sometimes spread to cattle when dogs or wild animals (coyotes, raccoons, foxes) defecate in feed. A farm dog is often the culprit in transmitting neospora. Dogs often follow a feed truck and defecate in fresh feed, in a feed bunk, or on a freshly opened bale of hay. The most common risk is when feed is piled on the ground, where carnivores may defecate on it, and the contaminated feed is mixed in a ration to put in feed bunks. The entire herd may be exposed to neospora and be at risk for abortions.

Neospora can also pass from cow to fetus. This disease can be picked up by cattle via contaminated feed or by the calf in the uterus of an infected dam, where it is passed from one generation to the next.

The affected calves are usually normal when born, but some of those calves, if kept as cows, will later abort their first or second calf. This is often the reason for ongoing sporadic cases of abortion.

Neospora is the leading cause of abortions in California dairy herds, and these problems are now appearing in beef herds as well. This disease has probably been prevalent in cattle for a long time, but the protozoan was discovered only 20 years ago. Researchers have found it to be a common cause of abortions in several countries. Healthy cattle seem to handle the infection fairly well, but protozoa may get the upper hand if a cow gets a big dose of fecal material in her feed.

There may be a continual low level of abortions year round (in a dairy herd) or during a calving season due to the cows having been infected with neospora before they themselves were born. The disease might also present itself as occasional outbreaks of abortions in which a group of cows might lose their calves within a week's time, due to contaminated feed.

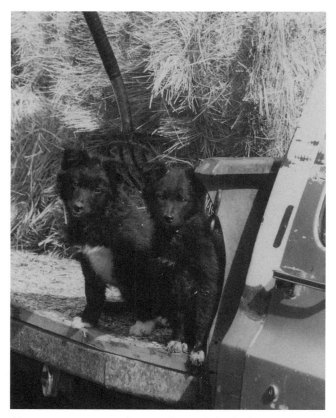

Neospora protozoa can be spread to cattle by the farm or ranch dog defecating in hay.

Cyst-Forming Diseases

Coccidia, neospora, sarcosporidia, and cryptosporidia are all fecal-oral organisms and are cyst-forming. With coccidia and cryptosporidia the cyst is in the intestinal tract. Sarcosporidia form cysts in muscle, including heart tissue. Neospora form cysts in brain tissue and create inflammation in the heart of the fetus, usually killing it.

We are still learning about neospora. Abortions are often misdiagnosed as something else. If blood samples are taken, some herds are all positive; all cows have been exposed, yet only a small percentage aborts. There must be other factors involved, and research is ongoing. One study in Canada, for instance, found that cows exposed to BVD virus abort more frequently from neospora than cows not exposed to BVD. The viral disease may hinder the immune system and put the cow at greater risk for neospora abortion.

Neospora affects the fetal brain and heart. Some calves are minimally affected, and some are born alive and normal. If a calf is sluggish at birth, you don't know whether it's due to a slow birth and oxygen deprivation or neospora in the brain. If a cow aborts from neospora, it's usually during mid- to late gestation (4 to 6 months). Unless she's culled, she may have a normal calf the next year, but there's a chance she'll pass infection to her calf.

Prevention

It may be impossible to keep dogs and wild canines out of pastures and pens, but you can fence off or protect stored and piled feed so they can't get to it. Since stored feed used in mixed rations is the most common route for infection, protecting your feed may reduce the risk considerably.

Blood tests can detect antibodies for the protozoa; a positive test means the animal is infected. An ELISA (enzyme-linked immunosorbent assay) blood test can determine the duration of infection. Because infected cows can infect their unborn calves, testing a herd and culling infected cows can help prevent this disease.

Trichomoniasis

Trichomoniasis is a subtle disease that may get into your herd without obvious signs. You may not suspect a problem until you test for pregnancy and find a high percentage of open cows. Or you may see cows in heat that were bred earlier. It's not unusual in newly infected herds to have up to 20 percent of cows open after breeding season. Trichomoniasis is transmitted from bull to cow at breeding, and the protozoa kill the developing embryo or fetus.

"Trich" can sneak into your herd if an infected bull breeds cows when they are in pastures shared by other cattle or if a fence breaks down and a neighbor's bull breeds cows. If you exchange or lease used bulls or buy any nonvirgin bull that has not been tested, you may discover trich on your ranch.

Trichomoniasis is most prevalent in western states, where ranchers must use rangeland pastures in common with other ranchers and have less control over the bulls being used, but it also exists in other parts of the country, including Missouri, Louisiana, Mississippi, Florida, and Texas. It's not as common in small herds with only one or two bulls, unless you buy used bulls or buy cows that came from an area where the disease exists.

This protozoan infects the sheath of a bull and the reproductive tract of a cow. If an infected cow is bred, she passes the infection to the bull. If an infected bull breeds a susceptible cow, he passes it to her. She usually conceives, but infection kills the developing *conceptus* at some point in the first 4 months of gestation. The cow returns to heat after losing the pregnancy, and if there is still a bull with the herd, she is bred again. Since she still has the infection, however, she won't settle or again loses the pregnancy early.

A bull often carries the infection for life, but a cow usually recovers after 5 to 12 months. Once she gets rid of the protozoa, she can carry a pregnancy. Occasionally, however, a cow develops a severe uterine infection and becomes permanently infertile. If a herd is infected, there will many open cows in the fall, especially if bulls were taken out of the herd at the end of a short breeding season. If bulls are left with cows year round, there will be some late-calving cows the next year, since they are finally able to become pregnant again late in the season.

After the cow's reproductive tract recovers, she usually has immunity and won't be infected again, even if bred by an infected bull, for about a year. A few cows carry the disease into the next year if they acquire it late in the season, but bulls are the main problem because they can be carriers for a much longer time.

Young bulls may become temporarily infected and spread the disease for a short while, then recover between breeding seasons. Older bulls generally remain infected for life. Most young bulls merely act as mechanical transmitters for a while (passing infection from cow to cow), whereas bulls older than 3 years carry the disease to the next season.

The causative protozoan thrives in airless places and lives in tiny pockets or folds that line the inner surface of a bull's sheath. It does not survive outside the reproductive tract. The high infection rate in older bulls may be because they have more folds in which the protozoa can survive for long periods. These carrier bulls can infect cows at the start of breeding season, greatly increasing the risk of exposing large numbers of cows to the disease.

Electron microscope enlargement of Tritrichomonas foetus

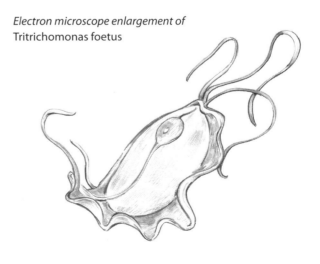

Symptoms and Diagnosis

You may not see disease symptoms other than repeat breedings of a cow that won't settle, open cows, or cows coming back in heat toward the end of breeding season. A few cows may have uterine discharge. Bulls and suspect cows can be tested; diagnosis requires microscopic examination or culture of mucus from inside the sheath of a bull, *pus* from an infected cow (taking mucus from the *cervix*), or tissues from an aborted fetus. Pregnancy testing is a good time to take a sample from any open cow that has an enlarged uterus (which may be full of pus) or shows a discharge of infected mucus.

Prevention

Virgin bulls that haven't bred cows are usually safe to use, but older bulls should be tested. Some states require annual testing well ahead of breeding season, and tagging of every bull. Virgin bulls are also tagged, so people will know that they are part of the program. Some states require testing of any bull coming into the state, and bulls must be tested before they change ownership. These programs help reduce the incidence of trichomoniasis.

To test a bull, the vet collects mucus from the deepest part of the sheath and cultures this material to allow any present *trichomonads* to grow and multiply. The culture is observed for 3 to 7 days. A heavily infected bull will show a positive culture within 3 days. Any bull that tests positive should be sold for slaughter. The best time to test is a few weeks after breeding season, but bulls can be checked any time before the next breeding season.

All bulls in the herd should be tested. Since protozoa may be intermittently shed, multiple tests a few weeks apart increase the odds of finding all infected bulls. Studies show that one test will find 80 to 90 percent of infected bulls; two tests will find 90 to 95 percent; and three tests will find 95 to 100 percent.

In herds or grazing associations, trich can be eventually cleared up by testing all bulls before the breeding season (so that no infected bulls are used) and by making sure all cows have calved by the time they are turned out into the breeding pasture. A cow that shows she can calve is generally no longer infected and will not spread infection to a "clean"

bull. If cows are always pregnancy-tested by a certain date, and any open cows are culled, this usually gets rid of the ones that are infected.

"Virgin" Bulls Can Spread Disease

A young bull may test positive for trich even though you think he's never bred cows. Bull calves mount and try to breed cows, and if there are infected cows in the herd, a young bull may become infected by trying to breed them.

A false positive may occur if a bull's sheath is contaminated with fecal material containing another

Trich Prevention Tips

- Buy only virgin bulls or heifers or pregnant heifers; avoid buying older cows or bulls.

- Test all mature bulls three times before using them, especially if you use community pastures and your bulls were breeding cows with unknown history the previous breeding season (in AI studs, the bulls are tested six times to make sure that they are free of this disease).

- If possible, use separate breeding pastures; when using a pasture with other stockmen, consider using that pasture just for yearlings to be sold for beef (not replacement heifers).

- Replace older bulls with young virgin bulls, but test all bulls coming into your herd, including young ones.

- Have a short breeding season, then do pregnancy checks and cull all open cows or late calvers, especially any that abort or have a discharge.

- Never put a cull cow in a pen with bulls, because she could infect them.

- After a short breeding season, keep bulls away from cows until next breeding season. The longer the period of sexual rest the better. Some young bulls eliminate the infection, but infected bulls over 3 years of age tend to become permanent carriers.

- Use artificial insemination, if practical.

type of trich. There are many kinds of tritrichomonas protozoa; some infect other animals, and some are harmless. A harmless type lives in the intestines of cattle and can be found in manure. When cultured, it is hard to distinguish it from the one that causes reproductive problems. A bull may have harmless protozoa in his sheath if he's been "riding" other bulls and "breeding" them rectally, as bulls confined in pens together will do. The intestinal protozoa grow in culture media and result in a positive test, even though the bull is not infected with the reproductive protozoa.

A different type of test — a polymerase chain reaction (PCR) test, that is done in only a few laboratories — can determine whether the protozoa are "reproductive" or "intestinal" trich. The PCR test is the surest way to know if a bull actually has the disease; you can find out with just one test whether or not the bull is positive or negative. If you ever decide to purchase or lease a mature bull, you can use the PCR test rather than having to test him three times.

There's no treatment for trich; prevention is the only recourse. If you have a closed herd (no new cows coming in) and use only bulls that have been tested and are free of this disease, you won't have problems. Even in an infected herd, trich can be eventually eliminated if you get rid of all carrier cows and bulls. Vaccinating the rest of the cows just ahead of breeding season can also give them some protection. Discuss this with your veterinarian if you suspect that you might have trich in your herd. When a herd has reproductive problems, proper diagnosis is important because there are other diseases that can lead to abortions and open cows. You'll want to know the nature and risk of the disease at hand as soon as possible.

CHAPTER SEVEN

Parasites

Parasitic organisms live in or on a host animal, depending on that host for their existence. Harm caused by parasites may not be noticeable in a well-fed, healthy animal that carries a small number of the freeloaders, but the damage becomes more obvious when a substantial infestation robs nutrients and blood and saps energy from the host.

Cattle are hosts for many internal and external parasites. Some coexist with the host without endangering her life, while others are far more damaging. Some, such as flies and ticks, spread diseases that can be fatal to the animals. Minimizing the introduction and effects of parasites is a vital piece of total herd health management.

Internal Parasites

Most internal parasites are "worms," but grubs are *larvae* of flies, spending part of their life cycle within the host. Most internal parasites are *host specific;* they live in just one type of animal and can't complete their life cycle in the wrong host. Most enter the host by ingestion, grow to maturity in the gut, and lay eggs that pass out with manure to be ingested with feed or water by a susceptible animal to start the cycle again.

Almost all cattle harbor internal parasites, but infestation levels vary with geography, climate, and pasture conditions. At least 85 percent of cattle are infected by *brown stomach worms,* and more than 67 percent are infected by large stomach worms. Heavy infestations cause weight loss, weakness, or even death, while light loads may not affect the animal's apparent health. Worms rob nutrients, however, and even a light infestation results in less feed efficiency and less-than-optimum growth or weight gain. An animal infested by stomach worms, for instance, has less appetite due to inflammation produced by larvae in the wall of the stomach and intestine.

All cattle are exposed to worm eggs or larvae. Calves are most susceptible. Adults have developed some resistance to parasites and may not carry such heavy loads yet can still pass a few eggs or larvae that may be picked up by other animals. Young, susceptible animals may get serious infections when first exposed, ingesting larvae in the infective stages once they've climbed onto forage plants.

Since pasture conditions that favor or inhibit the survival and spread of worms vary with climate, weather, and stocking rates in pastures, it's wise to consult your veterinarian periodically regarding the best deworming program and the frequency of treatment. Some herds should be dewormed regularly. In some instances it's not cost-effective to treat for worms, but in most cases it results in better body condition, improved milk production, weight gain, reproductive efficiency, less disease, and less feed needed to maintain proper body condition. Learn the parasite's life cycle so you can deworm at the most beneficial time of year.

Stomach and Intestinal Worms

Most stomach and intestinal parasites are round-worms; several types infest cattle. One species lives in the lungs, while others live in the digestive tract. The most common species, *Ostertagia,* lives in the fourth stomach (the abomasum) and part of the small intestine. In most species, the adults lay eggs in the intestine that pass out with manure and hatch into larvae on the ground. After *molting,* larvae migrate onto forage plants and are eaten by cattle. The larvae mature in the stomach and intestine and lay eggs, continuing the life cycle.

Eggs and larvae are fairly hardy and in some instances can overwinter on a pasture. Roundworm larvae may migrate into the soil or remain dormant under snow until warmer weather and new grass make conditions favorable for them again. Moisture is essential for their survival and migration. Rainy seasons, irrigation, marshy areas, and leaky water troughs all help create ideal conditions for parasite survival. Sunlight, heat, dry air, and *harrowing* pastures in hot weather when there are no cattle present to pick up scattered larvae all tend to inhibit or kill the larvae.

In most cases, 90 percent of the worm population inhabits the pasture and 10 percent is in the cattle. One way to reduce parasite infection is to reduce the numbers of eggs and larvae in the pasture. In some regions deworming in the spring before adult worms in the gut can lay eggs results in the greatest reduction of pasture accumulation.

HARROW WHEN IT'S HOT AND DRY

Moist manure pats protect larvae and keep them from drying out. If you harrow pastures in cool, damp weather you spread larvae all over the pasture. It's best to harrow during hot, dry weather, to break up manure and expose larvae to the dry conditions.

Common Stomach Roundworms

Some types of roundworm burrow into and form cysts in the stomach or intestinal walls, surviving in dormancy within the host during seasons they might not survive in the environment. These encysted larvae wait until ingested forage is lush and green again to emerge from the gut wall and continue their life cycle. Males and females mature, mate and produce eggs to contaminate pastures again, resulting in high levels of reinfestation in grazing cattle. The number of worm eggs shed is usually highest in spring and fall, if wet, and lowest in winter and midsummer.

▶ **Brown stomach worms,** *Ostertagia ostertagi,* are the most common of the worms that stay encysted and dormant in the gut awaiting favorable conditions for maturity. Larvae penetrate gastric glands in the abomasum lining, producing nodules. When young adult worms emerge, gastric glands are damaged, interfering with digestion. Irritation and disrupted digestion cause loss of appetite and weight, especially in calves 7 to 15

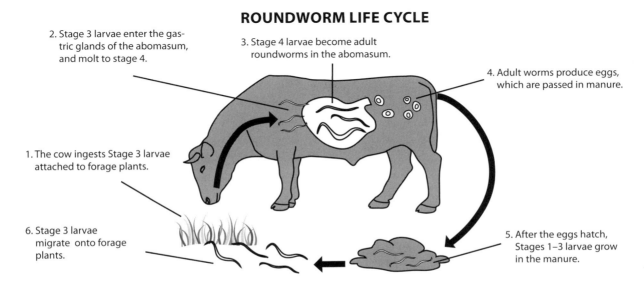

ROUNDWORM LIFE CYCLE

2. Stage 3 larvae enter the gastric glands of the abomasum, and molt to stage 4.

3. Stage 4 larvae become adult roundworms in the abomasum.

4. Adult worms produce eggs, which are passed in manure.

1. The cow ingests Stage 3 larvae attached to forage plants.

6. Stage 3 larvae migrate onto forage plants.

5. After the eggs hatch, Stages 1–3 larvae grow in the manure.

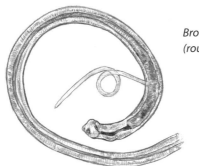

*Brown stomach worm
(roundworm)*

months old. Occasionally these worms hibernate for up to 6 months in the gastric glands, causing severe damage when they suddenly emerge in yearling cattle.

▸ **Large stomach worms,** *Haemonchus placei,* known to some as *wireworms* and barber pole worms, also live in the abomasum, puncturing small blood vessels in the lining and feeding on blood. Even small numbers of these worms can be very damaging. Affected animals suffer appetite loss, severe anemia, and sometimes edema under the jaw.

Small Intestinal Worms

Several species of *Cooperia* worms infect the small intestine and occur in all cattle. Heavy infections may cause diarrhea, appetite loss, and emaciation.

▸ **Hookworms,** *Bunostomum phlebotomum,* occur mainly in southern and midwestern regions. They enter the body by ingestion or through the skin and migrate to the small intestine. They feed on tissue and blood, causing weight loss and diarrhea.

▸ **Nodular worms,** *Oesophagostomum radiatum,* spend part of the larval stage in the wall of the lower small intestine after traveling through the gut. After 5 to 10 days (or longer if they go into a dormant phase) the larvae return to the rumen to finish development. Pea-sized nodules are created in the rumen wall by the damage they create. Nodular worms in young cattle result in poor appetite; persistent, dark, foul-smelling diarrhea; weight loss; and even death. Older animals may suffer from reduced gut motility. Because of this gut slowdown, less feed is eaten.

▸ **Thread-necked worms,** *Nematodirus helvetianus,* live in the upper one-third of the small intestine, creating damage while tunneling into the lining to feed on protein and blood. They are hard to detect in fecal samples because females produce fewer eggs than most other worms. The eggs are hardy and resistant to heat, cold, and drying, and often live from one season to the next in the environment. Infected cattle have rough hair and may suffer from poor appetite, diarrhea, and weight loss.

▸ **Threadworms,** *Strongyloides papillosus,* don't need male worms to complete the life cycle. Females embedded in the mucosal lining of the upper small intestine lay eggs passed with manure. Infected calves may show intermittent diarrhea, loss of appetite, weight loss, and occasionally blood and mucus in the feces.

▸ **Trichostrongylus worms,** *T. axae* and *T. colubriformus,* live in the abomasum and sometimes the small intestine, damaging the mucous lining. Signs of infection include poor appetite and watery diarrhea. Heavy infestations cause poor growth or weight loss.

▸ **Lungworms,** *Dictyocalus viviparus,* often appear when cattle are confined in dense numbers. Larvae are ingested and then migrate from the intestines to the lungs through the lymph system and blood vessels. They mature in smaller branches of the *bronchial tubes.* The resulting irritation leads to coughing and fluid secretion, which may cause lung congestion or open the way for pathogens that cause pneumonia.

▸ **Tapeworms,** *Moniezia expansa* and *M. benedeni,* primarily affect young cattle and require an intermediate host for their life cycle. This host is a *mite* that lives in soil and on forage plants. The mites ingest tapeworm eggs shed by infected cattle. After 6 weeks inside the mites, eggs become an infective form *(cysticercoids).* When infected mites are eaten with grass, the eggs within the mites can continue their life cycle in the new host.

The effects of tapeworm infection in cattle are usually minimal, but heavy infections that hinder digestion can be controlled with deworming products. Consult your veterinarian; some of the commonly used deworming products won't kill tapeworms.

Symptoms

Animals with low levels of worm infestation may show no symptoms. Animals carrying heavy loads may have a rough hair coat, diarrhea, weight loss, anemia, a swollen lower jaw (bottle jaw), or weakness, and may die if the infestation is severe. Heavily infested cattle are more likely to experience other diseases because the stress of worm infestation lowers their resistance.

The only sign in some cattle is less weight gain. They seem healthy but have less appetite due to inflammation in the stomach and intestine caused by worm larvae. Appetite depression accounts for most of the difference in weight gain. Worms also interfere with proper digestion and the movement of feed through the tract, which results in even less feed being consumed.

Prevention and Treatment

Manure can be checked for worm eggs, but the number of eggs may not be indicative of the infection level, especially if the sample is taken during a time of year when worms are encysted larvae rather than egg-laying adults. During fall and winter, cattle parasites in northern regions slow their growth and may not be detected in fecal samples. Deworming decisions can be aided by taking samples in the spring or by knowing the previous history of certain pastures

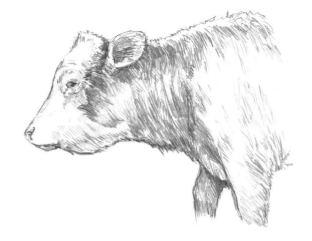

"Bottle jaw" swelling from fluid under the jaw is one sign of heavy worm infestation.

Obtaining a Fecal Sample

A sample can be taken from freshly passed manure using a plastic shoulder sleeve or glove.

1. Pick up fresh manure; invert the sleeve or glove as you remove it, keeping the sample inside the glove.

2. Tie a knot in the glove with the sample inside it, and put it into another plastic bag.

3. Label the bag with the cow's number, and refrigerate it until you can take it to your vet or send it to a diagnostic lab.

When checking a group of cattle, submit samples from 5 to 10 percent of the animals. When there's a choice, submit samples from the younger animals; they tend to be most heavily infected or shed the most eggs.

and infestations. Intensive grazing and pasture rotation increases parasite infestations. This should be taken into consideration when designing pasture-rotation systems and when determining the best times to treat for parasites.

Irrigated, wet pastures, where cattle are confined in small areas, generally present more risk of infection than large, dry areas, where cattle roam widely. In the large dry areas, conditions inhibit the worms' lifecycle, and cattle are not as apt to consume plants near manure. On dry rangeland the only places where worms thrive are wet areas along streams.

Infestation opportunities may be decreased if cattle are dewormed before putting them in a new pasture and if pastures are grazed for a short period rather than yearlong. Treating for parasites in mid-grazing season is often a waste of time and money unless cattle are moved into a new, clean pasture after treatment. If left in the old pasture, they immediately become reinfested.

Deworming cattle at the proper time of year increases weight gain. A study at Oklahoma State University compared three groups of calves: some dewormed upon arrival at a feedlot, some dewormed at the ranch while still on grass and again at the feedlot, and some that were never dewormed.

The group wormed at the ranch while still on grass gained 48 more pounds (21.8 kg) before going to the feedlot. The ones that were never dewormed were 96 pounds (43.5 kg) lighter than the calves that were dewormed at both the ranch and the feedlot.

Discuss parasite programs with your vet to determine the best time of year and what products to use, taking into consideration climate, pasture conditions, and pasture usage. Cattle fed hay and cattle in feedlots in feed bunks are not picking up worms from pasture plants. But calves coming into feedlots may carry a heavy load. Incoming cattle should be dewormed if they came from contaminated pastures and have not recently been treated for parasites.

Liver Fluke

The most common cattle and sheep liver fluke is *Fasciola hepatica*, which also infects wild rabbits and hares that spread and maintain these parasites on pastures. Another fluke, *Fascioloides magna*, is a deer parasite and can infect cattle when they occupy the same regions. Both parasites reside in the liver, where they cause damage and sometimes block the bile ducts. The life cycle requires two hosts: a grazing animal and a snail. An infected grazer sheds eggs in feces, which hatch and infect a small freshwater snail. This intermediate host, a *lymnaeid snail*, is found throughout the United States.

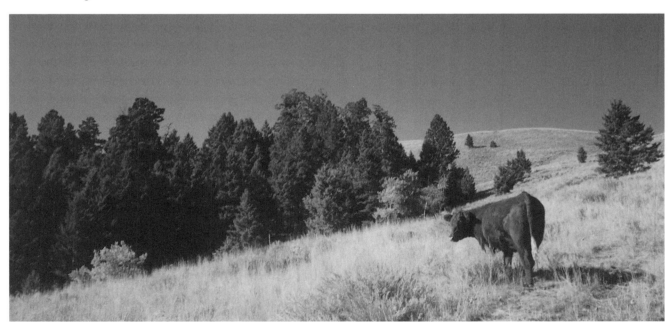

Cattle that are spread over many acres of dry rangeland are at much less risk for picking up worms.

When cattle graze in wet pastures or eat plants in or near springs or marshes where snails reside, they pick up fluke "eggs" (metacercarial cysts) attached to forage. Tiny flukes are freed from the cysts during digestion and are activated in the rumen, where they thrive in the concentrated carbon dioxide and a temperature of 102.2°F (39°C).

Young flukes feed on the mucosal lining, then bore through the gut wall into the abdominal cavity and migrate to the liver. After several days of migrating, feeding, growing, and destroying liver tissues, flukes enter the bile ducts while they are still small enough to get through. They complete their development and become adults, remaining there until they die. Adult flukes exist in the liver for years. Flukes are self-fertilizing; although there are both male and female flukes, they don't need to mate to reproduce. They feed on bile-duct linings, and their presence triggers inflammation and thickening of the lining.

Adult flukes lay eggs in the bile ducts; eggs migrate with the bile into the intestine and are passed in manure, appearing in feces 13 to 15 weeks after the host ingested the cysts. If manure ends up in water or wet pasture, free-swimming miracidia hatch from eggs after washing loose from manure. They hatch in 9 to 10 days at summer temperatures, taking longer at lower temperatures. If the temperature drops below 50°F (10°C), eggs remain dormant and survive for long periods, resuming development later.

Free-swimming miracidia live up to 24 hours in water after hatching, searching for a snail. If they find one, they penetrate its skin. The snail that serves as intermediate host is amphibious and lives on mud along the edges of small pools, marshes, and springs. If those dry up, snails burrow into the mud and emerge again in wet seasons to shed the next stage of flukes. Immature flukes undergo development in the snail. This takes 5 to 7 weeks in temperatures of 50 to 86°F (10 to 30°C) and longer in temperatures lower or higher. Then they emerge from the snail and migrate back into the wet environment, where they attach to vegetation and encyst, to be ingested by grazing cattle and start the cycle again.

Since development of immature flukes in a snail can take months, most new fluke infections in cattle do not occur until August or September in mild climates. Larval migration and maturation takes another 8 to 15 weeks, so eggs may not show up in manure until December or January, especially in northern regions. Conditions favorable to liver-fluke transmission vary regionally due to varying seasonal temperatures and quantities of moisture.

LIVER FLUKE LIFE CYCLE

2. The flukes migrate to the bile ducts in the liver, where they complete their development.

3. Adult flukes lay eggs in the bile ducts and the eggs migrate with the bile into the intestines.

1. The cow ingests metacercarial cysts attached to forage plants, and tiny immature flukes are freed from the cysts during digestion.

4. Eggs are passed in manure.

7. Free-swimming cercariae leave the snails, migrate onto vegetation growing in the water, and encyst.

5. If the manure ends up in water, the eggs hatch into free-swimming miracidia that search for mud snails to penetrate.

6. Immature flukes continue their development in snails.

Fluke infections in the United States were once thought to occur only in the southeastern coastal regions, areas with high rainfall, the Rocky Mountain region, and the Northwest, but are now found all over the country. Cattle are often transported from one area to another and, if infected, spread fluke eggs in feces. If conditions are right, the eggs infect snails and continue their life cycle, posing a risk for other cattle in the area.

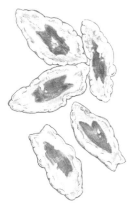

Liver flukes

It's not always easy to tell from a fecal sample if an animal has flukes; another way to tell if your cattle have flukes is to examine the liver of any animal that dies or is butchered on your place.

Symptoms of Fluke Infestation

There may be few outward signs of fluke infection, but a heavy load may have an adverse impact on reproduction. Cows or heifers may be slow to breed or may not breed at all. Heavy infestations may reduce milk production, growth rate, and weight gain, or cause diarrhea and weight loss.

As flukes migrate and cause liver damage, they open the way for infection by *Clostridium hemolyticum* (see chapter 4), the spores of which are often already present in the body, including the liver. When liver damage enables spores to proliferate and release toxins, they cause redwater disease and sudden death. Redwater is most common in regions where snails and liver flukes exist.

Harmful Effects of Flukes

Damage from flukes makes the liver unfit for human consumption and is a common cause for condemnation of beef livers at slaughter. It also causes trim loss in the diaphragm muscles attached to the liver. Flukes are also associated with slow onset of puberty in heifers and adverse effects on reproductive hormones. A study at Louisiana State University showed that when heifers were treated for both worms and flukes, their pregnancy rate was significantly higher

than that of the untreated control group. When gastrointestinal worms and liver flukes are both present, cattle do not have optimal fertility.

Prevention and Treatment

In some instances, fluke infections can be minimized by pasture rotation, using risky pastures at the times of year when there are no immature flukes on plants. If snails exist in just a few marshes or springs, fence these so cattle can't graze them. If there's no way to prevent exposure, treat cattle during the time of year they are most apt to be infected.

Many deworming drugs have no affect on liver flukes, but there are several products that will kill them. The best time to treat is late fall so cattle remain free of flukes over the winter. Cattle usually won't pick up new infestations from snails in winter except in a warm climate or from green forage that continues to grow in winter, such as in a marsh fed by a warm-water spring.

In areas where flukes are a year-round problem, spring treatment can be beneficial, especially if it's been a few years since you've used a broad-spectrum product that controls flukes as well as other internal parasites. A spring treatment reduces the population of flukes during the summer, reduces pasture contamination with eggs, and helps ensure a more successful fall treatment.

One way to tell if poor weight gains or poor reproduction rates are caused by fluke infestation is by trial and error. If you've treated for other parasites or other disease conditions and haven't seen improvement, try treating for liver flukes. If cattle improve, there's a good chance your herd is infected, and you should start a yearly treatment program.

Grubs

Grubs are the immature form of a fly (often called a *heel fly,* warble fly, *bomb fly,* or *gadfly*) that spends most of its life inside a host, becoming a fly just long enough to find cattle and lay eggs. Not only do grubs damage the hide and some of the meat (leaving holes in the animal's back where they emerge), but heavy infestations can reduce calf weight gains by a tenth of a pound (0.05 kg) or more per day. If you see or feel marble-size bumps or *warbles* on your cows' backs in late fall or early winter, they are infected by grubs.

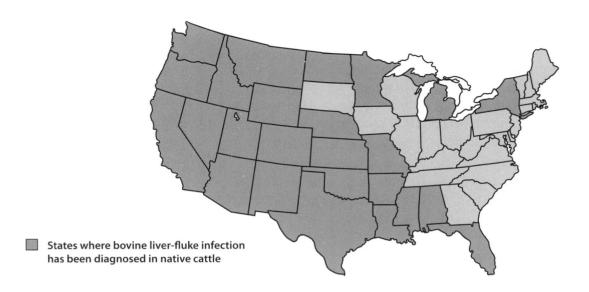

States where bovine liver-fluke infection has been diagnosed in native cattle

Warble Flies

There are two species of warble fly: *Hypoderma bovis* and *H. lineatum*. The latter is often called the southern cattle grub because it prefers a warm climate and is the only species found in the South. *H. bovis* is often called the northern cattle grub, but both species exist in the northern United States and Canada. Their life cycles are very similar, but *H. lineatum* tends to appear three to eight weeks earlier in the year.

▶ **The warble fly resembles** a honeybee in size and shape. They do not feed; they live only a week after emerging — just long enough to mate and lay eggs. They aggressively attack cattle, hovering and darting to lay eggs on hairs. *H. lineatum* deposits eggs on the legs or lower body of cattle. *H. bovis* lays eggs on the rump or upper part of the hind legs. Flies are active early in the fly season — late winter in the South, early spring in central states, and spring through early summer in northern areas.

The flies don't land on cattle, but the female hovers close to the legs or heels as she attaches eggs (500 to 800 of them) to individual hairs. This action tickles or irritates the animals, and, along with the buzzing of the flies, startles them. Cattle pestered by darting flies run wildly with their tails straight up, running into brush or water to try to get away from the flies or crashing through fences. This frantic activity in response to these flies is called *gadding*.

Life Cycle of the Grub

Once an egg is glued to the hair, it hatches in 3 to 7 days; the tiny first-stage larva crawls down the hair and burrows through the skin, then spends 2 to 4 months migrating up through the body. *H. lineatum* travels to the esophagus wall near the back of the throat, and *H. bovis* moves toward the spinal column, near the *pin bones*. First-stage larvae remain in these areas 2 to 4 months during fall and early winter. Then both species of larvae eventually travel to the back and spend their second and third (warble) stages in tissue beneath the skin. Upon arrival they cut breathing holes through the skin with their sharp mouthparts. The cow's body reacts to the grub by forming a fluid-filled cyst around it; this cyst under the skin is called a warble.

WHEN GRUBS APPEAR

Grubs first start showing in the backs of cattle in mid-September in the South and in January or later in northern regions. They start emerging through the skin in November in Texas but not until early March in Montana. Heel-fly larvae remain as warbles in the back for about 55 days and bomb-fly larvae about 75 days.

After 4 to 6 weeks of rapid growth in grub stage, larvae are ¼ to ½ inch (0.64 to 1.27 cm) long and emerge through the breathing holes and fall to the ground to *pupate*. Depending on the temperature, adult flies emerge from the ground 1 to 3 months later, completing the annual life cycle. Then the females seek out cattle so they can lay eggs.

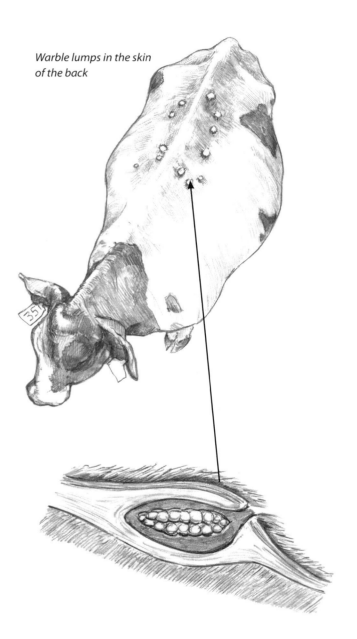

Warble lumps in the skin of the back

Cattle grub in its warble under the skin of the animal's back

Treatment

Control of adult flies is nearly impossible, since they live only a week or less; treatment is aimed at destroying the first-stage larvae in the body before they travel to the back. This prevents damage to the meat and hide and ensures that no flies hatch next season. In northern areas treatment can be given about 6 weeks after the first killing frost, when no more adult flies are present, and before larvae arrive at the esophagus or spinal cord.

Grubs can be eradicated by treating cattle once in the fall and again in spring before they leave the host, in case any were missed in fall treatment. The most effective treatment is a systemic product absorbed into the body to kill internal parasites; it kills grubs wherever they happen to be at that time. This can be sprayed or poured on or injected. Broad-spectrum products, such as ivermectin or moxidectin, kill grubs, and if a spring dewormer is given, this will kill any grubs that have reached the back.

Ideally cattle should be treated in the fall after there's no more risk for eggs to be laid and about 3 months before the expected appearance of grubs in the back. Treatment in northern regions should be given before December, and treatments in warm southern climates no later than mid-October (as early as August in the far South). All cattle on the ranch should be treated. Missing even a few will result in flies in the spring, to lay eggs on cattle.

Veterinarians recommend against treating for grubs during winter because of possible side effects due to grubs dying next to the spine or esophagus (though these reactions are rare). Treatment during the final 2 or 3 months of larval migration kills grubs in tissues of the esophagus or spinal canal, and their dying results in a localized inflammation caused by the body's immune response to chemicals released by the dying larvae. The resultant swelling could cause choking or bloat if larvae are in the lining of the esophagus, or temporary paralysis if larvae are in the spinal canal. If the animal's distress is noticed in time, these reactions can be halted and treated with anti-inflammatory drugs, but unobserved animals might die. Your veterinarian can advise you as to the best time of year and most effective products for treating grubs in your area.

Lice

Lice are tiny parasites that spend their entire life on the host. Heavy lice infestations are a common winter problem. Bloodsucking lice rob cattle of vital nutrition when they need it most. Biting and chewing lice irritate cattle and interfere with their grazing or eating. Infested cattle are itchy and restless and may spend more time rubbing on fences or trees than eating. Lice populations increase dramatically during cold weather, just when cattle need extra energy. If the animal rubs off patches of hair, natural insulation is lost and body heat is dissipated. The animal is more vulnerable to the effects of cold weather and requires more feed to create adequate body heat. Drain on the animal from severe infestation can cause weight loss, stress, reduced milk production, and general unthriftiness, making the host more susceptible to other diseases.

Biting lice *(Damalinia [Bovicola] bovis)* are most common, but *sucking lice (Haemotopinus eurysternus, Linognathus vituli,* and *Solenopotes capillatus)* are most damaging. Both types cause severe irritation and itching. Infested cattle lick or chew at themselves and rub on any available object, often damaging fences. Hair rubbed off contains *nits* (eggs) that can infest other cattle. The constant crawling, biting, and chewing of lice cause cattle to be restless. Normal feeding activities are disrupted.

External Parasites

Arthropod parasites hinder optimum milk and meat production and jeopardize animal health by feeding on body tissues such as blood and skin. These parasites include insects — flies and lice — and *arachnids,* such as ticks. The cumulative effect may reduce growth rate and cause general weakness and unthriftiness. The parasites may create skin damage that opens the way for infection. Some spread disease from one animal to another. Certain parasites are a problem in summer, and others are more of a winter problem. Knowing the life cycle of the parasite helps you to control them at the proper time before they multiply extensively.

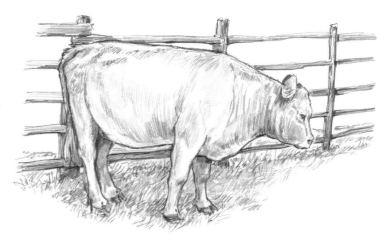

Cattle infested with lice rub and scratch themselves constantly.

Biting lice feed on upper layers of skin. Sucking lice bite deeper, to ingest blood. Lice migrate to areas of the body that meet their temperature requirement and usually stay in that general area. Sucking lice often congregate around the head, cheeks, neck, and shoulders of the host animal. Anemia and blood loss resulting from their activity can stunt growth in young animals and reduce weight gain. Continued heavy infestation makes cattle vulnerable to other diseases and can weaken the animal to the point where stress from disease or cold weather can cause death.

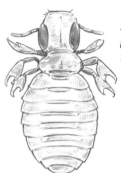

Sucking lice have mouthparts adapted for piercing the skin and sucking blood.

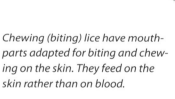

Chewing (biting) lice have mouthparts adapted for biting and chewing on the skin. They feed on the skin rather than on blood.

Lice Life Cycle

The entire life cycle (usually 20 to 30 days) takes place on the host, which makes lice an easy parasite to kill by applying pesticide to the animal. Eggs are attached to the hair and hatch in 4 to 14 days. *Nymphs* that look just like small adults emerge from eggs, molt three times, and become egg-laying adults in about 2 weeks. Though direct contact is the primary means of transmission, eggs and nymphs can be transmitted by the use of brushes, halters or other equipment, or contact with hair on feeders and fences. Also, when hair is rubbed off, dislodged eggs can hatch and infect other animals in the pen or pasture for about a week. If you put new animals in a pen where lousy animals have been rubbing, lice are transmitted to the healthy ones.

Certain animals harbor abnormally high numbers of lice, even in the summer, and serve as a continuing source of infestation for the herd. Young animals with little resistance and old, thin cows usually have the heaviest infestations. The latter can become carriers that reinfest the herd every fall or winter. Lice are continually spread from carriers to other cattle and from cows to their calves.

Evidence of Lice

If cattle have had lice for some time, you can easily tell that they are infected; they rub out patches of hair and may injure the skin. A close look at the animal — tied up or restrained in a chute (unless he's a pet that tolerates your touch) — reveals the tiny parasites. Part the hair on the head or shoulders with your fingers, so you can see the skin. Lice are easy to find on the face or withers. You can often see them with the naked eye, but a flashlight or handheld magnifying glass makes them easier to see. Check for nits, too. They are small white (sometimes yellow or black) barrel-shaped specks attached to hairs.

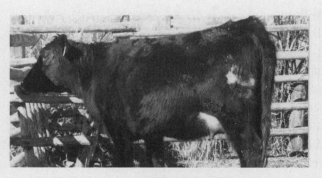

If the lice-ridden animal rubs off patches of hair due to scratching, keep in mind that insulation and protection from cold weather are lost.

Carriers

Most cattle develop resistance to lice after they have them. There's often a difference in severity of infestation in young ones with no previous exposure and an older animal that's encountered them before. The older, more immune animal has fewer lice. Young animals become infested more readily, and lice multiply quickly on them. Carrier animals usually have some deficiency in their immune system that makes them more susceptible to heavy lice infestations. (See chapter 1 for a detailed discussion of cell-mediated immunity and immune deficiencies.)

Carriers are usually older cows that always have high numbers of lice, even in the summer. They should be culled, since they serve as a continuous source of lice for the rest of the herd. Treating carriers for lice may not get rid of them all; the cow is carrying so many that some will lay eggs before they die. There is swift reinfestation on that animal. Unless you cull the carrier cow, lice in your herd can build up very quickly after you treat them, necessitating additional winter treatments.

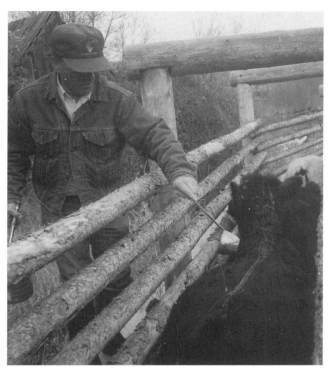

Treating for lice with a pour-on

Treatment

If one animal in a group has lice, the entire herd is probably infested and should be deloused before cold weather starts. Lice infest cattle all year, but numbers are lower in the summer because most are shed with old winter hair in the spring. Their reproduction rate also slows in warm weather. In the summer there is more heat on the animal's back, so lice tend to leave

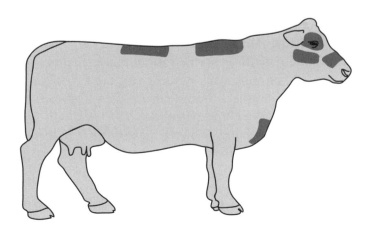

Areas on the body where lice are most easily seen

that area, slowing reproduction. Lice multiply much faster in cold weather; the time between egg laying and adult stages is much shorter, so there are more generations in a shorter time span, with numbers increasing astronomically.

Since lice populations build as the animal grows winter hair, you should delouse your cattle before this buildup, to minimize parasite load as the herd goes into winter. Increased body contact between animals, as when cattle are congregated for feeding or brought into corrals for weaning or vaccinating, aids in the spread of lice. Winter hair gives lice protection and an ideal environment for reproduction. Thus, lice control is more crucial in cold climates. Some stockmen in southern regions do not need to treat for lice.

Tips for Delousing

There are several treatments. Some are *topical* and some are systemic. Since there are often several species of lice on cattle at the same time, you usually need a treatment that kills both biting and sucking lice. Insecticides for lice are sprayed on, poured on, or applied by the cattle themselves via back rubbers or dust bags. Consider the following facts when choosing and applying a delouser:

▶ Sprays don't kill eggs, so a second application is needed 10 to 14 days later (no later than 18 days later) to kill lice that hatch in the interim.

▶ Spraying causes stress if cattle must be treated in cold weather; it should be done on a warm day to keep animals from chilling.

▶ Back rubbers or dust bags should be located where cattle will readily use them — on the way to water or feed — but not where any spillage might contaminate water sources.

▶ Dust bags and oilers (back-rubbing apparatus that spreads an oil-based insecticide over the animal when she rubs) take time to effectively reduce a high louse population; they are best used as a preventive to hinder lice buildup.

▶ Follow directions when applying any insecticide, and do not use it in conjunction with other insecticides, such as fly tags.

▶ If using pour-ons, do not exceed the maximum recommended dosage.

▶ Some pour-ons should be applied along the topline of the animal from shoulders to hips. Others need part of the dose applied to the top of the neck and down the face. Read the directions carefully.

▶ Oil-based pour-ons spread through the hair coat, down the animal's sides, and over the whole body.

Caution! Toxic Chemicals

Some systemic pour-on products are toxic to dairy cattle and to beef cattle of Brahman breeding. They may collapse and go into shock. Read labels, and avoid use of these products on susceptible animals. Some systemic insecticides must be used before winter to avoid toxic reactions to grubs being killed while migrating through the esophagus or spinal-nerve canal. Ask your vet for advice on insecticides and dewormers, including which products might be best for your situation and time of year. Be sure to follow carefully all label directions and cautions regarding human contact.

Lice eventually come into contact with the oil, which stays on the skin and hair for a while.

▶ Other pour-ons are systemic, absorbed into the body to kill lice, grubs, and internal worms at the same time.

▶ Injectable avermectin products (also effective against most internal parasites) kill sucking lice but not chewing lice. Newer ivermectin pour-on formulations are effective against both varieties.

▶ Whenever you treat for lice, treat all cattle on the farm. If you treat cows, also treat their calves and vice versa or the untreated animals will soon reinfest the treated animals.

▶ If treating one group at a time, put treated cattle in a "clean" pasture with no across-the-fence access to untreated cattle, so they won't be reinfested.

▶ Don't put treated animals back where they were rubbing and scratching.

▶ Treated animals should not be allowed contact with feed bunks, corrals, or other contaminated facilities for at least 7 days. Eggs on rubbed-off hairs are viable for up to a week.

▶ Never underdose an animal; if you don't kill all the lice, they serve as a source for the rest of the herd. Underdosing can also lead to resistant lice.

▶ Treat all new animals before adding them to your herd. Some delousing products have a two-treatment protocol; if this is the kind of product you are using, any new animals should be kept isolated until they've had both treatments.

Lice control can be attained with a systemic product that kills both lice and grubs in fall, before the cutoff date for grubs in your climate; then treat again for lice only, using nonsystemic products, late in winter if animals show signs of lice infestation, rubbing and scratching. Many ranchers treat for lice in the fall at weaning. In some regions this also kills the last of the *horn flies* (see page 150). But don't treat too early or you won't get winter-long control of lice; they will build up again by January or February.

A louse-free herd can be maintained if you treat every animal on the farm and treat all new animals before you add them to the herd, whatever time of year they're brought in.

GLORTIMER was a fat 2½-month-old calf when he and his mama, Glory Belle, went to range pasture in May of 1975. Late that month we saw Glortimer bawling for his mama, and we spent several hours looking for her but couldn't find her. The next day we moved the cattle to another range pasture, but by that time Glortimer was missing, too. We searched for him, hoping to bring him home and raise him on one of our milk cows, but it got too dark to keep looking.

We rode all the next day, searching, but he wasn't there. We thought he might have gone through a fence to our neighbor's cattle, so we rode through those pastures, too. We rode every day for a week, searching for him, and discovered his mother's hide. Glory Belle had been shot, skinned, and butchered, and the rustler had thrown her hide in the brush. Finally, we gave up on Glortimer. Our neighbor had seen a stray calf with his herd but he didn't stay. The little orphan kept on going — through more fences — searching for Mama.

Late that fall we got a phone call from a rancher farther down the valley. A skinny little calf with our brand had turned up with his cows when they came home from summer range. Lynn and I drove down and looked at the pathetic little creature in the corral. It was our calf; he had our brand, and his ear tag had Glory Belle's brisket tag number, but this poor little guy was a bag of bones with long, shaggy hair. He was smaller than when we'd seen him last. He'd survived but had not grown. He was weak and had diarrhea, lice, and worms.

We hauled him home and started calling him "the orphan." Our kids renamed him Orphy. He was too weak to be wild and didn't struggle when we lifted him out of the pickup and carried him to the barn. The weather was cold and windy, and we didn't want him to get pneumonia in addition to his other problems.

We put delousing powder all over him to get rid of the lice, dewormed him, and tried to feed him hay and grain. He didn't know how to eat grain and wasn't very interested in hay. He refused to nurse a bottle and was so weak that he didn't care whether he lived or died.

Being weaned so young, he hadn't had enough protein for growth; his bones were tiny. When he lost his mama, his digestive tract was not yet mature enough to handle a total roughage diet, and it's a wonder he survived. Now, four months later, he was so sick and stunted we weren't sure he could recover. We gave him our best hay, but he only nibbled at it.

One day that winter he just gave up. We found him lying in a corner in the barn, too weak to stand. We propped him up and hung a heat lamp over him and fed him milk with a stomach tube through the nostril and into the stomach. After that, we fed him milk every day by tube. When he was a year old in February, he was only as big as a 3-month-old calf. He still refused to nurse a bottle, so we continued the tube feedings all winter and spring.

Gradually he gained strength and ate more hay. When green grass came, we put him in a little pasture near the barn. I still fed him milk once a day, but he didn't like the stomach tube and always retreated to the far corner of his pasture. He *did* like the feeling of milk in his tummy, however. He'd stand there, resigned, and let me put the tube in his nose to the back of his throat, where he swallowed it as I pushed it on down into his stomach. With green grass and milk, he finally started looking like a calf.

Orphy lost a year of his life due to starvation and the effects of severe parasite infestation. We stopped feeding him milk when he finally reached the size and weight of a 6-month-old calf. By the time he was 2 he looked like a yearling. Tender loving care — and ridding him of the parasites that nearly killed him — helped make up for the lost time he'd spent wandering in the mountains without a mama.

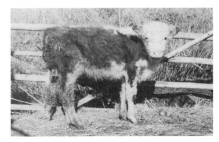
"Orphy," a few days after we brought him home. He's been deloused and dewormed but still has a lot of dried manure stuck to his tail.

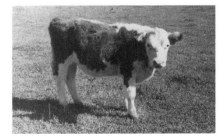
Orphy at 1½ years, looking like a 6-month-old calf. He's finally starting to grow and fill out.

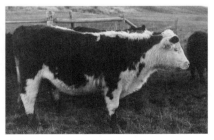
Fully recovered but still growing and making up for lost time, here is Orphy at 2 years, the same size as our yearlings.

Mites

Several kinds of mites live on or in the skin of cattle, causing a skin condition called scab or *mange.* Most mites are tiny and hard to see with the naked eye. Mange mites *(Psoroptes, Sarcoptes,* and *Chorioptes)* feed on the skin surface or burrow just beneath it, creating tunnels up to an inch (2.5 cm) long. Mites prick the skin to feed on tissue fluids (not blood), making itchy, oozing wounds. The most serious type of mange is called *scabies;* it causes great discomfort.

Sarcoptic mites burrow inside the skin. Fluid seeps from the tunnel openings and dries to form tiny bumps. A secreted toxin causes intense skin irritation and itching. The host animal continually scratches, rubbing out hair in affected areas and damaging the skin, often rubbing it raw. Hides from infected animals may be severely damaged and of little value. Mites may spread over the entire body, creating large, cracked, scabby areas on the thickened skin. They are transmitted from one animal to another by direct contact.

Scabies

Sarcoptic mites cause scabies, a reportable disease; animals with scabies must be quarantined and treated. Scabies mites are very active on the host and easily spread from one animal to another by direct contact. Due to extensive control efforts, cattle scabies is now rare in North America.

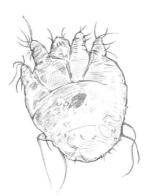

A Sarcoptes *scab mite (female) has a rounded body and backward-projecting spines on the back, blunt mouthparts, and long, unjointed leg stalks. The third and fourth pair of legs do not extend beyond the rim of the body.*

A Psoroptes *mange mite (female) has an oval body, sharp, piercing mouthparts, and long, jointed leg stalks.*

> **SIGHTING MITES**
>
> Psoroptic mites appear first on the withers, spread along the neck and back, invade over shoulders and brisket, and eventually move in on the belly and flanks. Adults and nymphs feeding on the skin surface cause fluid to ooze from breaks in the skin and form a scab.

Symptoms

When you first detect a scabies problem, you may think the animal has lice; she's kicking and scratching, with patches of hair rubbed off. Scabies lesions appear first on the head, neck, and withers; then bare spots rapidly spread over the body and may become raw. Serum oozing from skin mixes with dirt to form an infected, thick scab that hardens to a yellow-gray color. Skin is nearly twice as thick as normal and has a heavy crusting and elephant-hide appearance.

The animal constantly tries to relieve the itch, rubbing on fences, feeders, and trees, or lying down and rubbing on the ground. Mites may attach to any part of the body from nose to tail tip, and some animals become denuded of hair. The animal is so preoccupied with the itching that she spends little time eating and rapidly loses weight. Debilitation may increase susceptibility to other diseases.

Prevention

Never expose your herd to animals infected with mites. Do not buy any animals that are itchy and scratching with patches of hair missing. If one animal in a herd becomes infected, treat them all to halt the spread of this damaging condition. A vet can take a skin scraping from the outer edges of the scabs to check for mites and assist with treatment.

Mange Mites

Other mites include chorioptic, psorergatic, and *demodectic* mites. These cause itchiness and discomfort but not the severe lesions of scabies.

Symptoms

Affected animals lick and scratch, constantly swish their tails, and may lose hair due to continual rubbing. Small *papules* (tiny lumps) may appear on the withers. Mites may concentrate on the pasterns (below the *dewclaws*), inner surfaces of the legs, in front of the udder, and the tail head. Typical signs are flaky skin, occasional scabs, and hair rubbed off. Demodectic mites live in dense colonies inside hair follicles and cause tiny swellings that may grow to pea size or larger.

Signs of mange usually show up in late fall and winter. The lesions may heal in spring, and hair grows back, but there are still a few mites on the animal, and the problem recurs the next fall. The life cycle is completed in 10 to 20 days, depending on the species and environmental conditions. Mites and their eggs are spread by close contact but may also spread via contact with infested bedding, feed, and objects that infected cattle have rubbed against. Unless treated, an affected animal loses weight and drops in milk production.

Treatment
Treatment with the proper products will generally kill mites; consult your veterinarian. There are pour-ons, sprays, powders, dips, and injectable products that control mites.

Flies
These winged parasites reduce cattle weight gain by sucking blood and causing discomfort and irritation that interrupts grazing. Cattle pestered by flies expend energy stomping and swatting; they stay in the brush swatting flies, stand belly deep in a pond, or bunch in groups when they would otherwise be grazing. Lost grazing time means poor weight gain, less milk production, and sometimes lower conception rates during breeding season due to poor body condition. Cattle may try to run from flies and may suffer injury or bruised udders. Many types of flies affect cattle, including horn flies, stable flies, horse flies, deer flies, face flies (which also spread pinkeye), black flies, and gnats.

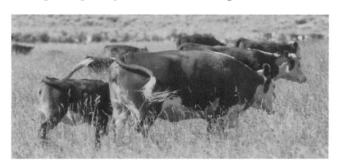

Cattle swat and swish their tails and sling their heads around to dislodge flies on the shoulders and withers.

Pesticide Disposal

Jugs of deworming or delousing products need meticulous disposal, since contents are generally hazardous to humans and other animals. Some are especially toxic to fish and aquatic life and should not be used or disposed of in areas where spillage might contaminate water sources. Most pesticides have an expiration date on the label but are still effective after those dates, and remnants do not need to be discarded; the product can be used until the jug is empty. But the empty containers need to be disposed of safely.

Some pesticides, such as the pour-on delousing product Atroban, carry a caution label, with instructions to keep the product away from food and animal feed and directions for disposal, such as triple rinsing with water, then recycling the jug or puncturing it and disposing of it in a sanitary landfill or incinerator, or by burning at home if allowed by state and local authorities (caution: stay out of the smoke).

Skull and Crossbones
A hazard label on any product indicates that it is extremely poisonous to humans and animals. Unused product and empty containers must be disposed of according to applicable federal, state, and local laws. Safer classes of pesticides that are not as environmentally hazardous have replaced most of the older, more hazardous products, such as organophosphate dewormers and delousers.

When in doubt about proper disposal methods for a certain product or its container, consult your veterinarian or county Extension agent. He or she will know the applicable rules and regulations regarding veterinary pesticides and proper container disposal.

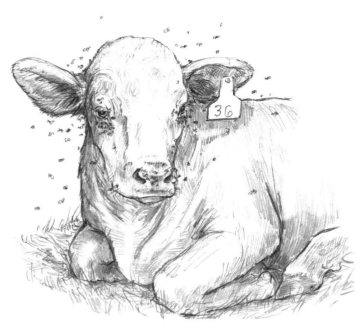

Flies are a constant annoyance during summer months.

Buffalo Gnats and Blackflies

Flies in this family *(Simuliidae)* are small and dark-colored, with a hunchback appearance. They hover around the eyes, ears, and nostrils of cattle and puncture the skin with painful bites to suck blood. Large numbers of gnats cause weakness from blood loss and even anaphylactic shock or death. Blackflies may suck blood from more than one animal and transmit bloodborne diseases. These flies often appear in swarms near rivers or swift-flowing streams that provide well-aerated water for their larval development. Other related gnats, including biting *midges* and *sand flies,* are also serious pests in some regions. It is difficult to protect cattle from these insects.

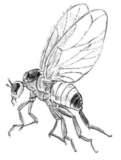

Buffalo gnat   *Blackfly*

Houseflies

These flies don't bite, but they feed on manure and secretions around eyes, nose, and mouth, and spread disease. They multiply dramatically wherever there's manure or rotting organic matter such as wasted feed or wet bedding to use as breeding sites.

Stable Flies

These gray-and-black flies are similar to houseflies in size, shape, and color, but are vicious biters with long, sharp mouthparts that stick out like bayonets from the head. They slice skin to drink blood, then rest on barn walls, feed bunks, and fence posts. They can travel miles from their breeding sites in wet debris like rotting hay, straw, or silage. A female fly may lay 500 to 600 eggs, and larvae develop into adults in 3 to 4 weeks. Old bedding or wasted hay around big bale feeders make ideal conditions for stable flies. In years past, stable flies were a problem just in confined cattle areas (dairies, feedlots) with manure buildup. But they are now a problem on farms that use bale feeders, because of the buildup of manure and organic matter around the feeders.

Stable flies bite cattle on the front legs. Animals may be restless, but generally bunch up in tight groups to protect themselves from these flies. Cattle may trample and beat out the grass when bunching and jostling. Usually the dominant cow is in the middle of the group where she's most protected.

Stable flies remain on the animal only long enough to get a blood meal. Since they primarily bite the legs, and most insecticides are applied to the animal's back, they rarely come in contact with insecticide for long enough to be killed. Even if you put insecticide on the legs, walking in a pasture tends to rub it off, especially if grass is wet with dew.

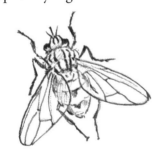

Stable fly (similar in size to a housefly)

Control of Stable Flies

Stable-fly control involves removing old bedding from barns and calving areas and properly composting it. It's also necessary to remove manure and wasted feed around bale feeders or scatter it so it dries. Unroll big bales around the pasture and rotate feeding areas to reduce buildup of organic matter.

▶ **Premise sprays** are helpful because stable flies spend more time in the surrounding environment than on cattle, but their use requires repeated spraying and is costly. If you don't want to use chemicals, biological control can be effective.

▶ **Parasitic wasps** don't sting and are no threat to humans or animals, but they can control stable flies, houseflies, *face flies,* and horn flies (all of which lay eggs in manure) if enough of them are present. The wasps lay eggs in fly *maggots,* and then the immature wasps feed on the maggots, eventually killing them.

These fly-managing wasps can be purchased from companies that raise them. They should be released in spring when flies first appear. New batches must be released every 2 to 4 weeks for continuous protection. Follow directions regarding the number of wasps needed for your herd. It usually takes at least 500 wasps per animal per month. Since the wasps affect only larval stages of flies, you may still need other methods to reduce a high population of biting flies, such as flytraps, dust bags, oilers, and sprays. If these methods are aimed at nonmanure areas where flies congregate, you won't kill wasps that are laying eggs in manure.

Horse- and Deerflies

Tabanids, horse- and deerflies, range from ⅓ inch to 1 inch (0.85 to 2.5 cm) in length. They have a painful bite, slashing skin with sharp mouthparts and drinking blood that flows freely from the wound. If disrupted, they may fly to another animal carrying bloodborne diseases with them. These flies breed near water or mud and are prevalent around ponds, lakes, marshes, or wet ground. The larvae develop in mud or water and feed on immature forms of other insects in the mud. After hatching out during the first hot days of summer, adult flies may travel as much as 5 to 10 miles (8.1 to 16.1 km) from their breeding sites to find a blood meal.

Drawbacks to Chemical Control of Parasites

Routine use of chemicals for controlling parasites leads to resistant strains of parasites. After so many years, the dewormer or insecticide no longer works as well because a high percentage of the parasite population has become resistant. This resistance problem can be minimized or delayed by not using the same chemical every year and by not exposing parasites to low levels of the chemical. Always use a sufficient dosage to kill all the parasites.

Another drawback to chemicals is that they may kill or hinder beneficial insects or other organisms that play a role in killing flies or breaking down manure and hindering fly and worm life cycles. Constant use of chemicals also threatens to promote increased numbers of cattle with little natural resistance to parasites.

Before pesticides came into use, cattle with low resistance carried heavier loads of parasites and were dragged down more than an average animal. Under natural conditions, individuals with less resistance were too thin and less fertile and did not reproduce as well. Over time, nature selected for resistant animals — animals that were better able to survive and perpetuate their genetics. Some breeds, such as Brahman and certain African cattle, have more resistance to flies than English and European cattle.

Within any breed, there are also some individuals with more resistance than others. In any herd, you'll find some animals bothered by fewer flies and others that always have more parasites or flies. It's also common to find more flies on black cattle than on red or light-colored cattle in early summer, perhaps because the black hide is warmer.

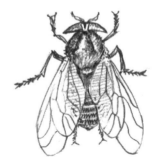

Horsefly/deerfly (larger than a stable fly)

Mosquitoes

Mosquitoes are gnatlike insects (*Culicidae* family). Several species attack livestock and may transmit disease as well as cause painful bites. Large numbers cause excessive blood loss, loss of weight, and decreased milk production.

Face Flies

Face flies, *Musca autumnalis,* are the same size and shape as houseflies and stable flies. They feed on eye secretions, nasal mucous, saliva, and serum oozing from wounds, rather than bite to ingest blood. Face flies cause eye irritation and are instrumental in the spread of pinkeye from one animal to another.

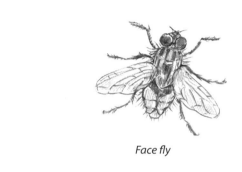

Face fly

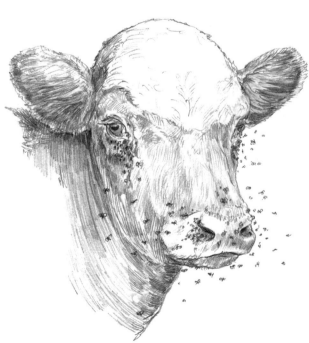

Face flies are the most important vector in the transmission of pinkeye. They congregate near the moist areas of the face.

It was once thought that face flies had mouthparts similar to a housefly's that sponge up nutrient material from objects they land on. With the use of an electron microscope, Kansas State University researchers discovered in 1993 that the face fly has sharp microscopic teeth on the end of its tongue to scratch and irritate the animal's eye, making it water. This gives the fly access to protein-rich eye secretions, the mainstay of its diet. Animals bothered by face flies produce more tears than normal, and the eye is irritated. Pinkeye bacteria (see chapter 9) gain access to the eye via tiny wounds in the cornea. If flies scrape an infected eye and then move to another animal, they carry bacteria to that next animal.

Face flies don't travel far from where they hatch (less than a mile [1.6 km]), spend a short time on one animal, then move on to another. At any given time only 5 to 10 percent of the local face-fly population is on the cattle; the rest are in the pasture. When they're on cattle, they stay just long enough to feed on eye secretions. They are not as exposed to pesticides applied to cattle as are horn flies (see below). Systemic pour-ons won't kill face flies because these flies don't eat blood. Since they congregate around the eyes and face, however, insecticide ear tags will control them.

Horn Flies

Of all the flying parasites, horn flies, *Haematobia irritans,* probably cause the most problem for cattle. Infestations can result in great economic loss for the rancher, with cows producing less milk and calves not gaining the proper weight. They are also a cause of summer mastitis; when they feed on cows' teats, the resulting lesions enable pathogens to get through the skin.

Horn flies spend most of their time on the animal — day and night drinking blood 20 to 30 times in a 24-hour period. During the peak of fly season, an animal may have thousands of these flies covering neck, shoulders, and back (enduring up to 60,000 bites per day). Smaller numbers may cluster on the rest of the body or along the underside and belly midline. During the heat of the day, flies group on the shady underside of the body. They leave the animal just long enough to find fresh cow manure to lay eggs.

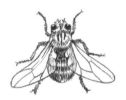

Horn fly (smaller than the stable fly)

Cattle covered with horn flies try to rub them off by slinging their heads over their backs or walking under low trees or bushes to brush them off. The result of these efforts: flies rise up in a black cloud and settle right back down on the animal again.

Studies have shown that horn flies reduce daily weight gain in calves about ⅛ to ¼ pound (0.06 to 0.11 kg) per day or more. Research in Auburn, California, showed that calves from herds with fly control gained ½ pound (0.23 kg) more per day than calves from unprotected herds. In Nebraska studies, where fly season is 3.5 months long, horn-fly control resulted in 14 pounds (6.35 kg) more weight per calf at weaning time. In Georgia, where fly season is 5 months long, fly control can give as much as 40 more pounds (18.1 kg) per calf. In mountainous regions of the Northwest, heavy fly infestations can reduce weight gain by ¼ pound per day, which translates into 10 to 20 pounds (4.5 to 9.1 kg) less at weaning. For the stockman this means many dollars lost — many more than the cost of fly control!

Horn-Fly Life Cycle

Horn flies have a short 11-day life cycle in warm weather. Many generations live and die during fly season. Adult flies spend most of their time on the host, sucking blood; females leave the host only to deposit eggs on fresh manure. A fly may lay several hundred eggs in its lifetime. Eggs hatch in 24 hours or less, and maggots become pupae in 4 to 8 days if temperatures are between 75 and 80°F (23.8 and 26.7°C). Fly populations peak in early summer; however, the life cycle from egg to adult may take 2 to 3 weeks in cool conditions. Horn flies may breed continuously in regions with a warm climate; in a cold climate they overwinter in the pupal stage under manure piles, emerging as adults the next spring.

Control Horn Flies, and Face Flies Will Flee

Any tag will control face flies and help to prevent pinkeye. Face flies don't seem to develop resistance. Horn flies are a larger economic problem (affecting every animal on your farm) than outbreaks of pinkeye. Choose a tag that will adequately control horn flies, and it will also control face flies. To know if tags are working, check the number of horn flies on the backs and shoulders of cows. If you have recently installed insecticide tags and still see large numbers of flies, they are resistant.

Horn-Fly Control

Horn flies can be controlled with insecticides, which can be applied in several ways. Sprays are a quick way to get rid of all flies on the animal and may have a residual effect for 2 to 6 weeks, depending on the timing of the next rainstorm. Back rubbers and dust bags are effective in gateways through which cattle travel each day or on their way to water. This is more effective than hanging an oiler or duster under a tree in the pasture; it must be located where cattle rub under it daily. The applicator should not be too close to a water source, to avoid contamination of the water. Insecticide spilled into a stream could harm aquatic insects and other invertebrates. Insecticides for flies do not harm mammals but kill flies and other insects by affecting their nervous systems.

Any device that sprinkles insecticide dust on the animal when he rubs will control flies. Dust bags or devices employed where cattle reach in to lick salt or minerals and brush the applicator with their neck and shoulders are effective. If the applicator is recharged regularly and protected from moisture to prevent caking and the product is changed from year to year so flies won't develop resistance, these methods do a good job of killing horn flies.

▶ **Oral larvicides** added to feed or mineral mixes or given in a bolus by mouth kill fly larvae when flies lay their eggs in manure. The larvicide goes through the digestive tract intact (with no harm to the animal), ending up in manure. There, it inhibits growth of the larvae, and they eventually die. For this kind of "feed-through" product to work, each animal must consume the proper amount. The drawback in a mineral mix is that some animals don't eat it and others eat more than their share. Giving it to each animal in a time-release bolus is more effective.

This method can break the life cycle and can keep cattle free of horn flies most of the summer unless they come from neighboring untreated herds. Horn flies can easily fly a mile (1.6 km) in a day — and up to 5 miles (8 km) if necessary — to find a host. Unless your cattle are isolated, or your neighbor is also controlling flies, a feed-through product won't give adequate protection.

▸ **Pour-on chemicals and sprays** give good control for a month or so, reducing fly populations to less than 100 flies per animal, but these must be repeated. Be sure to select insecticides that flies are not yet resistant to. Most control methods must be repeated or used in conjunction with other methods, for season-long control. Many stockmen also use insecticide-impregnated ear tags. These can be put into the ears at the start of fly season, and the animal rubs insecticide over shoulders and body as she slings her head at the flies.

▸ **Ear tags** must be effective through the peak of fly season. Don't tag too early or the protection will run out by late summer. Cattle can tolerate low fly populations in early spring. Reserve your most effective control weapon for later in the season when large numbers of flies take a toll on unprotected cattle. Start your fly-control program when you can count at least 50 flies on one side of a cow. Count during a cool part of the day; during warmer hours the horn flies move under the belly, making them harder to count.

Fly tags should be installed in late spring or early summer when there are 50 to 100 flies on each animal. If cattle go to spring range pastures, waiting this long to put in tags is not possible; cattle are already out on the range by the appropriate time, so all tagging, treatments, and vaccinating must be done before they are turned out in the mountains. However, the later you can put tags in, the more of the fly season they'll cover. Several types of tags are designed to be effective for up to 5 months but are most effective during the first 60 days. If you wait until May or June to put them in, the better your season-long fly control will be.

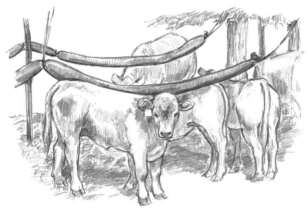

Back rubbers and other devices allow cattle to self-apply insecticide and are often an effective way to control flies or lice.

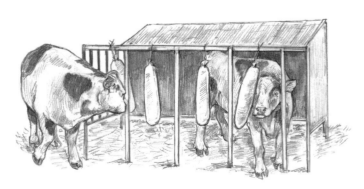

Dust bags apply insect powder when cattle rub on the bags.

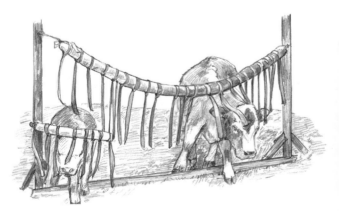

Face strips apply insecticide to the head.

EAR-TAG RESISTANCE

THE FIRST INSECTICIDE ear tags became available in the 1970s. The first pyrethroid tag came into use in 1980, but some five years later, horn flies began to develop resistance to pyrethroid insecticides. Next came organophosphate tags, to which flies were slower to develop resistance. Resistance occurs because a small percentage of flies in any given fly population can survive the insecticide's effect on their nervous systems or they produce an enzyme that breaks down the chemical before it can kill them. These flies survive, and though they are a minority at first, they are soon the majority, since they live to produce offspring. As survivors, their resistance is passed to succeeding generations.

With susceptible flies killed off, the resistant flies soon increase dramatically. This occurs faster in regions that have a long fly season and many generations of flies per year. In northern climates with short fly seasons, it took several years before resistant populations were noticed, whereas in southern areas this happened much sooner. Companies marketing fly tags came out with different formulations to give adequate control. Stockmen should periodically switch to a different type of insecticide.

There are several ways resistance is hastened, including the use of insecticide at levels that are too low. Most tags work best with two tags per animal, one in each ear.

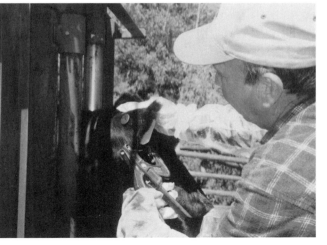

Installing insecticide ear tags

But few stockmen want to spend that much for tags. Some put one tag on each animal, and some use only one tag per pair (in either the cow or the calf, which means only 25 percent of the recommended dose of insecticide). Dosage that low can result in accelerated development of fly resistance.

Some companies developed organophosphate tags approved for adequate control at the rate of one per animal. Tests showed these tags perform well at this dose but not for as long; fly control using just one tag drops dramatically after 12 to 14 weeks. Protection may run out about the time it's needed most, in late summer. Best results are still obtained using a tag in each ear.

Some stockmen put two tags in either the cow or the calf (rather than four tags for both). It's better to put both tags on the cow. A cow has more flies (larger body surface), so more flies are killed if tags are in her ears, and she does a better job of spreading insecticide onto the calf than her calf can do spreading it onto the cow.

Fly resistance may be hastened by leaving tags in the ears all year. After about 5 months insecticide level in a tag drops below what's needed to kill flies and continues to drop until there is no insecticide left. If flies are still active after the tag has lost effectiveness, these low levels encourage development of fly resistance. It's best to remove tags in the fall.

Use of the same insecticide for many years results in fly resistance. Eventually you must rotate between synthetic pyrethroids and organophosphate insecticides. In southern regions with long seasons (20 to 25 generations of flies per season), this alternation should be done yearly or even more often. In northern areas (15 to 18 generations of flies per season), the same class of tag can be used for 2 or 3 years before switching, to allow time for resistance to one type to disappear from the fly population before that type is used again. If you used organophosphate tags for 2 or 3 years, you may be able to switch back to a pyrethroid tag; the second- or third-generation pyrethroids may work as well as the early ones did when first introduced.

Most veterinarians recommend using organophosphate tags for 2 years, then pyrethroids for a year, then back to organophosphates. Flies develop resistance to organophosphates more slowly. Rotating among various pyrethroids won't give adequate control because if flies have become resistant to one, they are resistant to the others. You must switch classes of insecticides when you change to a different tag. Many veterinarians do not recommend tags that contain both classes of insecticide, since eventually horn flies develop resistance, and then you'll have nothing to switch to.

The crucial time to control horn flies is while the cow is raising her calf. If you can protect the pair until the calf is weaned, it can make a difference in weaning weights. If you wean in late summer or early fall, put tags in during early June. Use pour-on insecticides or dust applicators earlier if you need to start protection sooner. If calves are weaned midsummer, tag the cows earlier. If the tags' effectiveness wanes by late summer, use a different insecticide starting early August (though this won't be feasible if cattle are still on the range). Using a pour-on or oiler late in the fly season will kill any that started building resistance to the tags and will knock out any buildup of flies that is due to fading effectiveness of the tags. This will reduce the number of resistant flies going into their overwintering phase, making fly control less difficult next year.

Many producers in southern areas with long fly seasons get the most complete horn-fly control by using ear tags in spring, then a follow-up treatment with a good systemic product (that kills both internal and external parasites) about the first of August, when the tags' effectiveness wanes. The systemic product gives a few more weeks of control for adult flies, ensuring that there won't be a lot more eggs laid.

In one study of the effectiveness of insecticide tags for horn fly control, a flight of dung beetles moved in and the study had to be started over because the control group of cows (with no insecticide tags) had no horn flies. The dung beetles had eliminated the horn flies in the fresh manure. A large population of beetles can control horn flies because, even though the beetles are active only a few months of the year, this is the same time horn flies are active.

Biological Control of Horn Flies with Dung Beetles

Aware of the problem of growing insect resistance to pesticides and not wanting to negatively impact the environment, many farmers and ranchers are trying to use less chemical pesticide and are seeking natural ways to control damaging parasites. One alternative for horn-fly control is the use of dung beetles. These amazing insects spend their entire lives in manure. Adult beetles use the liquid contents of manure for nourishment and also lay eggs in it. Hatching larvae consume the manure. The beetles help control parasites that depend on manure for part of their life

cycle. Some beetles also remove and bury manure, which helps fertilize soil and get rid of large accumulations of manure.

Beetles that feed on cattle manure are not active during cold months but are active year-round in warm regions. Native beetles are relatively small compared to species imported from Africa. The latter do a better job of manure management and fly control. Today there are more than 90 species of dung beetles in North America, including some that were imported during the 1970s and 1980s.

Of these species, three varieties exist:

▸ **Dwellers** live in manure pats, laying their eggs in them.

▸ **Rollers (tumblebugs)** are larger, about the size of a thumbnail. They cut out balls of manure, lay an egg in each "brood ball," and roll it away to bury it, pushing it with their hind legs.

▸ **Tunnelers** dig below the manure pat and put manure into the ground, leaving just its dry shell.

Dung beetles remove manure from the ground surface, preventing buildup that smothers grass. Tunnelers are most beneficial, burying manure, churning up soil, and fertilizing it. In Australia dung beetles are used for horn-fly control. Beetles bury 95 percent of horn-fly eggs and larvae and 90 percent of internal parasites that are passed in manure. A high percent of cattle parasites that depend on manure are inactivated or destroyed by dung-beetle activity. Dung beetles are attracted only to fresh manure, where horn flies lay their eggs and also where eggs

DUNG-BEETLE TUNNELERS AND ROLLERS

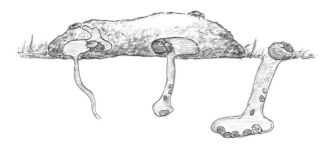

Some types of dung beetles shape manure into brood balls and roll them away to bury them (right). Others tunnel under the manure pat and deposit the manure in their tunnels (left).

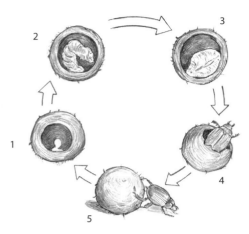

1. Female lays a single egg inside each brood ball.
2. Larva hatches a few days later.
3. Larva pupates 1–4 weeks later.
4. Young adult emerges and digs its way to the surface.
5. Adult beetle shapes dung into brood balls that will nourish growing larva. He may bury the brood balls in tunnels under the dung pat.

Why Use Beetles?

Today's cattle producers face the challenge of trying to stay profitable while being good stewards of the land and conscientious caretakers of the environment. Dung beetles can be allies in this challenge by making soil and vegetation healthy while at the same time helping to control internal and external parasites. A single pat of manure without dung beetles can generate 60 to 80 adult horn flies. Long-term control of flies is better achieved by using dung beetles to degrade manure than by sporadic application of chemicals.

Fly resistance is a problem when relying on chemical control; mechanical breakdown of manure by beetles is a more dependable control. Dung beetles are a help to agriculture as well — they bury manure, add nitrogen to the soil, increase grazing acreage by eliminating areas around manure piles that are often not grazed, reduce the effects of parasites, and improve control of flies.

of internal parasites can be found. Even if those eggs hatch, they can't get back up to the ground surface after beetles bury the manure.

Dung beetles help reduce the numbers of any flies or internal parasites that pass eggs in manure. Birds are attracted to the site, tearing manure pats apart to eat beetles, which helps spread manure and disrupt parasite development. But some types of dewormers and pesticides destroy dung beetles, killing the larval stage. Ivermectin products, for instance, will eventually decimate beetle populations because fresh manure of treated cattle is toxic to beetle larvae.

If you want to use deworming/delousing products without affecting the dung-beetle population, use products other than ivermectin and use them only in early spring or late fall, so there will be several months during summer when beetles can reproduce and keep horn flies at bay. If you've inadvertently killed off your local dung-beetle population, they can still move in from surrounding areas; some species can fly distances up to 10 miles (16.1 km). It may take 3 to 4 years for native beetles to reestablish after heavy use of ivermectin products. Although Australian stockmen have been able to purchase dung beetles for their pastures for many years, there are currently no commercial sources of dung beetles in North America. They may become available in the future, however.

Biological Control with Ducks

Some stockmen with small herds control flies with Muscovy ducks. This breed is not a water duck; it eats insects and doesn't need commercial feed. The ducks range freely in pens and pastures and are prolific breeders. They follow cattle around, searching through manure and scattering the piles so thinly that no fly larvae survive. It takes about four ducks per cow to adequately control the fly population. The ducks also eat adult flies and pick flies off cattle when they are lying down chewing their cuds. Cattle become accustomed to the ducks and stretch their heads and necks lower to the ground while lying there resting so the ducks can reach more flies.

Muscovy ducks are readily available for purchase for your ranch. Check out ads in farm and poultry magazines or on the Web if you're interested in purchasing these animals.

The battle against flies is constant, but there are several ways to reduce the numbers of these costly pests without using pesticides and toxic chemicals. Pesticide chemicals are a short-term solution because eventually the pests develop resistance and new pesticide must be created. These manufactured poisons can sometimes have harmful effects on species other than the targeted pest. A growing number of stockmen are seeking other solutions. Biological methods of fly control such as dung beetles, predator wasps, and fly-eating birds can help.

Now there are also some innovative flytraps that don't depend on pesticides for killing flies. One product that controls biting flies (especially horse flies and deer flies that can come to your place from miles away, and can't be controlled by dung beetles or predator wasps because they don't lay eggs in manure) is the Epps Biting Fly Trap, invented by Alan Epps, a cattleman in Oklahoma. His trap is now made and marketed by Horseline Products in Henderson, Tennessee.

Since biting flies are attracted to the shape and silhouette of an animal, Epps made a framework of wood with a large contrasting surface area, utilizing a dark portion and transparent panels to simulate air space above the animal and under the belly — the areas flies normally circle before landing to bite. When flies hit the transparent sheets, they ricochet into trays of water below, and drown. The only maintenance required is to periodically dump out the dead flies and replenish the water (the trays hold 3.5 gallons) and add about 8 drops of dishwashing soap to each tray. The soap breaks the surface tension on the water so the insects can't float on it. They are immediately wetted, sink, and drown.

Research studies showed that one of these traps kills about one pound of flies each day (the actual number depending on your fly population) and draws horse flies from more than 20 acres of the surrounding area. All biting flies (including horse flies, deer flies, stable flies, black flies, and mosquitoes) are attracted to large, dark objects, and tend to fly around the animal 2 or 3 times before landing to bite. The flies run into the trap panels thinking they are flying over the animal or around its legs.

Ticks

Ticks are arachnids, like spiders, with eight legs. They have mouthparts that protrude forward from the head, and when ingesting blood, the headlike structure is inserted into the skin, fastening to the host animal with strong teeth so the tick can fill its saclike body with blood. These small parasites affect cattle adversely by sucking their blood, causing discomfort and hide damage (that may open the way for invasion of the body by other parasites and pathogens), and spreading disease.

Several types of ticks feed on cattle; some are hard-bodied and very flat (until they engorge with blood), and others are soft-bodied. The latter may appear wrinkled, leathery, raisinlike or spiny. Some species — the Rocky Mountain wood tick, the lone

FOUR TYPES OF TICKS

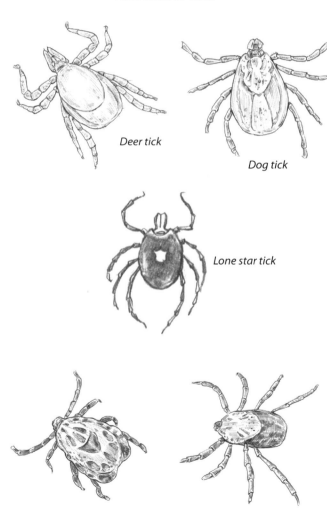

Deer tick

Dog tick

Lone star tick

Male (left) and female (right) Rocky Mountain tick

star tick, the black-legged tick, the American dog tick, the soft-bodied tick, the Gulf Coast tick, and the spinose ear tick — are more common in certain geographic areas. In any one location there may be one to six species, and each has a preferred feeding site on the animal. Some species attach around the head, some feed in the ears, while others feed around the *anus,* under the tail, around the udder, and on the underside of the animal.

The life cycle of different species is variable, but it takes one to two years for most ticks. Some species require two or three hosts, spending their immature stages feeding on different animals between when they hatch and the time they become adults. The adult female tick must engorge with blood before she lays eggs. In the life cycle of a three-host tick, larvae hatch from eggs laid on the ground and attach to a small mammal such as a rodent. After feeding on blood, engorged larvae drop to the ground to molt and become nymphs, which attach to a different host. After engorging on blood, nymphs drop to the ground and molt again to become adults and attach to yet another host. After filling with blood (some ticks becoming as large as a plump blueberry when full), females drop to the ground to lay eggs and die. A female may lay from 2,000 to 18,000 eggs.

The tick inserts anticoagulant into the host to thin the blood (making it easier to suck through its tiny mouth), which causes itching, swelling, and inflammation at the site of the bite. Host animals can have a serious reaction to the secretion of a toxin in the "saliva" of some species of hard-bodied ticks, especially if there are many ticks attached at the base of the skull. This toxic reaction produces a slow wasting disease called *tick paralysis.* The animal may not be able to stand and may die if the ticks are not removed from the base of the skull. Removal of ticks results in immediate recovery.

Ticks can transmit serious diseases, including anaplasmosis, bovine *piroplasmosis,* and *Lyme disease.* Boophilus ticks spread the highly fatal protozoan disease known as Texas cattle fever. This disease affected cattle in 14 southeastern states before a federal eradication program was begun in 1906. After an intensive program of dipping cattle, the United States was declared free of these ticks in 1943, but they are still a problem in Mexico.

A quarantine zone is maintained along the Rio Grande River in Texas for livestock and whitetail deer, the tick's main hosts, to keep from bringing these ticks into the United States. Any animals found that come from Mexico are captured and checked for ticks, then dipped with insecticide and sent back to Mexico. Ranchers who raise cattle in the quarantine zone must have cattle checked and dipped before they can be moved out of that zone.

Tick control along the border is very important. Agricultural scientists have estimated that if this tick becomes re-established in the United States it could cause the death of up to 90 percent of the cattle. It would be extremely difficult to eradicate this tick if

NATURAL HABITAT OF THE CATTLE-FEVER TICK

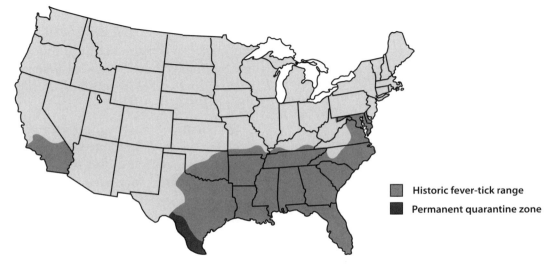

Historic fever-tick range

Permanent quarantine zone

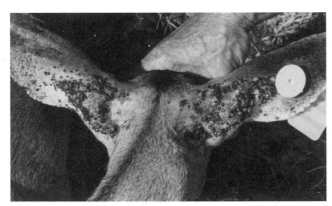

Ticks on a whitetail deer in Texas

it becomes established again, since the whitetail deer population (which was very low in the early 1900s, when the first eradication program was begun) has now expanded tremendously.

Treatment and Control

Ticks on cattle can be killed with various sprays, dips, and pour-on products. Read labels, and follow directions for use. Consult your vet for the most effective way to treat the varieties in your region.

Diseases Spread by Ticks

Many parasites feed on more than one host, acting as mechanical *vectors* physically transmitting pathogens from one animal to another, or they serve as part of the life cycle of a certain disease. In the latter situation, because the pathogen lives within its body in these instances, the parasite is also a host,

To remove a tick from a cow or a person, do not pull on its body, because the head and mouthparts could remain embedded in the skin.

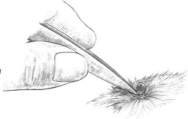

Instead, grasp the tick's head with tweezers as close to the skin as possible and pull straight out.

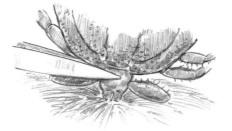

and it spreads the disease to cattle in the act of injecting "saliva" while sucking blood. Diseases currently spread by ticks in the United States include anaplasmosis, Lyme disease, and foothill abortion.

Anaplasmosis

Also called *yellow fever,* this disease is caused by *Anaplasma marginale,* a rickettsia, which is a genus of gram-negative bacteria that typically infect ticks, lice, fleas, and mites and can be transmitted to animals by the bites of these parasites. The anaplasmosis organism infects ticks and can be passed from one generation of tick to the next. It can be transmitted to susceptible cattle in two ways: biologically (from infected ticks) and mechanically (by the transfer of infected blood from one animal to another by flies or by hypodermic needles, dehorners, and other tools). Transmission is always via infected blood. There is no direct transmission between animals.

Incubation time is from 2 weeks to more than 3 months but is usually 3 to 4 weeks. Adult cattle are most susceptible. The disease is usually mild in calves or yearlings because young animals rapidly produce new red blood cells to replace the ones that are destroyed. The disease is sometimes fatal in animals up to 3 years of age and frequently fatal in older cattle. After recovery, an infected animal may carry and spread the disease for the rest of her life, even if she shows no more symptoms.

Anaplasmosis occurs in most states and is a large problem in Gulf Coast states and many western regions. Since ticks and insects spread the disease, animals in large pastures and range conditions are most at risk, though occasionally it can be passed from a cow to her unborn calf via the placental blood exchange. The Rocky Mountain wood tick is a common culprit, though other ticks may be involved. Most new disease cases crop up in late spring and early summer after flies and ticks become active.

▶ **Symptoms.** *A. marginale* infects red blood cells of cattle; the cow's immune system rejects her own red blood cells and destroys them. This causes severe anemia, increased pulse and respiration, pale mucous membranes, jaundice, weakness, depression, fever, loss of appetite, decreased milk production, and, in serious cases, change in disposition, abortion, and sometimes death. If lack of oxygen to the brain is severe, the animal will become aggressive and belligerent and may attack horses, people, and vehicles. Anaplasmosis can be diagnosed with a blood test.

▸ **Treatment.** Some broad-spectrum antibiotics are effective if administered together with supportive therapy such as fluid and electrolytes. If the animal is given antibiotics immediately, before the disease is advanced, she will generally recover. But in severe cases, the stress of catching and treating the animal may push her over the edge into aggressiveness or may kill her.

If susceptible cattle are brought to an area where anaplasmosis exists, they will become infected and get sick — and half of them will die unless treated. If you live in a region that has anaplasmosis, make sure any cattle you purchase were raised in an anaplasmosis area (and are likely to have natural immunity) or were vaccinated as young animals, before they come to that environment.

▸ **Prevention.** Control of insects is helpful but difficult. Proper disinfection of veterinary instruments and equipment can help prevent spread of the disease. Feeding antibiotics in grain during fly season can help keep susceptible animals from getting the disease and may eliminate the pathogen from the blood of carrier animals.

Vaccination may be helpful, if you live in an area where this disease is a problem. The first vaccines (available until 1998) were effective in preventing losses from anaplasmosis but had some serious drawbacks. Made from the killed pathogen harvested from cells of infected cattle, the vaccine stimulated some cows to produce antibodies that would later attack their calves' red blood cells and cause severe anemia when the newborn calf ingested colostrum.

Today there's modified live vaccine that's safe and effective for cattle less than a year old and that gives them a controlled infection so they become immune carriers. The vaccine cannot be given to adult animals, however, or it may sicken or kill them, just as the actual disease can. Base the decision to vaccinate on whether or not you live in a region where cattle and deer are often infected and there are ticks that transmit the disease. If you live in an area where some adult cattle become ill every year, routine vaccination of young cattle can prevent losses. This is a complicated disease, and since the need to vaccinate can vary from herd to herd, consult your vet.

Lyme Disease

The *Ixodes* deer tick spreads this disease. Cattle become infected after being bitten. Once infected, an animal can transmit the disease directly to other cattle via infected urine. Infected cows may also pass the disease to their unborn calves. In herds where cattle are in close contact (such as a dairy) the entire herd may be infected.

TICK AREAS IN THE UNITED STATES AND SOUTHERN CANADA

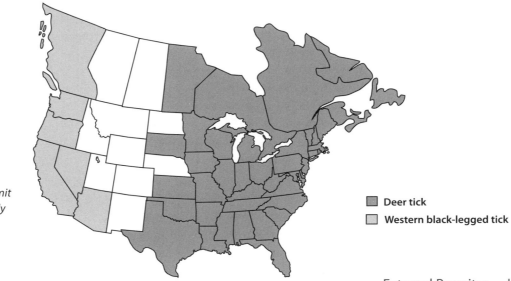

Regions where the two types of tick that transmit Lyme disease commonly occur

■ Deer tick
■ Western black-legged tick

Signs of Lyme disease include fever, lameness, and arthritis. Diagnosis is usually based on symptoms, history, exposure to *Ixodes* ticks, or exposure to infected herdmates. Broad-spectrum antibiotics (such as penicillin) can be used to treat Lyme disease. Although it is rare for humans to contract Lyme disease from cattle, it might be possible if someone were to come into contact with urine from an infected animal. Consult your veterinarian regarding treatment and transmission.

Foothill Abortion

Foothill abortion was first recognized as causing abortion in cattle that grazed foothill regions of coastal and central California, but it also occurs in southern Oregon and western Nevada. The pathogen is transmitted by the bite of a soft-bodied tick, *Ornithodoros coriaceus,* and may be similar to the one that causes Lyme disease.

Cattle with no prior exposure (and no immunity) may abort if bitten by a tick during the first six months of pregnancy; abortion generally occurs three to four months after the bite. The greatest risk for exposure is during warm weather. Pregnant cattle should not be brought into regions inhabited by these ticks.

Exposed animals usually have some immunity for a year or two. Some ranchers avoid abortions by exposing yearling heifers to tick-infested pastures before breeding to establish immunity before they are bred. Abortions can also be avoided by using tick-infested pastures after cows are past six months of pregnancy. Other ranchers have changed their breeding season to avoid overlapping of the susceptible gestation period with tick exposure.

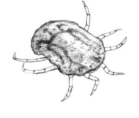 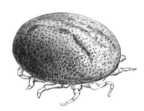

(Left) A tick before feeding on blood.
(Right) Engorged pajahuello (O. coriaceus), *the soft-bodied tick that transmits the pathogen that causes "foothill abortion."*

PART THREE

Body System Disorders

CHAPTER EIGHT

Digestive Problems

THE COW HAS A UNIQUE AND COMPLEX digestive system; she depends on microorganisms in the rumen to ferment and break down the fibrous portions of forages into usable nutrients. The four stomachs of the ruminant are more efficient at digesting a wide variety of food than the simple stomach of a human. The complexity of the system also makes it vulnerable to a great number of digestive problems, however. Some ailments arise due to factors that affect the workings of the beneficial microbes that reside in the rumen to facilitate fermentation of forages. Others are the result of the introduction of nonfood foreign objects into the digestive tract. All of theses conditions can cause discomfort, ill health, and in some cases, death if not discovered and treated in time.

Normal Digestion

Cattle have no top teeth in front, just a hard *dental pad* at the front of the upper jaw. They can't nip plants off close to the ground. Cows break off grass and other plants by biting against the dental pad with the lower teeth or by wrapping the tongue around the plants and using a swing of the head to break off a mouthful of feed. The strong tongue pulls food into the mouth. Because they swallow without much chewing, cattle produce lots of saliva to moisten feed and help it slide down the throat. They also produce and sling extra saliva over their backs on a hot day, to help cool themselves.

Cattle eat until the first stomach is full, then lie down and chew the cud, belching it up again in small increments and grinding it with their rear teeth (molars). Each belch contains liquid as well as food, which helps the mass come back up more easily. The cow then swallows the liquid again and chews the food mass more completely before swallowing it and burping up another mouthful. The twice-chewed food goes into the third stomach, where excess liquid is squeezed out. It then continues into the fourth stomach where it is further digested and passed on into the intestines.

A cow may spend only 8 to 10 hours grazing (compared to a horse that may graze up to 18 or more hours per day) or 5 to 6 hours eating hay, but spends

Why Belch?

A cow must burp to get rid of gas produced by fermentation of feed, but she also uses part of the gas before it gets away. Gas from digestive fermentation contains ammonia and volatile fatty acids. As the cow belches, the gas comes up the esophagus, and much of it goes into the windpipe and down to the lungs, where these nutrients are absorbed. A cow gains additional food value from her meal by inhaling her burps!

another 8 to 10 hours daily chewing her cud. This requires strong molars and may take up to 40,000 jaw movements each day.

Because a cow's natural diet is forage, which is high in fiber and low in nutrients, a great deal of feed material passes through after nutrients are absorbed. Cattle generally pass manure 10 to 12 times in a 24-hour period for a total of about 50 pounds (22.7 kg). When pasture plants are green and lush with high moisture and low fiber content or when cattle are fed rich low-fiber alfalfa hay, manure is soft and loose or even runny. Manure is firmer if cattle are eating mature pasture plants or high-fiber hay such as grass hay or coarse, mature, stemmy alfalfa.

Four Stomachs

Ruminant animals have a four-chambered stomach.

▸ **The rumen (first stomach)** is the largest compartment. It is a huge storage area in a mature animal, enabling her to process a lot of feed quickly. It's also a fermentation vat where microbes break down fibrous forage into usable nutrients. Thus cattle and other ruminants can utilize plant material humans can't digest. A ruminant eats a lot at one feeding and then chews the hurriedly eaten meal again to break down feed so it can be thoroughly digested by the fermentation process.

▸ **The reticulum (second stomach)** is a small compartment just ahead of the rumen. It is like a subdivision of the rumen — they work together — with the rumen being the major component. Feed must go through it to get to the rumen. The reticulum is called the honeycomb stomach because its lining is covered with small pockets to catch and hold any foreign material that might injure the digestive tract. For this reason it is also called the hardware stomach and is the place where foreign objects that lead to *hardware disease* are usually lodged (see page 174). The rumen and reticulum work together to break down roughage via fermentation by bacteria.

▸ **The omasum (third stomach)** is a small compartment that helps grind feed. It is also called the *manyplies;* the walls are lined with many folds and rough surfaces that aid in grinding coarse food. This is where any excess liquid is removed from the food (absorbed through the lining and into the bloodstream) as it passes through.

▸ **The abomasum (fourth stomach)** is also called the true stomach and is comparable in structure and function to the human stomach or that of any non-ruminant animal. It contains gastric glands that secrete gastric juice. The same enzymes and acids that digest our food are found in the abomasum.

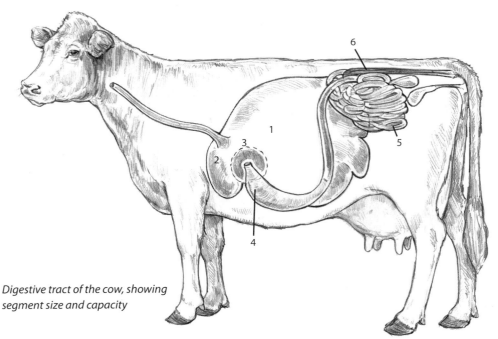

1. Rumen – holds 15–30 gallons
2. Reticulum – 3 gallons
3. Omasum – 5 gallons
4. Abomasum – 3–5 gallons
5. Small intestine – 14 gallons
6. Large intestine – 8 gallons

Digestive tract of the cow, showing segment size and capacity

In a young calf, this is where milk is digested. The fourth stomach lies underneath the other stomachs; milk has to go through the reticulum (via the *esophageal groove*) to get there (see page 163).

Once a calf starts eating solid food, the rumen is enlarging, and microbes start fermenting feed there and in the reticulum, even though milk continues to be digested in the abomasum. If milk goes into the reticulum, it is altered by microbes and can't be properly digested. Digestion of milk in the "true stomach" (instead of the reticulum/rumen) is so important that nature makes sure the milk goes into the abomasum even after the rumen is fully developed. When the calf nurses, his sucking action and the raised udder-reaching position of his head sends a signal to the brain that causes a fold in the front part of the reticulum to roll over and form a tube that becomes a temporary extension of the esophagus. Milk flows down this esophageal groove into the abomasum, bypassing the reticulum and rumen completely.

A newborn calf can be fed colostrum with a stomach tube or esophageal feeder probe. But a calf with a functional rumen gets less food value from milk or milk replacer fed by these methods or by drinking it from a bucket, since much of the nutritional value of milk is lost when processed by rumen microbes. If you feed with a nipple bucket or bottle, his sucking reflex and head position creates a direct pipeline into the true stomach.

Solid Feeding

The rumen of a young calf is small and nonfunctional. It starts to enlarge and acquire gut bugs for fermenting forage after he starts eating grass or hay. Calves often start nibbling solid feed by 2 or 3 days of age, following Mama's example. They obtain microbes for fermentation from the environment, ingesting them with feed.

Some calves start burping and chewing the cud when they are as young as 2 weeks of age. A bottle-raised calf, with no mother to mimic, may not start eating solid feed as quickly. You might have to stick food into his mouth to get him started eating it.

Rumen Microbes at Work

In a healthy rumen, microbes thrive in a fluid environment. They break down and digest feed, creating usable byproducts. For certain feeds, microbe populations change, because some types digest fiber and some digest starches. When grain is added to the diet, this limits the viability of microbes that digest cellulose. They need a more neutral pH and can't tolerate the acid environment of a rumen with more grain. When the animal is fed grain regularly, however, cellulose-digesting microbes are replaced with starch digesters that thrive in the acidity.

For efficient digestion and fewer digestive upsets, cattle need a healthy population of the proper kind of microbes to use the type of feed being eaten. When adding grain to a forage diet to fatten a steer or to supplement dwindling pasture with grain or high-energy pellets, the change should be made gradually, feeding only a small amount at first, so the microbes can adjust. It can be detrimental to add a lot of grain all at once or to change back and forth between a forage diet and a high-concentrate diet. If cattle eat fiber and starch intermittently, the microbe population is in constant turmoil. There won't be enough of either kind. This results in inefficient utilization of both types of feed.

Gas Production Is Normal

Gas in the rumen is a normal result of the digestion and fermentation required to break down fibrous feeds. Under normal conditions gas separates from the solids and liquid and rises to the top of the rumen. Pressure from this gas bubble stimulates the animal to belch; the rumen contracts and pushes the gas to the front where it collects around the esophagus opening. This valve is controlled by receptors in the rumen wall that can differentiate between liquid and gas. If covered by liquid (or foam), the valve remains tightly closed, and the animal cannot burp. This may be a protective mechanism to keep rumen fluid from coming up the esophagus and overflowing into the windpipe, which would be fatal.

Belching occurs when receptors around the esophagus sense gas is present. The opening relaxes, and the animal takes a deep breath that draws gas up the esophagus. More than half of this gas enters the windpipe and lungs (where some is absorbed as nutrients), and the rest is expelled through the mouth. Since most of the gas enters the lungs (and is exhaled), you rarely hear the animal burp, unless he is belching a large volume. Normal belching occurs about once a minute, except during peak fermentation periods, 2 to 4 hours after the animal has eaten, when the volume of gas produced increases. During this period the animal belches three to four times a minute.

Acidosis

The digestive disorder known as acidosis is most common in grain-fed cattle that eat too much starch or sugar in a short time and subsequently suffer from rapid production and absorption of acids from the rumen. This can occur in feedlot cattle or dairy cows on a high-grain diet or when cattle are pastured on cornstalks and consume corn left on the stalks. Grain is an unnatural feed for cattle; they evolved eating forage, which is digested more slowly in the rumen. The microbe population in the rumen is best suited for digesting fibrous forage plants by fermentation. If an abrupt change is made to grain, this disrupts the rumen environment, and acidosis is a common result.

Effects of subacute acidosis may be slight (mild indigestion, appetite loss, lowered weight gain, or drop in milk production). In acute cases, the effects may be so severe that the animal dies. Problems related to acute acidosis include sudden-death syndrome in feedlot cattle, *polioencephalomalacia* ("blind brainers" that wander aimlessly or can't stand up), *founder* (inflammation of the hoof attachments called laminitis), liver abscesses, inflammation of the rumen, and clostridial infections. Dairy cattle may have "low-milk-fat syndrome."

Acute Acidosis

In feedlots many of the cattle that go into shock and die suddenly are affected with acute acidosis, the result of the overwhelming increase in acid content of the body. They often die so fast that the illness is not noticed; they are simply found dead. The cattle that don't die quickly but wander aimlessly or can't get up often recover if given an injection of thiamine (one of the B vitamins). Thiamine is important to proper brain and nerve function, but under normal conditions cattle never need supplemental B vitamins because bacteria produce them during feed fermentation and digestion. But during an attack of acute acidosis, when rumen microbes are disrupted, production of thiamine via digestion is halted. This results in acute thiamine deficiency, which causes sudden nervous disorders.

Acute acidosis can also have less obvious effects, resulting in belated health problems. During an episode of acidosis and the change in microbe activity, the pH of the rumen may drop as low as 4 or 5, much more acid than normal. A pH of 7 is neutral — neither acid nor alkaline — and the cow's body usually tolerates a pH range of 7 to 7.8, which is slightly alkaline. When pH drops and the rumen contents become more acidic, the rumen lining is damaged. The lining of the abomasum and intestines are also inflamed, and the inflammation destroys the *villi* (tiny fingerlike projections that absorb nutrients). This may result in poor feed efficiency, slow growth, and poor weight gain or a drop in milk production.

Occasionally, acidosis is responsible for suppression of the immune system, which may halt an animal's ability to resist infection with a disease for which she has been vaccinated. In feedlots, some epidemics of sudden death are due to BRSV and severe lung impairment, despite proper vaccinations.

Founder (see chapter 12) is a common sequel to acidosis. Damage in the feet becomes obvious 40 to

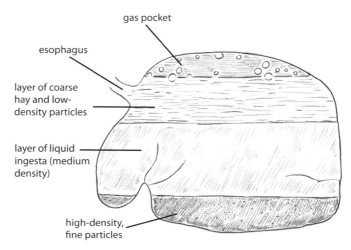

esophagus

gas pocket

layer of coarse hay and low-density particles

layer of liquid ingesta (medium density)

high-density, fine particles

If the layer of less-digested material (floating on the fluid) expands and covers the opening to the esophagus, the animal can't burp to get rid of the gas pocket and gas builds up, causing bloat.

60 days after the acute acidosis. Changes in the body result in inflammation of the laminae (interface between the hoof-horn and inner-foot tissues) and a disrupted blood supply to the hoof horn. Damage is often permanent, and the animal is lame. Overfeeding young bulls on grain (for fast growth) is the biggest cause of foot problems and unsound bulls.

Treat acute acidosis immediately. *Bicarbonate* of soda (baking soda) can be used. Ask your vet about dosage, which will vary with the size of the animal, and work with your vet for additional treatments. The soda can be added to water and given via stomach tube.

Subacute Acidosis

This happens more frequently than acute acidosis and may not be noticed, since affected animals may simply eat less. Other signs include kicking at the belly due to indigestion and discomfort, drooling, panting, eating dirt, and diarrhea.

Feedlot cattle, animals being fattened for slaughter, young bulls on feed tests to see how fast they gain, and dairy cows fed a lot of grain almost always experience some degree of acidosis when started on grain because it takes awhile for rumen bacteria to adjust. Most cattle recover from subacute acidosis without treatment.

Preventing Acidosis

Changes in the ration should never be made all at once. To prevent acidosis, high-energy feeds should be introduced gradually. Even when cattle are on a high-grain diet, the ration should include roughage. The more fiber in the diet, the less incidence of acidosis. If roughage is too finely chopped or ground, however, problems may still occur. It must be coarsely chopped so the animal will do more chewing and still *ruminate*. Chewing, belching, and cud chewing stimulate more saliva production, which helps buffer the acid in the rumen and prevent acidosis. Saliva contains bicarbonate, which is alkaline.

Acidosis can occur whenever feeding is disrupted, since cattle tend to overeat when they start eating again. Any interruption in normal eating or feeding patterns can cause acidosis. Storms, excessive heat, and extreme weather can put cattle at risk for the condition if they stop eating a while and then overeat. If weather is very hot they may not eat much during the day and then overeat at night when it's cooler. Try your best to stay on schedule and feed several times a day, if possible. This should keep cattle from going hungry between meals and overeating when the food arrives.

Remember: The safest diet is forage. If you feed grain to increase weight gain or milk production, do it carefully. Work with a cattle nutritionist to design a safe diet and proper feeding schedule for feedlot animals or high-producing dairy cattle.

Bloat

Bloat is simply the distension of the rumen by gas that won't pass. Carbon dioxide and methane gases form during the fermentation process that breaks down certain feeds in the rumen. Bloat may occur if the animal can't get rid of gas in an efficient manner. If the belching mechanism is impaired or hindered for any reason, bloat can develop rapidly, because large volumes of gas are produced. An obstruction in the esophagus from a blockage (as when animals eat whole potatoes, beets, apples, or a chunk of frozen feed) can cause acute bloat. If gas builds up faster than the animal can belch it out, the rumen may get so full that it puts pressure on the lungs, leaving no room for intake of air. In untreated cases of severe bloat, the animal suffocates.

There's a lot of fluid mixed with partly digested material in the rumen. A mass of foamy, less-digested material floats on top of the fluid, with a gas pocket above it that is regularly let off by belching. Some plants cause the foamy portion to expand and take up more space, covering the opening to the esophagus. This traps the gas; it can no longer be belched out. Once that happens, bloating can quickly increase, and the animal may die.

Bloat was described in historic writings as early as 60 A.D. Some early theories about why cattle developed "gas in the belly" blamed poisonous plants or blockage due to dense feed. Some early attempts at treatment seem strange today — holding burning feathers under the bloated animal's nose; dashing cold water over the body; administering lime, ginger and cold water; or giving a pint (0.5 L) of gin to the bloated animal.

As early as the 1890s, however, stockmen were using a *trocar* (a sharp tool with rounded handle, for stabbing a hole in the rumen) to let out excessive gas. This procedure was recommended if passing a hollow tube into the stomach was not successful in letting off the gas. Another useful treatment that has been practiced for many years is standing the bloated animal on a mound, with front feet higher than the hind. This elevates the juncture of stomach and esophagus so gas can escape more readily. Another remedy was to make the animal walk; this can be effective if done before bloat reaches acute stages and if exercise is slow and gentle (no jostling of rumen contents). Another treatment involved putting a broom handle or rope through the animal's mouth to encourage production of saliva (due to the animal's chewing on the object), which helps break down foam in the rumen.

It wasn't until experimental research in the middle part of the twentieth century that animal nutritionists learned how to control feedlot bloat with careful diet formulations and proper feed processing. Pasture bloat, however, continues to be a problem on many farms and ranches.

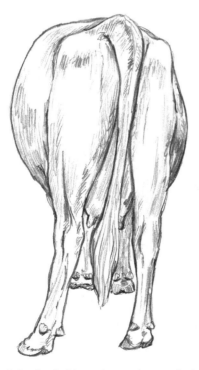

The entire left side of a bloated animal is greatly distended due to excessive gas in the rumen.

Two Types of Bloat

Free-gas bloat is generally caused by interference with normal belching, which can be due to such causes as damage to the vagus nerve or esophageal blockage. Enlargement of lymph nodes between the lungs, which can occur in the aftermath of a respiratory infection, may compress the esophagus or put pressure on the vagus nerve, making that animal a chronic bloater. Free-gas bloat can also occur with a heavy grain ration.

Frothy bloat may occur with grain feeding due to proliferation of certain slime-producing bacteria but is usually associated with forage plants — specifically legumes, such as alfalfa or clover pasture, green chop, or hay under certain conditions.

Frothy Bloat

Foamy rumen content resulting from *legume* or feedlot bloat can hinder proper belching. Gas is trapped in fluid, forming an emulsion of tiny bubbles. Pressure of the frothy material inhibits nerve endings that control the opening into the esophagus. If pressure becomes severe, it halts all rumen contractions. If a stomach tube is passed to try to let off gas, the tube fills with froth and plugs up. If the rumen is distended with free gas, however, the gas pocket can be located (by moving the tube around a bit, when it is inserted down the throat and esophagus), and the gas will come rushing out — giving the animal immediate relief (see Emergency Bloat-Relief Efforts, page 172).

Pasture Bloat

In cases of pasture bloat, frothy gas was once thought to be caused by soluble proteins in rumen fluid, produced by fermentation of legumes. Alfalfa is notorious for causing bloat. Research in Canada in the 1980s and 1990s proved that soluble proteins alone do not account for the extreme viscosity of frothy rumen content. Current theories point to microbial activity and involvement of small particles. Young low fiber alfalfa plants are rapidly digested. The resultant burst

Some Animals Tend to Be Bloaters

Bloating tendencies can be inherited. Some cattle have a lower esophagus; the juncture between stomach and esophagus is not as high on the rumen and is more easily covered with fluid when the rumen is full. This inhibits belching. In other instances, bloat-prone individuals have a slower rate of food passage through the rumen. If fermentable material is in the rumen longer, there's more microbial activity and gas production, which contributes to foam formation. By contrast, more rapid passage of feed decreases the amount of microbial action and hence the chances for bloat.

Body type may also predispose cattle to bloating. Animals that are smaller and short bodied with big bellies are more susceptible to bloat than long-bodied cattle with more stretch and trimness of middle. The short-bodied animal may not have as much room for the rumen and may also have more problems with the placement of the juncture at the esophagus and stomach.

Cull any cows that bloat repeatedly, and don't keep offspring from cows or bulls that tend to be bloaters.

of microbial activity produces large quantities of gas and bacterial slime, creating the froth.

Some farms have more problems with pasture bloat than others, depending on the makeup of plants and soils. In New Zealand it was noted that pastures near the ocean produced very little bloat. Tests of forage plants taken from farms near the sea where no bloating problems occurred and from inland farms where bloat was a constant problem showed the *sodium* levels in "no-bloat" pastures were three times higher than those in the bloat-causing pastures. The conclusion: Salt inhibits bloat.

Cattle may bloat within 15 minutes or up to an hour after being put in a bloat-producing pasture (like lush green alfalfa), but there's often a lag time of 24 to 48 hours before bloating occurs in a new pasture. Cattle may bloat on the first, second, or third day. Sometimes cattle can be in a certain pasture weeks before they bloat, which is often a surprise to the stockman and vet. In a group of affected cattle, many will have severe bloat, and the rest may have mild to moderate distension. The latter may be uncomfortable and graze for only short periods.

Factors That Increase Pasture Bloat

If cows are hungry when they go into a new pasture, they may eat too much too quickly and bloat more readily. Pasture that is moist from dew, rain, or frost is more likely to cause bloat than dry plants because less saliva is needed for swallowing and not enough bloat-inhibiting saliva is mixed with feed. Plants with low energy and low fiber content predispose cattle to bloating because of the resultant lowered rumen pH and poor digestion. Short, lush pasture with too little fiber (such as immature alfalfa plants) can cause bloat.

Legumes are the main cause of pasture bloat, yet bloat can be unpredictable. Even when alfalfa is young and at a stage most likely to cause bloat, the risk is variable. The incidence of bloat on certain pastures can vary from year to year. Clover can be a culprit, yet some clover pastures rarely cause bloat. A few grass pastures cause bloat. Perennial ryegrass has that reputation; it needs a high level of fertilization to grow well, and bloat risk increases with high fertility and fast growth. Ryegrasses are also softer and more palatable than some other grasses and can be eaten faster. The type of fertilizer used on a pasture can affect whether or not cattle bloat. Any fertilizer that stimulates fast growth can make forage more apt to cause bloat, but potassium fertilizer seems to be the worst culprit.

KEEP 'EM SPITTING

Anything that decreases saliva production or swallowing can make an animal more likely to bloat, because saliva contains sodium and bicarbonate, both of which help prevent bloat.

Preventing Pasture Bloat

Minimize bloat on pastures by carefully timing grazing and paying attention to plant maturity, soil moisture, and weather. Choose a dry day, and wait until any dew is off before putting animals in a new pasture. Feed a full ration of hay before allowing them to graze so they don't overeat on lush pasture. Cattle may experience mild bloat when first put in a new pasture, but the problem usually disappears after a few days as digestion adjusts — unless weather conditions change and feed is wet or frosted.

▶ **Disruption of normal grazing patterns** results in more intense feeding activity afterward and may increase bloat risk. It is often safer to leave cattle on a pasture (unless they start bloating severely), rather than take them out and in again to graze it intermittently. Avoid taking them out of the pasture for the night and returning them the next morning. Other disruptions such as those caused by storms or biting flies can also affect eating habits and bloat risk.

▶ **Plant maturity** is one of the most important considerations when hoping to minimize pasture bloat. Bloat potential is highest when alfalfa plants are in prebud stage and decreases as plants mature to full flower. In studies at Kamloops Research Station in British Columbia, Canada, alfalfa 8 to 10 inches (20.3 to 25.4 cm) high produced twice the amount of bloat as alfalfa 20 to 30 inches (50.8 to 76.2 cm) high, though plants more than 20 inches tall still carried some risk.

▶ **Soil moisture** makes a difference; plants with adequate moisture for optimum growth are more likely to cause bloat. Bloat-risky stems are soft rather than dry and fibrous, and the leaves are tender and easily crushed between your fingers. The bloat potential of alfalfa is reduced if the soil's moisture is not sufficient for healthy growth and the plants are dry.

▶ **Weather** plays a role; bloat occurs more frequently following a cool day. Moderate temperatures (68 to 78°F [20 to 25.6°C]) promote optimum plant growth. Cool nights in combination with moderate daytime temperatures may increase the risk for bloat in the fall. Lower temperatures delay plant maturity and extend their growth phase.

Cattle in a seven-year test at Kamloops bloated twice as often in October as during summer months, in four different years. At the other temperature extreme, days that were hot enough to cause moisture stress to plants and drying reduced the risk for bloat. Researchers didn't find a significant seasonal change in bloating incidence when cattle grazed irrigated alfalfa, where plants always had plenty of moisture. Bloat occurred spring through fall and increased with cool weather and frost.

▶ **Heavy dew or frost** contributes to a higher incidence of bloat in the fall. In dry, nonirrigated conditions, the worst seasons for bloat are spring and fall. Stockmen generally think alfalfa is safe to graze after a killing frost, which slows plant growth and dries them, but there is still a risk as long as plants are green. The first frosts actually increase the risk for bloat, preserving the immature stage of plant growth. Frost also disrupts plant cells, releasing bloat-causing agents and increasing the rate of cell breakdown, thereby hastening the fermenting process and the possibility for bloat. It usually takes many hard freezes to render plants safe to graze.

▶ **Seeding grass-legume mixtures** with alfalfa or clover only 50 percent or less of the mix can minimize pasture bloat, except in soils and terrain where it's impossible to maintain a uniform stand. Cattle may selectively graze the alfalfa and avoid the grass. Bloating has been reported in pastures where the proportion of legumes was less than 15 percent. Legumes also grow faster than grasses after being grazed, so use of faster-recovering grasses such as orchard grass and timothy helps reduce the bloat potential of a pasture. If areas of a mixed grass-legume pasture get trampled out, reseed them with a balanced pasture mix so these bare spots won't be colonized by clover.

GOING UP?

In rolling or mountainous pasture, cattle often stand with their heads uphill to relieve bloat. In a level field or pasture, provide a mounded area near a water source that cattle visit every day. This will allow them to stand with their front legs higher than their back legs for easier belching.

Mow the Bloat Down

If bloat is a problem in a pasture-rotation system, mow about a quarter of the fresh paddock in afternoon or early evening when plant sugars are higher and nitrates are lower, and graze it the next day. Use a portable electric fence to make the animals eat the mowed part first. This will generally stop the bloating, even in alfalfa pastures. Each time you put them into a new pasture in your rotation system, mow part of it the day before. Gradually increase the mowed area for each new paddock, to about a third of the paddock. Once they get used to it, cattle often eat the mowed portion first when they are turned into the new paddock; you may no longer need the temporary fencing to keep them in that part.

LOSING BOZO AND BILLY TO BLOAT

WE HAVE OFTEN KEPT a few yearlings on our pasture, choosing not to put them on the range, but allowing them to grow faster on irrigated pasture, giving us the option of selling them midsummer. One year, this group included a handful of calves we'd kept over the winter because they were too small to sell the fall before. We decided we'd grow them bigger and sell them the next fall. We had a small pasture for them and also let them graze regrowth on our hayfields.

That fall we let the yearlings out for a short time in a small alfalfa field at midday and herded them back to the other pasture the rest of the time to avoid overeating and bloat. One day we had to be gone most of the day, so we put them in the alfalfa earlier than usual and rounded them up before we left home. When we returned, we found two of the biggest steers, Bozo and Billy, had bloated and died. We realized that letting them into the alfalfa field early in the morning, when they were empty and hungry and dew was still on the plants, was a serious mistake.

Supplements to Reduce Bloat

A variety of minerals have been promoted or tried for bloat control, including phosphate, calcium, and potassium, but none has actually controlled bloat under test conditions. Antifoaming agents such as oils and detergents that break down froth in the rumen are more effective for prevention and treatment.

Most vegetable oils work, as do a few detergents such as *poloxalene,* the active ingredient in products like Bloat Guard. The latter can be mixed with grain and is effective if cattle are eating two daily feedings. It is also marketed in salt-molasses blocks and in liquid-molasses supplements for lick feeders. The blocks work best if they can be scattered around the entire field, with one block for every 10 animals. Blocks are more effective in small fields than large ones and not very effective if placed only near water sources; cattle must consume the preventive continually through the day.

Ionophore antibiotics such as *monensin* and *lasalocid* are used for bloat protection (added to feed or supplements) because bloat can't develop without a large, active population of microbes to produce fermentation. These products alter microbial populations in the rumen. Monensin may reduce severity of legume bloat by as much as 73 percent; lasalocid effectively controls grain bloat but not legume bloat. If used, they should never be given in doses higher than recommended because they will be toxic to cattle. Also be aware that even tiny amounts are deadly for horses; supplements containing monensin should never be placed in pastures where horses might find

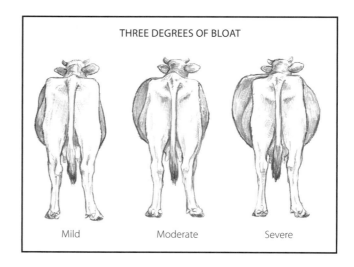

THREE DEGREES OF BLOAT

Mild   Moderate   Severe

them. Ionophore antibiotics cannot be used if you are raising natural or organic beef or milk.

Many New Zealand stockmen use salt to reduce bloat. Some put salt in the drinking water as soon as bloat shows up in cattle grazing certain pastures, and they claim it stops the bloating. Many farmers have fertilized their pastures with salt for decades.

Forage That Causes Bloat

Some forages are considered risky, some are considered safe, and a few are in between (causing bloat under certain circumstances). Grasses are usually safe, but legumes may not be. However, some of the less-popular legumes can be grazed without causing bloat (see chart on page 171). Studies in Canada tested many types of alfalfa for bloat potential and found all types can cause bloat. This disproved claims that creeping varieties are safe to graze.

The bloat-causing potential of pasture forage is related to the ease with which rumen microbes digest it; the forage that causes bloat is digested rapidly, whereas bloat-safe forage is digested more slowly. The lower-risk group takes a medium amount of time to digest.

Tannins in a plant bind with soluble proteins (foaming agents) and inhibit the activity of rumen microbes. Plants that contain tannin do not cause bloat; other plant characteristics that inhibit bloat are leaves with thick, strong cell walls and veins that keep rumen bacteria from quickly invading the inner structure of the leaves. Forage with thin-celled, tender leaves is more vulnerable to rumen bacteria and fast breakdown.

Emergency Treatment for Bloat

Acute bloat must be treated immediately to keep the animal from suffocating. In the final stages of severe bloat, a few seconds of delay can result in death. If the animal is not yet in danger of suffocating, a tube can be passed into the stomach via the nostril and down the throat or a larger hose put directly down the throat, making sure the animal does not chew on it or make a hole in it. A block of wood can be put between the jaws so the animal can't chew. If not much free gas comes out the tube, pour an antifoaming agent down it. A gallon (3.8 L) of mineral oil can be used for an adult cow, but it's also wise to keep a good defoaming agent on hand; ask your vet about products to use. This will often break down the foam and allow large amounts of gas to come back out the tube.

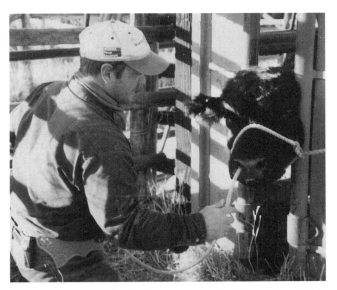

Inserting a nasogastric tube into a cow to administer mineral oil to break up foamy bloat

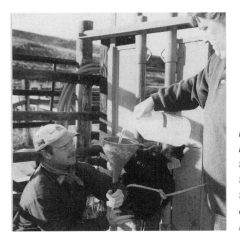

Pouring a gallon of mineral oil into the funnel attached to the nasogastric tube, to put it directly into the rumen

If the animal is in immediate danger of suffocation, don't try to insert a tube. Instead, jab the highest part of the distended rumen with a trocar to let out gas. The area to "stick" is midway between the last rib and the point of the hip on the left side of the animal, a few inches below the edge of the back (loin area). The full rumen will be pressed tightly against the abdominal wall, and the trocar will go through all the layers at once; it should be pushed clear through the abdominal wall of an adult cow. Most trocars come with a cannula (flexible tube) that can be placed in the hole to keep it open. If the rumen contents are too frothy, and not much gas comes out, you can administer an antifoaming agent directly into the rumen through this cannula.

If the foam is so thick that the trocar opening immediately plugs with foam, and there's not time to pour in the antifoaming agent, make a larger hole using a sharp knife. Open a slit 3 to 4 inches (7.6 to 10.2 cm) long and spread it apart with your fingers to let out the foam. Keep your fingers in the incision until bloat is completely relieved or the rumen may move as it becomes smaller, shifting the opening away from the slit through the skin and abdominal wall. Call your vet to come and stitch up the knife wound afterward. A simple hole made by a trocar will heal quickly on its own.

EMERGENCY BLOAT-RELIEF EFFORTS

USING A TUBE

Use metal speculum to pass a stomach tube through the mouth.

USING A TROCAR (OR KNIFE)

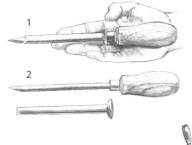

1. Trocar inserted in its cannula.
2. Trocar and cannula taken apart

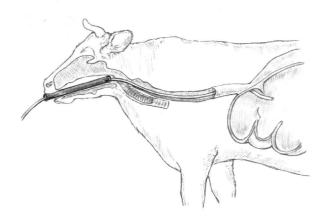

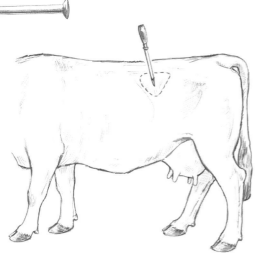

A metal speculum is ideal to protect the tube from being crushed by the cow's molars as you try to insert the tube down her throat. A wooden block can be stuck between her jaws on one side of her mouth while you insert the tube down the center of her throat.

The location for insertion of the trocar is shown here in a normal cow with no bloat extension. The area to "stick" will be much higher (the level of the backbone or higher) when the rumen is full of gas.

Grain Overload and Bloat

Cattle overfed on grain may bloat, but this doesn't happen as frequently as bloating on fermentable forage. Most cases of grain overload cause milder signs; the animal is very full and uncomfortable but is not as apt to suffocate. The animal's overload may be due to disrupted feeding and subsequent overeating.

Symptoms are the same as for pasture bloat; the animal is very full, with a distended rumen. The cow may be panting (taking rapid shallow breaths) or may show signs of labored breathing due to pressure on the lungs. Urination and defecation may be frequent, from the increased abdominal pressure and unease. Discomfort may cause restlessness.

Treatment is the same as for pasture bloat. If the animal is in danger of suffocation, the rumen must be punctured to let out excess gas. If the animal is not yet at this stage, mineral oil or a defoaming agent can be put into the rumen with a long hose or tube. It can also be put directly into the rumen if you must puncture the rumen to let out gas. Don't pour mineral oil or an antifoaming agent down the throat; if some goes down the windpipe the animal will be at risk for immediate death or *aspiration pneumonia.*

Prevention of feedlot bloat can usually be accomplished by adding more roughage to the ration, such as coarsely chopped hay mixed with the grain. If the roughage being fed is alfalfa, exchange it for lower-quality forage. If feeding rolled barley or *milo* (sorghum grain), rolling the milo more coarsely or adding moisture to the barley a few hours before rolling may help. Substituting whole corn or coarsely rolled corn for part of the other grain can be another option, if corn is available. Consult your county Extension agent or a cattle nutritionist when devising a grain ration, to make sure it's balanced for protein, vitamins, and minerals and to avoid problems with bloat, acidosis, and other digestive ailments.

Impaction

Cattle that don't drink enough water have insufficient fluid in the digestive tract to keep the contents moist and readily traveling through the gut. When this happens, they become impacted. Impaction may occur during times of drought if water sources become inadequate and especially if feed is also very

---

Grain Bloat Symptoms May Be Enterotoxemia

Some feedlots have problems with cattle dying of sudden bloat; the lungs of these cattle will be full of froth at necropsy. At first thought, the death of the animal might be attributed to bloat. But sometimes bloat is due to gas formation caused by bacterial toxins created by a gut infection. In a number of feedlots, when the cattle were vaccinated against *Clostridium perfringins* (the bacteria that cause enterotoxemia), the bloating episodes ceased. The two problems may be interrelated. This can also occur in young calves that develop enterotoxemia from Clostridium perfringens or other toxin-forming bacterial gut infections.

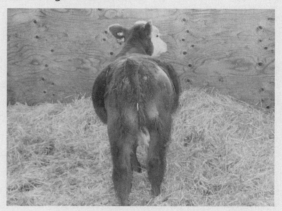

Two-month-old calf with gut pain and severe bloat due to bacterial infection

---

dry. It may also occur in winter if water supplies freeze up and there is no snow. Cattle can learn to get the water they need by scooping up snow with the tongue between mouthfuls of food. This works best if snow is powdery and not crusted (see chapter 3).

Eating coarse, low-protein forage (such as that on dry pastures during winter or drought) is the most common cause of impaction. Rumen microbes need adequate protein to function properly. If there is not enough protein to "feed" these microscopic gut bugs that bring about efficient fermentation and digestion, food breaks down and goes through the tract too slowly. The cow can't eat enough food to supply the nutrients needed by her body because she's

IN THE FALL, after our cattle come home from their Bureau of Land Management summer range and their calves are weaned, they spend two months on our private upper pastures. There is usually enough native grass on those mountainsides to feed the herd until the pastures are snowed under in late December.

Dry bunch grasses are more nutritious than dried-out tame grasses, and our cattle generally do fine without any supplemental protein or minerals. Cows thin from milking heavily all summer typically gain weight on that grass. The biggest problem is always cold weather and thick ice on the water troughs and creek. Some of the cows learn to lick snow, but some years we have to hike or ride up there daily to break ice.

One year after a very dry summer, there wasn't as much grass as usual. Cows were eating the last of the grass before we brought them home to the fields to feed hay. Most of the good bunch grasses were gone, and they were eating coarser plants that didn't have much protein. One of our black cows, named Red Devil because she had a red streak down the center of her back, became lethargic, wasn't grazing much, and was losing weight. Her manure was scanty and very firm, so we brought her home. She didn't poop much at all during the 3-mile trip down the road.

During the next few days we gave her mineral oil and water several times a day by stomach tube to try to relieve impaction, but her condition had been worsening for some time. She would not eat or drink, and her stomach contents were impacted and dry. We could not get things moving through. We discovered the seriousness of her impaction at postmortem after she died a few days later.

already full of undigested roughage, so she loses weight and may also become impacted. If cattle are eating dried-out or overly mature forage, there's not enough protein to meet the needs of the microbes, and some of them die off. When this happens, the cow's ability to digest low-quality forage decreases, and the feed piles up in the digestive tract.

The best way to prevent impaction is to add protein to a diet of grasses from poor pasture or low-quality hay or straw. Feed the cows a protein supplement or small amount of alfalfa hay. Protein allows the microbe population in the rumen to increase and thrive, enabling a cow to digest more fiber. Then she can eat more total roughage and turn it into energy. Since the material is being processed and moving through the gut more normally, the risk for impaction is eliminated.

Animals with a protein deficiency will drop to about 66 percent of their normal feed consumption; this leads to weight loss and, in some instances, digestive problems and impaction. In any situation where you've had drier than normal seasons or a multiyear drought, the forage may be too short on protein to facilitate proper rumen digestion. If the protein (or phosphorus) level drops low enough, the cattle need a supplement.

Hardware Disease (Traumatic Reticulo-Peritonitis)

Cattle eat quickly and can consume large amounts of food in a short time. Since they grab wads of grass or hay with the tongue and pull it into their mouths, they don't sort their feed carefully and occasionally swallow foreign material such as small rocks or pieces of wire chopped up by a baler. Cattle grazing near junk piles or old buildings may pick up nails, roofing tacks, and other sharp objects. Hardware disease occurs when a sharp object penetrates the gut lining and damages other abdominal organs or creates infection in the abdomen (*peritonitis*). Unless quickly corrected, this mishap may kill the cow.

Consuming foreign material with feed is more common than most people realize, probably because the ingested object does not always cause trouble. Only occasionally do sharp pieces penetrate the stomach. More than 70 percent of slaughtered cull dairy cows have some form of hardware inside them but exhibited no symptoms while living. (Dairy cows are culled when they no longer milk enough, become infertile, or have udder problems of some sort, not necessarily because they are "sick.") This is likely because they were given a magnet to hold any metal objects safely inside the stomach or the ingested objects were not sharp enough to penetrate the stomach.

Often the stomach absorbs and eliminates a metal object. When performing postmortems on cows, one of our local veterinarians has found rusty nails that were almost completely dissolved and disintegrated by digestive fluids in the reticulum. He's also found many rocks and other heavy objects. Roofing nails are the most common objects found in dairy cows, now that most balers no longer use wire.

Silage cutters and balers may chop up wire in a hay swath, however. Some equipment manufacturers put strong magnets on feed wagons, silage choppers, and other livestock feeding equipment to catch and hold any metal passing through. If these collect a lot of metal pieces, they should be cleaned off periodically to allow room for more to be attracted. Despite these measures, some metal pieces are eaten.

For beef cattle, the biggest cause of hardware is usually wire and other junk that ends up in baled hay. If a hayfield has old, fallen-down fences or is next to a junk pile, pieces of wire and other foreign material may get chopped up by the baler into a size that fits perfectly in the cow's wadded mouthfuls. Cattle generally eat more foreign material in hay and other harvested feeds than they do when grazing, unless the pasture is strewn with junk.

Symptoms of Hardware

When a cow eats a sharp foreign object, stomach action during digestion may push it through the stomach wall. The reticulum (second stomach, with honeycomb compartments) is where heavy material usually ends up. In an adult, this stomach is about the size of a volleyball. If a nail, a piece of wire, or a sharp rock goes through the stomach wall, it may puncture another organ or go into the heart cavity. If it pierces the diaphragm, the animal usually dies of heart failure.

The most common signs of hardware disease are discomfort and abdominal pain. The cow stands humped up with elbows out away from her body. Head and neck may be extended. She may be breathing hard, grunting with each breath. One way to see if her pain is due to hardware is to pinch her withers firmly. Usually when you pinch a healthy cow's withers, she will sink down a bit, lowering her back and

> ## HARDWARE IS NOT ALWAYS METAL
>
> **I**N 1967 WE LOST FLOPSY, a middle-aged cow who was pregnant and due to calve in about a month. One day when we moved the cows to a new pasture, several of them gobbled up some loose hay that was lying along the edge of the road on top of the gravel. We didn't think much about it until a couple days later when we saw Flopsy standing by herself with head and neck thrust forward, panting and grunting. She was reluctant to move and very weak and trembling. She let me walk right up to her and take her temperature.
>
> Thinking she had an acute respiratory infection, we tried to bring her to the corral to give her antibiotics, but she collapsed and died. We called our vet to do a postmortem and find out what killed her, and his search through her "innards" revealed bleeding in the heart cavity and a sharp rock shaped like an arrowhead. She had apparently licked up some gravel with the loose hay she'd eaten, and digestive action (along with the gut being crowded by her large pregnant uterus) had pushed the rock through the stomach wall and into the heart.
>
> We have reversed hardware disease in several animals over the past 42 years by giving them a magnet, but this was one case of "hardware" in which a magnet would not have helped.

belly to get away from the pinch. But if she has hardware she won't do this because it hurts too much to move away from your touch. Another test for diagnosis is to put a pole under her belly, just behind her front legs, and lift it up under her breastbone (sternum). If she has hardware, she will usually grunt or show some other sign of discomfort.

She may also have a fever of 103 to 105°F (39.4 to 40.6°C), depending on the stage of the disease. If a wire or nail is just starting to migrate through the stomach wall and the contents of the abdomen are becoming infected (peritonitis), she may have a fever of 104 to 105°F (40 to 40.6°C). With a chronic case, the fever may be about 103. Her respiratory and rate is usually elevated. She is dull and eating less or not at all, and rumen contractions may be decreased.

A cow with hardware moves reluctantly. She may grind her teeth — a sign of abdominal pain — and often she'll grunt as she breathes, audible from some distance away. At this stage you might mistake the problem for pneumonia, especially if the foreign object has penetrated through the diaphragm and into the chest cavity. She may actually have pneumonia, caused by infection from the wire or nail.

Hardware may also be confused with ulcers. An abomasal ulcer can show very similar symptoms. With an ulcer, however, you will usually see some blood in dark, tarry manure. But she generally does not have a fever.

If peritonitis is severe, she may die in a couple of days, but chronic peritonitis may go on for months and cause liver damage. She may just seem to be doing poorly, and you might mistake this for some other problem. On rare occasions a wire or nail may migrate through the liver, creating the same type of damage as might be done by liver flukes or a liver abscess, making the cow susceptible to redwater infection (see chapter 4).

Some cows recover from hardware without treatment. The body may wall off the foreign object so it can't keep poking the stomach. But this can lead to other problems: If the walled-off foreign body creates an adhesion, the reticulum may adhere to the abdominal wall, so the rumen can't function

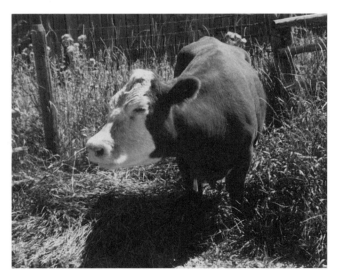

A cow with hardware disease may stretch her head and neck forward, breathe hard, and grunt with every breath.

> **HASTY EATING**
>
> The cow chews food just enough to mix it with saliva, wadding it into a mass that can be swallowed. This minimal chewing often leads to ingestion of foreign material such as small pieces of wire baled in the hay. These objects generally end up in the lowest part of the tract, the second stomach (reticulum), and may perforate the stomach wall.

normally. Sometimes the cow becomes a chronic bloater due to *vagus indigestion,* which means the cow can't belch to chew her cud properly (see page 183). The stomach adheres to the body wall and can't slide around or contract as it should. A chronic bloater may actually have a case of chronic hardware.

A cow with a sharp object in her stomach is more at risk for hardware disease in late gestation, due to the extra pressure on abdominal contents from the enlarging uterus. There's also risk for problems during labor. When she strains there is added intra-abdominal pressure from uterine and abdominal contractions, and this may push the sharp object through the stomach wall.

Prevention

If cattle are at risk for eating metal objects with their feed, the best prevention for hardware disease is a magnet. A cylindrical magnet is put in the stomach with a plastic or nonmagnetic balling gun — a long probe for pushing a bolus down the throat to where the animal will swallow it. The magnet usually comes to rest in the reticulum (second stomach), where it attracts and holds any metal objects churning around in the stomach or pushed by with feed by the contractions of the rumen. This magnet helps keep objects more in the center of the reticulum so they won't be pushed through the wall. Digestive juices gradually erode and disintegrate the metal pieces. The magnet usually stays in the stomach for the life of the animal and generates an ongoing process of metal being attracted and degraded.

Many dairymen routinely put a magnet into heifers when they enter the breeding herd. Beef raisers rarely give magnets to cows, but it's always a good idea if cattle are fed questionable feed that might have wires or other junk in it or when cattle are grazing pastures with old fences, dumps, junk piles, old machinery parked in the pasture, or other situations where they might pick up bits of sharp metal. Older animals are more likely to develop hardware disease than calves or young cows, mainly because they've had longer to accumulate sharp foreign objects.

When using magnets, make sure each animal gets only one. Keep track of which animals have been given magnets. Putting another one in the stomach defeats the purpose; magnets attract one another and line up together and won't collect metal. Some farmers who feed processed feed from a feed truck into feed bunks install a magnet on the dispensing unit of the truck, to pick up any metallic material before it gets to the feed bunk.

Treatment

After a cow shows signs of hardware disease, and if it's plausible that a foreign object has migrated out of the stomach and may penetrate another organ, your veterinarian must do exploratory surgery to find and remove it. This can be frustrating, however, because by the time the decision for surgery is made, the object may have migrated a long way, causing a lot of damage and severe infection, and it is too late to save the cow.

If the object can be removed, the abdomen flushed with sterile fluids, and the cow given antibiotics, she may recover and do fine. But even if surgery to remove the object is successful, if damage and infection are too severe, the cow may die. To be truly successful, surgery must be done soon

enough to resolve the problem. If a cow is just starting to show symptoms, however, many veterinarians advise giving her antibiotics and a magnet and waiting to see if it will pull the nail or wire back into the stomach. If this works, the damage to the stomach wall usually heals, the metal stays safely in the stomach (adhering to the internal magnet), and surgery isn't needed.

Digestive Tract Blockage

Complete blockages of the tract sometimes occur in cattle. In young calves, a blockage may occur when a calf has eaten a large amount of dirt or hair, or if they ingest baling twine or plastic bags that plug the tract. If blockage is complete, the calf will be dull and off feed, and will eventually die from a ruptured gut, shock, or peritonitis, unless surgery is performed to remove the foreign material.

A blockage consisting of dirt in the stomach can often be "washed out" by repeatedly flushing the stomach with water. This entails putting water into the stomach via nasogastric tube and allowing it to come back out of the tube, carrying some of the dirt with it. For this procedure the calf should be laid on his side on a table, or some other elevated surface, that allows your end of the tube to be held below his

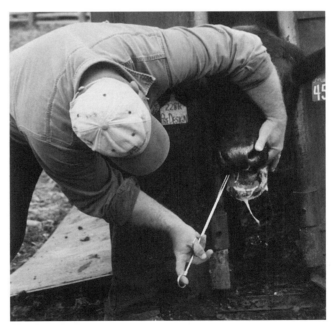

Giving an animal a magnet for hardware disease, using a nonmagnetic metal balling gun

stomach level in order to effectively siphon the water back out. When the condition is detected early, this method for removing dirt is generally successful.

Small amounts of dirt and small hairballs can often be moved on through the tract by giving the calf a large dose of castor oil. This substance not only lubricates the material but also stimulates the gut to contract and move the material past the narrow portion where it is lodged, such as the valve between stomach and intestine. Larger and more solid foreign objects such as twine, or large hairballs, however, must be removed by exploratory surgery. This is most successful if done early on, before the calf goes into shock or the plugged area ruptures.

Adult cattle that eat foreign material such as baling twine or plastic may not die if the material does not completely block the tract. Because the adult animal is large, and the gut so spacious, indigestible material may in some cases pass on through or wad up in the rumen without actually blocking a valve.

Baling twine is especially troublesome for causing indigestion and subsequent poor performance. It often ends up in a ball that looks like an octopus with tentacles. If one of the stray ends of twine gets sucked down through the valve into the abomasum, the main mass gets pulled against the opening and plugs it, interfering with proper digestion. The cow may not die, but she will definitely lose weight and may be mildly uncomfortable.

If baling twine pieces are left in the field or pasture, calves will chew on them just because they are curious, and usually end up swallowing them. If twine is mixed in with hay (as when a broken bale is rebaled without first removing the original twine), cows will ingest it. Rather than spitting out the twine when it gets in the mouth, they continue to chew it and end up swallowing the whole thing.

One year we saw a cow starting to eat a twine, but before we could catch up with her to try to pull it out of her mouth, she had ingested it. That summer she had mild diarrhea and was thin; it was several months before she was in peak health again, and in hindsight we suspected that the twine might have been to blame. It was probably caught in her stomachs until digestive action and juices eventually broke it down and disintegrated it.

Plastic bags can be deadly. The large bags that enclose silage and other feeds are just as dangerous to cattle as small bags released from human garbage that blow around the field. In one case of plastic ingestion, a dairy culled about 50 cows that were losing weight, and at slaughter it was discovered that their stomachs were full of plastic from old silage bags. Even well-fed cows seem to like chewing on anything that may have contained feed, and they may do it just from curiosity. Leaving any kind of plastic within reach of cattle, or where it might blow into their pen or pasture, is asking for trouble.

Ulcers

An ulcer is an open sore in the surface of an organ or tissue caused by sloughing of damaged, dead tissue. In the digestive tract — the long tube consisting of the esophagus, stomachs, and intestines — any ulcer that becomes deep may penetrate the lining and wall and make a hole. Whenever the stomach or intestinal wall is perforated, it becomes a life-threatening situation, as contents of the digestive tract may leak into surrounding body cavities. This contamination of an otherwise "sterile" environment creates serious infection.

Ulcers in Adults

Cows sometimes develop abomasal ulcers. If the ulcer is deep, there may be blood in the manure. The cow may have indigestion; fresh blood or tarry, black clots in manure, indicating hemorrage in the stomach; or chronic indigestion with minimal evidence of blood. If the ulcer eats through the stomach wall, a cow may develop acute local peritonitis or a diffuse infection throughout the abdomen that causes rapid death.

Ulcers may occur as a primary problem or secondary to another disease (viral diseases like BVD may erode the mucous lining), or as trauma to the abomasum, such as displacement or impaction. The cause of primary abomasal ulcers is unknown, but they occur most frequently in high-producing, lactating dairy cows.

There may be correlation between stress and ulcers. Abomasal ulcers in dairy cows in early lactation (producing peak levels of milk) sometimes occur following prolonged illness (pneumonia) or the stress of a sale or cattle show. Ulcers sometimes occur in bulls after the stress of transportation, prolonged surgery, or painful chronic lameness. Abomasal ulcers are also a cause of sudden death in yearling feedlot cattle; there may be a correlation between high-grain diets and gastric ulcers.

Symptoms and Treatment

Signs of abomasal ulcers include abdominal pain, grinding the teeth, blood in manure, and anemia (resulting in pale mucous membranes), due to the bleeding. The animal may go off feed, have a drop in milk production, scanty feces, or suffer from periodic diarrhea. If an ulcer perforates, the animal may die suddenly without much evidence of illness.

In other instances, the cow will have blood in the feces for 4 to 6 days, after which she starts to recover if the ulcer begins to heal, or she may develop chronic indigestion if the ulcers do not heal. In some instances the abomasum is distended with fluid and gas and makes a sloshing, splashing sound if the animal is jostled or trots.

Giving the cow antacids is the best treatment and is usually aimed at buffering and protecting the damaged stomach lining from gastric juices and acidosis. Your veterinarian may try to inject the medication directly into the abomasum via a cannula through the abdominal wall. Oral administration of keolin and pectin twice a day to coat and soothe the raw tissue is sometimes helpful. If the animal is severely anemic due to loss of blood, a blood transfusion may be needed. Consult your veterinarian.

Ulcers in Calves

In calves, a common cause of digestive-tract ulcers is erosion of the gut lining by infection and inflammation due to acute gut infection. It's usually a bacterial infection in which toxins are formed that severely damage the gut lining to the point that some of it sloughs away. Even if a calf is successfully treated and the toxic condition halted before it kills the calf, the damaged lining may slough away a few days later. The calf, who may have seemed to be recovered from the acute infection, then becomes dull and goes off feed. He may grind his teeth (a sign of pain and discomfort), start to nurse his mother, and then quit or just fiddle at the udder instead of nursing.

> ## Determine the Cause
>
> Each farm or ranch has its own set of circumstances and conditions that predispose calves to various problems. In order to prevent a problem or treat sick calves successfully, it's important to work with your vet to find the cause of death losses. Symptoms in animals are often similar but sometimes due to different kinds of illness.
>
> A colicky calf may be suffering from a perforated ulcer or in the acute stage of a clostridial (*C. perfringens*) infection or some other bacterial disease that causes rapid proliferation of toxins that compromise and shut down the gut (see chapter 4). In these latter instances the calf can often be successfully treated if you find him soon enough and administer the proper antibiotic and a large dose of castor oil to get the gut moving again. If you find him before he goes into shock, this emergency treatment can quickly reverse the condition.
>
> If the problem is due to *C. perfringens*, there is a vaccine that can prevent this infection. If it's an unknown type of bacteria, which plague some farms and ranches, the only solution is diligently checking calves to find and treat any sick ones before they go into shock. Once they slip into shock, administration of large amounts of IV fluid and treatment to reverse shock may save some of them, but they die very quickly in this condition — it's always an immediate emergency.

In these instances, supportive care (gut soothers like mineral oil or keolin/pectin to coat the raw tissue) and feeding by tube during the time he isn't nursing enough can usually keep him going until the gut lining heals. Otherwise, some of these calves lose weight and become weak — or starve themselves to death — because it's too painful to eat.

Often the cause of ulcers is a mystery. Stress may be one factor, along with mineral deficiencies and feed quality. Some affected calves don't even seem sick. Every spring some herds experience sporadic cases of sudden death in otherwise healthy-looking calves at 6 to 8 weeks of age (sometimes up to 4 months), and these are often the fastest-growing calves in the herd. Some herds average a 1 to 2 percent death loss, losing a few calves almost every year. Postmortem examination reveals a perforated ulcer in the abomasum; the erosion eats through the stomach wall, spilling gut contents into the abdomen.

The calf usually dies within 24 hours after the rupture, due to severe peritonitis. If you're not observing the herd closely, you may simply find the calf dead. If you see him while he's still alive, he may be weak and going into shock. If you find him early enough, not yet in shock and merely suffering gut pain (colic), he may survive if you take him to your veterinarian for emergency surgery and subsequent antibiotics to combat abdominal infection.

Eating Dirt

Calves that eat dirt may ingest small rocks that penetrate or wear holes in the gut lining, killing the calf. Some stockmen feel that calves may be trying to get the minerals they need by eating dirt and sometimes get ulcers in the process. Some ulcers are thought to develop when cattle have copper or selenium deficiencies. Deficiencies certainly may play a role in some cases or be factors that lower resistance to disease, since these trace elements are important to the immune system. There's an ongoing debate about whether dirt eating is really an effort to counteract nutritional deficiency, especially because mineral supplementation doesn't always halt the dirt eating. Calves that consistently eat dirt, sand, or fine gravel often scrape and damage the gut lining.

Calves may eat dirt out of boredom or curiosity (not unlike a small child reaching to put things in his mouth to taste) or eat dirt because they already have an irritated gut. When they are off feed, they nibble on strange things. On some farms, stockmen feel that using a mineral supplement slows or halts incidence of dirt-eating, whereas on other farms it doesn't seem to make much difference.

Green Grass Is the Best Prevention

Whether calves feed on green pasture or hay may have some bearing on their dirt-eating behavior. Early-born calves, whose dams are on hay rather than pasture, tend to eat dirt more regularly than calves on good pasture. Calves at pasture always have green grass to eat, whereas calves in a herd being fed hay once or twice a day may nibble hay with their mothers and have nothing much else to do the rest of the day. They're more likely to chew on baling twine, lick hair off fences, nibble dirt and sandbars, and cause themselves problems.

Green grass is the most natural feed for a calf. It contains more of the nutrients he needs to augment his mother's milk than does hay. It's also softer to eat and not as irritating to the gut. Ulcers, in general, rarely occur in calves that are eating lush, soft green pasture, but tend to be a problem in herds fed hay or silage. When the calf's digestive tract is changing from reliance primarily on milk (digested in the abomasum) like a single-stomached animal to relying more on forage (digested in the rumen), this is the point in his life when he's more susceptible to ulcers. They don't occur as often, though, if he's on pasture. There are multiple factors involved in the development of digestive-tract ulcers, but feed quality may have the greatest influence, since winter-born and early-spring calves have the most problems.

Choking

Because cattle don't always take time to chew feed when it's first ingested but chew more thoroughly later when they chew the cud, they sometimes *choke* on apples, turnips, whole potatoes, and other foods. The object becomes stuck at the back of the throat or at the top of the esophagus. A cow can also choke on her placenta after calving, since most cows quickly eat these membranes as soon as they shed them. This may be an instinctive action to protect the newborn calf from predators that would be attracted to the birth site by the smell of the afterbirth.

Occasionally, a cow will suffocate if the placental mass shuts off her airway as well as her esophagus, and this is an emergency. In other instances, as when a medium-size potato or apple gets stuck at the top of her esophagus (but isn't blocking her windpipe), she is not in immediate danger of dying. But the foreign object blocks the esophagus, and she can no longer burp up gas from the rumen. She becomes anxious and uncomfortable due to pain from the blockage but also from gas building up; she soon bloats.

HOW TO SAVE A COW FROM CHOKING ON AN OBJECT

1. Restrain the cow in a chute or stanchion.

2. Grab her nose with one hand, fingers in her nostrils, to help hold her head still.

3. Carefully insert your other hand into her mouth, with your palm facing upward and fingers cupped closely together and pressed firmly against the roof of her mouth, as you move your hand back toward her throat.

4. Try to keep your hand and fingers away from her agile tongue.

5. Take care to keep your hand safely out of the way of her back molars; otherwise, she can crush your hand with her teeth. Although there's really not room to put something in her mouth to keep her from biting you, holding her by the nostril with fingers from your other hand will help.

6. Once you get to the back of the throat, you can twist your wrist, turn your hand over, and feel for and then reach and grasp the object.

7. With it safely grasped, turn your hand over again and bring it slowly back out, pressing the object and your hand firmly against the roof of her mouth so she can't manipulate it with her tongue and grab it with her teeth.

8. If the object is too far down into the esophagus to reach, wait for your vet, who may be able to safely push the object on down into the stomach with a probang — a long flexible rod with a ball or sponge on the end designed specifically for removing obstructions from the throat.

Don't Try to Force It Down

Choking animals have sometimes been saved by carefully pushing the obstruction on down with a shovel handle or broom handle, but this is risky because the stiff, straight handle is apt to damage or puncture the esophagus or windpipe or penetrate the back of the throat unless the cow's head and neck are stretched far forward and kept perfectly straight. You are better off waiting for the vet, if possible, unless the cow is gasping and struggling for air and about to die.

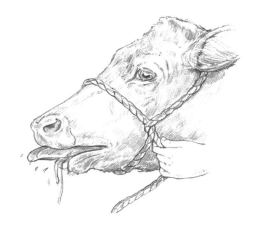

When a foreign object is stuck in the back of the throat or the top of the esophagus, the animal will slobber and cough continually.

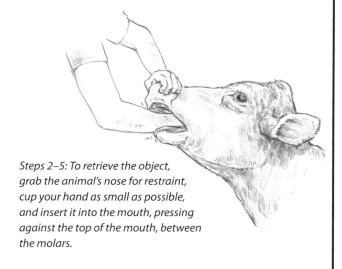

Steps 2–5: To retrieve the object, grab the animal's nose for restraint, cup your hand as small as possible, and insert it into the mouth, pressing against the top of the mouth, between the molars.

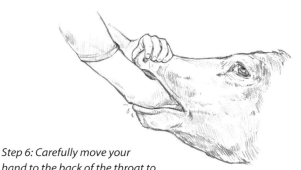

Step 6: Carefully move your hand to the back of the throat to try to reach and grasp the foreign object.

If the foreign object is not removed fairly soon, she will die. If she's unable to breathe and is collapsing, there's no time to call a vet. If she's choking on afterbirth, grab the part still hanging out of her mouth and pull it out, or reach in her mouth to get hold of the mass. If it's a piece of apple, potato, or some other object stuck in her throat and she's bloating, you may have time to have the vet come to your place, but if it might be a while before he or she gets there, try to get the object out yourself.

Calf Scours

Scours is diarrhea. Runny feces in calves can be caused by indigestion, change in feed, and lush green feed. But the most common cause is intestinal infection, which may be caused by viruses, bacteria, protozoa, or a combination of these pathogens. These infections are transmitted by ingestion, as when a calf eats contaminated feed; nurses a dirty udder; or licks a dirty, contaminated hair coat.

Symptoms and Treatment

Most cases of intestinal infection develop loose, watery feces progressing to dehydration and weakness unless treated in early stages. A vet's proper diagnosis is vital so you know whether you're dealing with a virus, protozoa (see chapter 6), or a bacterial infection, which is treated with antibiotics.

When you treat for intestinal infections, your goal to halt the infection (using antibiotics for bacterial infections or coccidiostats for coccidia), but the most important treatment is supportive

---

READ UP AND BE READY

Successful treatment of calfhood intestinal infection is a large and complex topic covered more fully in *Essential Guide to Calving* (Storey Publishing, 2008), the companion volume to this book. Because the causes of infections and specific treatments can be varied, be sure to get a proper diagnosis from your vet, who can advise you on treatment and prevention of certain types of scours.

— giving the calf fluids with electrolytes added, to replace what's lost through diarrhea. Gut soothers given to slow and coat the intestinal tract may help. If the calf is so dehydrated he's unable to stand, oral fluids are of no benefit; he'll need IV fluids. If his circulation is compromised by dehydration or shock and is no longer adequately servicing the muscles (cold extremities, calf too weak to stand), it is no longer servicing the gut, either. Oral fluids will not be absorbed. The only way to save the calf is with IV fluids.

The key to treating scours successfully is to detect illness early and begin treatment while the calf is still strong and able to absorb oral fluids. If the condition can be reversed before much gut damage is done, the calf will recover much more quickly. Early treatment can often mean the difference between a short course of mild illness and an extended battle that sometimes results in the death of the calf.

Prevention

Maintaining a clean environment for baby calves so they don't pick up pathogens soon after birth is the best way to prevent scours. Cows should be well fed, and their vaccinations should be up to date (especially the vaccines that protect against certain scour infections, if your veterinarian advises this), so they have high levels of antibodies in their colostrum. If calves ingest plenty of colostrum soon after birth, they'll be protected against most of the pathogens that cause scours. Cows should be in clean areas before and after calving, so calves won't be exposed to pathogens by nursing a dirty udder.

It is also very important to control the pathogen load in the stomach of the cow. *Clostridium perfringens* type A can be a big issue (see chapter 4). If you can keep the cow in a clean environment, thereby protecting her from too many pathogens, she won't be passing so many infection-causing bacteria to young calves.

Group calves by age, so older calves won't spread scours to younger ones. Put cows with new calves in a pasture that's separate from older calves. Always immediately remove sick calves from any group so they don't spread disease to other calves.

Use of Probiotics

Microbe cultures, called *probiotics,* are sometimes given to cattle to enhance appetite, digestion, and health or to restore a normal population of microbes after illness or some other factor has disrupted digestion. When treating a sick calf for scours, for instance, prolonged use of oral antibiotics, sometimes necessary to save a seriously ill calf, may destroy normal gut flora. The calf is unable to effectively and efficiently digest food and may continue to do poorly. Restoring normal gut flora with the use of a probiotic product after completion of antibiotic therapy can help him recover faster.

Microbe populations in the gut can change dramatically when subjected to antibiotics, stress, illness, or an abrupt change in feed. Prolonged stress or illness results in overproduction of cortisol in the body (see discussion of the immune system in chapter 1). The excess cortisol hinders appetite and adversely affects the epithelial lining of the intestine, which may allow pathogenic bacteria to attack it. Inflammation of the gut lining is less likely to occur or result in intestinal infection if the proper balance of microbes inhabits the tract.

If most of the "friendly" microbes die off, this not only interferes with optimum digestion and fermentation but also opens the door to opportunistic, harmful microbes that can then multiply more rapidly and move into the void. Antibiotics to treat disease may kill beneficial bacteria as well as the disease-causing bacteria, resulting in proliferation of *yeasts* and fungi that are not affected by antibiotics. To restore proper balance for health and efficient digestion, probiotics can be beneficial by innoculating the gut with natural, helpful bacteria.

In a healthy animal, the majority of microbes in the gut are beneficial. They live in the digestive tract and maintain a good environment for digestion and nutrient absorption, inhibiting competition from pathogenic organisms. Beneficial bacteria lower the pH of the intestinal environment, which creates unfavorable conditions for harmful bacteria. Some of the "friendly" microbes create B vitamins, and others are necessary for proper fermentation breakdown of fibrous feed into usable nutrients.

Administering probiotics (cultures of friendly bacteria) to a recovering sick animal helps restore production of volatile fatty acids, which also help regulate intestinal yeasts and fungi. The introduced cultured bacteria multiply faster than most pathogenic bacteria and outcompete, restoring the balance. The animal starts eating again, and the digestive tract resumes its task of converting and absorbing nutrients for body function and growth.

There are many probiotic products available, including cultures of *Streptococcus faecium, S. lactic, S. thermophilus, Lactobacillus acidophilus, L. bulgaricus* and *L. lactis.* Ask your vet for advice about whether to use probiotics for a certain animal, which products to use, and for what purpose. Some have a longer shelf life, or multiply faster after being introduced into the gut. This enables them to lower the intestinal pH more rapidly, which can be an advantage when competing for space *(adhesion sites)* to help crowd out more harmful microbes.

Restoring the Cud

A cow that's been ill or hasn't eaten for several days because she's been sick or injured may lose her ability to properly ferment and digest forage and cannot belch up feed to chew again. She's lost her cud. Without daily addition of nutrients into the rumen, some microbes die off. The balance between various microbe species is changed. In some instances, after a long or severe illness, there are not enough of the right kind of microbes left to re-establish the needed population for proper digestion.

The traditional remedy for a lost cud is to obtain the "cud" or its juices from a living animal or to collect some rumen content or fluids from a freshly butchered animal and put it into the stomach of the malfunctioning cow to reinstall proper microbes in the rumen. This material can be administered orally or by stomach tube. The simplest way to do this is to open the mouth of a gentle cow (or a dairy cow restrained in a stanchion) while she's chewing her cud, grab the wad she is chewing, then put it immediately into the mouth of the cow that's lost hers. When she swallows this material or its juices, she regains the needed rumen microbes.

CHAPTER NINE

Eye Problems

Occasionally a cow or calf has an eye that needs care. Some problems resolve on their own, such as foreign matter washing out with tears or a minor infection clearing up without treatment. But in other situations, you must help remedy the problem.

You may need a vet to help diagnose and treat the condition, as several ailments can look the same. A runny eye, for instance, could mean something is caught in the eyelid and causing irritation or that pinkeye, a viral infection, or, in some instances, cancer is the cause. Among other things, a cloudy eye can be a sign of infectious bovine rhinotracheitis, injury, or sensitivity to sunlight due to photosensitization, which would also cause skin damage. Looking for symptomatic clues in other parts of the body will help you with the diagnosis, but there's no match for the experienced eye of a veterinarian for diagnostic accuracy.

Eye Injuries

Cattle rarely suffer direct injury to an eye. They have good reflexes and close the eye if anything threatens to strike it. Eyelid skin is thick and tough and can protect the eye from most things that brush it. Eyeballs are recessed in the skull with a pad of fat behind them and can withstand a direct blow without bursting. When you see cattle fighting head to head, often hit on the side of the face by a herdmate, you realize how tough and well protected their eyes are.

Eyes may still be injured by running into something sharp or by a severe blow. If the animal is temporarily blind in one eye because of an infection like pinkeye, she may run into something solid or sharp that might injure or puncture the eyeball.

Pinkeye

Infectious bovine keratoconjunctivitis (IBK), commonly called pinkeye, is an infectious disease that

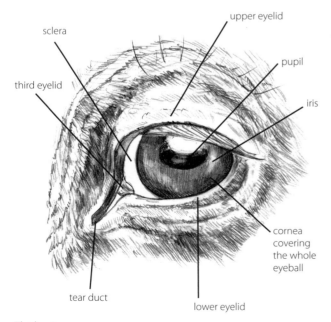

The bovine eye

sclera

third eyelid

upper eyelid

pupil

iris

cornea covering the whole eyeball

tear duct

lower eyelid

causes inflammation of the eye covering (cornea), the exposed white of the eye around the edges of the colored part *(sclera)*, and the delicate membrane that lines the inside of the eyelids and sclera *(conjunctiva)*. The animal holds the painful eye shut and may not spend much time grazing. She may be temporarily blind in that eye if it becomes cloudy.

Pinkeye can have a serious economic impact if many animals in the herd are affected. Ranchers must endure lost production, time and expense of treatment, and decrease in value of any animal that ends up with a permanently scarred or blind eye. Cows with pinkeye eat less, and milk production drops; this in turn affects the growth rate of their calves. Not only will the cow give less milk, but if you treat a dairy cow so the eye can heal quicker, her milk must be discarded for a number of days. It can't be used for human consumption until no antibiotic residues in the milk remain.

Calves suffering from pinkeye have a poor growth rate. They don't eat well because of the pain. In research trials, calves with one eye affected gained 17 pounds (7.7 kg) less, on average, than their unaffected herdmates, and calves with both eyes affected were 30 to 65 pounds (13.6 to 29.5 kg) lighter. Severe infections permanently damage the eye, leaving a thick, scarred area on the cornea, or rupture it, causing blindness. An animal temporarily or permanently blind in one eye can be dangerous to handle. She may run over you or crash into gates and fences on her blind side.

Cause of Pinkeye

Dealing with pinkeye is complicated at times; there are several causes of eye lesions in cattle, which are all lumped together and called pinkeye. A bacterium, *Moraxella bovis,* is the infectious agent most commonly involved, but other pathogens can also cause the eye infection. Pinkeye may start in two or three animals and quickly spread through the herd. In most cases eye lesions result from the spread of contaminated eye secretions from an infected eye to a noninfected animal, which can happen in several ways. Flies, especially face flies that feed on eye secretions, physically carry bacteria from one animal to another. *M. bovis* survives only a few hours on a housefly but may remain viable for up to three days

on a face fly. These flies go from animal to animal to feed on eye secretions (see chapter 7) and carry bacteria from infected animals to many others in the herd or even from neighboring herds to your animals.

Pinkeye is generally a summertime problem when flies are active, but the condition existed in the United States before we had face flies; this disease was first identified in the 1890s. Face flies didn't enter this country until 1952 from Nova Scotia, gradually moving south and across the country. Incidence of pinkeye increased with the spread of the face-fly population. Face flies definitely contribute to the problem but are not the only reason for the existence of this disease.

It's not known how long *M. bovis* can survive in eye and nasal secretions or on contaminated surfaces, but since it can survive for up to three days on the feet of a face fly, we can assume that surfaces touched by infected animals may be infective for several days. Chutes, barn walls, fences, trailers, human hands, clothing and instruments may be potential sources of disease spread.

Some cattle are carriers of *M. bovis,* retaining a few bacteria in eye tissues even after they overcome the infection and the eye heals. Bacteria are often found in eyes and nostrils of healthy animals and serve as a source of infection for a new herd outbreak. Bacteria are shed in the tears and nasal fluid of noticeably infected cattle, as well as of carrier animals with seemingly healthy eyes. Individuals with active infection shed higher numbers.

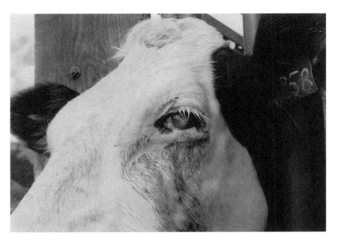

Pinkeye is eye inflammation caused by bacteria. The condition creates excessive tears, ulceration of the cornea, and temporary blindness.

Most animals that recover from pinkeye develop some immunity to *M. bovis*, but immunity is of short duration and not very strong. There are at least seven different strains of these bacteria, with several subtypes in each strain. Immunity to one does not protect the animal against the others; she may get pinkeye again the next year or even later the same season if a new strain comes along and conditions are right for bacteria to multiply.

Cows usually have more resistance to pinkeye than calves do, just because they've had more exposure to the bacteria and may have some immunity. Carrier animals may retain the bacteria over winter, however, and pinkeye crops out again the next fly season when it's spread to other animals by face flies, by direct contact, or by cattle rubbing the same objects. Even if cattle are spread out in large pastures, they still congregate at water sources or shaded areas during the heat of the day, thereby spreading bacteria to one another.

Just having *M. bovis* in the eye is not enough to cause pinkeye. There must be trauma or irritation to allow bacteria to establish an infection. The bacteria tend to stay in the lubricating fluid of the conjunctiva. Unless there is a scrape, bacteria cannot bind to the cornea and cause infection. Anything that disrupts the protective covering of the eye (such as being switched in the face by the tail of another animal) can open the way for bacteria to start a new infection in a carrier animal.

Dusty feed, blowing sand, plant pollens, weed seeds, virus infection, fly bites, tall grasses scraping

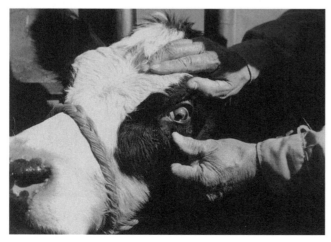
Cattle with dark skin around the eyes may still get pinkeye.

the eye as the animal grazes, or UV rays in sunlight — combined with a face-fly population — can create a herd outbreak of pinkeye. Other flies, such as horn flies, houseflies, or stable flies, may play a minor role in physically carrying bacteria from one animal to another, but face flies are the primary culprits; they not only fly from animal to animal, taking bacteria on their legs, but also scratch the animal's eyes to make them water so they can feed on the secretions.

Face flies are difficult to control except via insecticide ear tags, dust bags, or other applications that apply the insecticide directly to the animal. Though flies lay eggs in fresh manure, removing manure from pastures is impractical, especially since eggs hatch quickly and larvae immediately move into the soil. A large, healthy population of dung beetles is a more effective measure for minimizing fly populations than trying to remove the manure. Use of dung beetles is also a less toxic choice than insecticides for fly control. See chapter 7 for specific approaches to external pest regulation.

Cattle Color Doesn't Matter (Much)

Solid-colored cattle with dark skin around the eyes have traditionally been thought to have less pinkeye. In fact, Angus breeders claimed for a long time that their breed does not get pinkeye at all, but this is not true. The color of skin around the eyes and the irritation from ultraviolet light affecting nonpigmented skin (such as a white-faced animal with pink eyelids and more light reflected into the eye) is one factor, but because of the variety of other causes, color is not the only determining element in whether or not an animal will get pinkeye.

Symptoms

Infection with *M. bovis* is highly contagious. Under the right conditions, nearly half the calves in a herd may be affected during the course of a summer. The first signs of pinkeye appear suddenly, 3 to 5 days after bacteria enter the eye. The animal blinks frequently, holds the eye shut, rubs the eye, and seeks shade to get away from painful bright light. At that point, small ulcers may already be developing on the cornea surface. The face is wet from excessive tears running from the inner corner of the eye. Within a day, you'll usually see a pit (ulcer) on the surface of the eye if you look closely and red swollen membranes around the eye. A few days later, the ulceration on the transparent cornea becomes a white spot up to a half-inch (1.3 cm) in diameter.

About 48 hours after tears streak down the face, the cornea becomes cloudy, and the entire eyeball appears blue. The animal is temporarily blind, unable to see through the ulcerated tissue. The lining of the eyelids is red, and there may be secretion of mucus and pus. There may be an outwardly protruding blood red border around the ulceration. In severe cases the cornea looks white. The ulcer deepens, and blood vessels grow toward the ulcer, finally reaching the center of it in 14 to 16 days. By then the entire ulcer bulges outward. White blood cells gather in the area to ingest and destroy the bacteria. These white blood cells release enzymes that increase the depth and size of the ulcer, which perforates the cornea and allows the iris to prolapse through the damaged area, creating an obvious bulge.

After a time, this defect usually heals, but in some instances the damage can lead to rupture of the eyeball. Rupture is rare but may occur with a severe infection or from trauma when the blind animal runs into objects. Otherwise, the eyes of most infected cattle will generally heal within about 2 months, leaving a permanent scar (a white or blue spot) on the cornea. Once healed, the eye surface may be somewhat enlarged or misshapen.

Make Sure It's Pinkeye

Other diseases and conditions mistaken for pinkeye include chaff and foreign bodies in the eye such as cheatgrass seed heads, sharp awns of foxtail (see page 192) or microscopic *burdock* slivers caught beneath an eyelid (see page 193). These irritants make the eye sore and runny, and it won't heal until the foreign particle is removed or works itself out.

IBR and Pinkeye Distinctions

Infectious bovine rhinotracheitis (IBR) can also cause eyes to be inflamed and watering and to develop lesions that look very much like infectious pinkeye (see chapter 5). IBR is a herpes virus that causes recurring ulcers for life and does not respond to antibiotic therapy. Eye lesions that do not improve with pinkeye treatment may be the eye form of IBR.

BLIND CALF ON THE RANGE

WE HAD SEVERE PINKEYE in our first crops of calves when we started ranching in 1967. We were young and naive and didn't know much about this disease. We took an Angus calf who was blind in one eye from pinkeye to a new vet, and he removed the eye. This was a costly procedure that was tough on our small, struggling budget. We didn't use that vet for long; another vet showed us how to treat serious cases and sew the eyelids shut. In the years since, we've successfully treated many eyes that were much worse than the eye the other vet removed. They all healed, regaining vision.

During the 1970s and '80s, before the advent of pinkeye vaccine, we had several cases of pinkeye most summers, especially in calves. We rode the range often to check cattle in the mountains, but some cases of pinkeye were well advanced by the time we saw them. Some cleared up on their own, but a few animals had cloudy eyes or were blind, so we brought them home to treat them and sew their eyes shut.

One of the worst cases was a calf whose mother, Brown Eyes, died on the range from eating larkspur. The orphan was blind in both eyes from pinkeye when my daughter and I found him. He was stumbling around, running into trees. We needed to bring him home before he fell down a mountain or into a gully. Since he had no mother to follow, we selected a gentle cow named Grendel as his "seeing-eye cow" to bring him slowly home.

We patiently kept the blind calf with Grendel and her own calf, taking the little trio 5 miles through the mountains. We tried to select the easiest route through the best canyon crossings to avoid thick brush and steep hillsides. We got them most of the way home — to a small corral where we could load the blind calf in our pickup and haul him the rest of the way home for treatment and care. He eventually recovered sight in both eyes and was sold with the rest of our calves that fall.

During the acute early stage of IBR, some cattle develop cloudy corneas similar to pinkeye, but the opacity travels inward from the outer edges of the cornea, rather than starting in the center in the manner of a pinkeye infection.

That pinkeye almost always occurs during warm weather when flies are active and IBR can occur any time of year is another diagnostic clue. Pinkeye infection usually peaks in July and August when fly populations are highest, sunlight is most intense, grass is tall, and the weather is dry.

Prevention

Conditions that lead to pinkeye outbreaks fall into three categories:

1. Circumstances that reduce the animals' ability to fight off infection, such as stress and vulnerable immune status

2. Factors that help spread the bacteria that cause pinkeye

3. Conditions that produce trauma to the eye, enabling the bacteria to enter the tissues

Age of the animal can affect immune status. Calves with less experienced immune systems are often more susceptible than adults. Cows that have some immunity already, due to previous exposure or to vaccine, may pass some protection to their newborn calves via colostrum.

As with many diseases, a window of opportunity for infection occurs between the time a young calf's antibodies from colostrum start to decline and when he starts generating his own immunity. This is another reason most pinkeye outbreaks in calves occur on summer pasture, when spring-born beef calves are between 4 and 8 months of age. Stress during this time, including that from other disease infections and mixing of cattle from different sources, may also make calves more vulnerable.

Eye trauma gives bacteria access. Management efforts to help minimize situations in which eye trauma might occur include dust reduction, clipping tall pastures with sharp seed heads, providing shade, and controlling flies. None of these practices is 100 percent effective. It can be difficult to control dust and pasture height in many situations and almost impossible to control the effects of ultraviolet light.

Face-fly control is probably the most important antipinkeye measure (see chapter 7). Insecticide ear tags help, because face flies are only attracted to head and eyes. Since calves are most vulnerable to pinkeye, it is important to put tags on them as well as on cows. Insecticide dust bags and rubbers also help, and larvicides added to grain feed can kill larvae in manure before they become flies.

Overall Herd Health

Focus on total herd health and diet before you reach for antibiotics and pinkeye vaccines. A lot of people start at the top, thinking that a certain drug or vaccine will solve all the problems, but they never address some of the basic underlying causes of poor herd health.

Vitamin A is essential to the health of skin and mucous membranes, including eyes. Inadequate trace minerals or basic deficiencies in mineral and vitamin content of the diet may be factors in immune status. If you have a pinkeye problem, look at your soils, grasses, protein levels in forage, and other feed.

Maintaining strong immunity to other diseases (especially viral diseases such as IBR and BVD) can help prevent pinkeye. Viral diseases can hinder the immune system and lead to a higher incidence of other health problems, including pinkeye. When cattle are vaccinated annually with modified live-virus IBR-BVD vaccines, for instance, this can dramatically reduce the incidence of pinkeye, foot rot, diphtheria, and "summer pneumonia" of calves on some farms.

There are many ways to try to prevent the spread of pinkeye via trauma to the eyes. Some of these methods work on some farms but not on others. On one farm the main problem might be dust, and even if the stockman has a good fly-control program, there are still cases of pinkeye because the flies are not the only cause of eye trauma. On another farm it might be long grass, nicking the eyes. During a bad fire year, smoke and ashes may be the culprits.

If cattle are being fed grain (as in a feedlot), tetracycline in feed helps with prevention, but the levels in feed are not high enough to be 100 percent effective. It can be challenging to determine the most appropriate and affordable treatments. If an outbreak occurs, however, aggressive treatment for bad eyes and immediate isolation of infected animals or other control measures taken to prevent the infection from spreading are always a better choice than waiting to see if things get better.

Vaccination

There are vaccines that can help control pinkeye in certain instances, by boosting an animal's immune response to *M. bovis*. Results from vaccination are variable, however, since there are several strains of these bacteria. Select a vaccine that contains as many strains and substrain isolates as possible. In some vaccinated herds, even though a few animals still get pinkeye, the incidence of this disease is much lower than in unvaccinated herds. If a vaccinated animal does get pinkeye, the disease is often less severe than in an unvaccinated animal.

Some vaccines are given as a single dose, and other products must be given twice, 2 to 4 weeks apart, for effective immunity. Always follow label directions. Calves can be vaccinated in the spring when they are handled for other vaccinations, dehorning, and other procedures. Vaccinate the entire herd at the same time.

The vaccine is most effective if given 6 to 8 weeks before fly season. If you wait and use it at the start of an epidemic later in summer, it will be much less effective because many animals will already be exposed and in the early stages of the disease. They'll get pinkeye in spite of vaccination because they can't develop adequate immunity quickly enough.

Not All Vaccines Are Equal

M. bovis binds to the eye by means of filament-like appendages (pili). These pili contain some of the antigenic properties of the bacteria. Vaccines that contain the pilus antigens are thought to be more effective than vaccines that do not. But pilus antigens of these particular bacteria seem to change and can change more rapidly than vaccine manufacturers can test new vaccines and have them approved.

When the vaccines finally get to market, they'll work if used on a farm or herd where pinkeye bacteria have that particular antigen. But if the bacteria's pilus antigens change or if another pilus antigen is introduced to the farm from new flies or new cattle, the vaccines may not work on the animals. There may be some cross-protection between the different types but not much.

Custom-Made Vaccine

Trying to build robust immunity in the eye is difficult, and stockmen must realize that in many instances the vaccine will not prevent an outbreak of pinkeye. If the commercial vaccine does not seem to be helping enough for prevention, there may be other pathogens involved besides *M. bovis* or its binding appendages *(pili)* have changed, requiring a different vaccine formulation. Some veterinarians take swabs from affected eyes and culture the causative organism to make an *autogenous vaccine* for that herd. There hasn't been a scientific trial to affirm that a custom-made vaccine does or doesn't work. Some farms claim it does, but this is hard to prove because the conditions that create a pinkeye epidemic may change from year to year.

For instance, one year you might have a bad pinkeye problem and administer the autogenous vaccine your vet created to take care of it for the following year. The next year there might not be any pinkeye, so you attribute this improvement to the vaccine, but it might be due to other conditions. The first year might have been very dusty, for instance, and the next year it rained. You might have less pinkeye due to less dust, fewer flies, or some other condition that changed. The vaccine may even work for a couple of years in a row, and then a face fly or new cattle on the ranch might bring in another strain of *M. bovis* with a different pilus antigen, and now your vaccine doesn't work.

Treatment

Pinkeye treatment can be a frustrating undertaking. If it is indeed pinkeye, and not another affliction with similar symptoms, timely isolation and treatment can help halt the spread and prevent an epidemic. Early treatment will also clear up a bad eye much quicker, reduce pain and the detrimental effect on milk production or weaning weight, and prevent permanent eye damage.

Pinkeye is easily spread, so take care not to spread it inadvertently. If you corral cattle to treat those with pinkeye and then run them all through the chute, you may put them all at risk. Often it's better to treat affected animals individually. If you handle an animal with pinkeye, wash your hands before you touch the eyes of another animal or you'll be just as likely to spread the disease as any face fly.

Cases treated in early stages respond very well to antibiotic treatment, but even eyes that are badly ulcerated and blind will recover if treated. Be sure to not only use an antibiotic to combat the infection but also protect the eye from dust, sunlight, flies, and other irritants while it heals.

Antibiotics

M. bovis is susceptible to many commonly used antibiotics, including penicillin, oxytetracycline, florfenicol, sulfonamides, and tilmicosin. When dealing with *M. bovis,* early treatment with injected tetracycline is very successful. Intramuscular injections often halt the infection, since the antibiotic is taken into eye tissues by the bloodstream. It is simpler to give an IM injection than to treat the eye itself.

EARLY PINKEYE TREATMENT

Twice-daily application of a topical pinkeye antibiotic for a few days may be adequate if the infection is caught early, when the eye is simply watering and held shut. But if pinkeye has several days' start and the eye is already turning blue or ulcerating, injecting the eyelid and protecting the eye for 2 weeks gives much better results.

Topical Ointment

Giving systemic antibiotics may not be feasible for a lactating dairy cow, however, due to lengthy withdrawal time before there are no longer any residues in the milk; the milk must be discarded for a certain number of days (see label directions on the antibiotic) because it cannot be used for human consumption. The milk can be fed to calves being bottle fed because residue won't hurt them. When treating a dairy cow, use a local antibiotic within the eye itself, since these have shorter withdrawal times.

Some antibiotics are marketed as topical treatments for pinkeye. Unfortunately, it's hard to maintain adequate levels of the antibiotics when they are applied topically (as ointments, powders, sprays, or liquid squirts) because they don't stay in the eye long enough. To be effective, they must be put into the eye at least twice daily (for 3 to 5 days), since tears wash medication out of the eye within a short time. Normal cattle produce slightly less than an ounce (29.6 mL) of tears daily, but cattle with pinkeye produce many more times this amount of tears (due to eye irritation), which rapidly washes away antibiotic preparations applied to the surface of the eye. A topical antibiotic may work fine for a dairy cow you are handling twice daily to milk, but most people don't want to capture and restrain a beef animal this often.

Eye Injections

Penicillin injected under the conjunctiva, beneath the membrane lining the inside of the eyelid, is more effective and longer lasting than a topical antibiotic. It's a good treatment choice for a dairy cow, as the method has a much shorter withdrawal period (during which milk must be discarded) than that of a systemic intramuscular or subcutaneous antibiotic injection. To give the eye injection:

1. Restrain the animal in a chute or stanchion, with her head tied around to one side with a halter.
2. Roll back the upper eyelid of the infected eye.
3. Direct the needle just under the surface of the membrane and into the inside of the eyelid.
4. Inject 1 cc of antibiotic with a small-diameter (18 gauge) needle.

Penicillin mixed with dexamethasone is often used for this inner-eyelid injection. The steroid helps reduce pain and swelling. This mix not only lasts longer at the site than any topical medication applied to the eyeball (being gradually absorbed over 2 to 3 days to provide a constant source of medication) but also provides pain-killing and anti-inflammatory effects. One injection is usually sufficient to treat a serious case, but you can repeat it a few days later if necessary.

Studies have shown that antibiotic residues in milk from an eyelid injection can be detected as early as 4 hours after the injection, peak at 10 hours, and disappear by 28 hours. The recommended withdrawal time for injecting 1 mL of penicillin into an eye is 36 hours. By contrast, withdrawal time for a systemic injection of oxytetracycline is 96 hours after the final treatment (for milk), and most types of penicillin are not allowed for systemic use in lactating dairy cows.

Systemic Injections

If you are not planning to sell or butcher an infected beef cow right away, antibiotics can be given systemically to combat pinkeye. Treat cattle with intramuscular or subcutaneous injections of long-lasting oxytetracycline, given according to label directions for dosage and administration (withdrawal time before slaughter is 28 days). A single injection of LA-200 or Biomycin, for instance, is often effective, and both are labeled for pinkeye (see chapter 2 for injection steps). This treatment can be

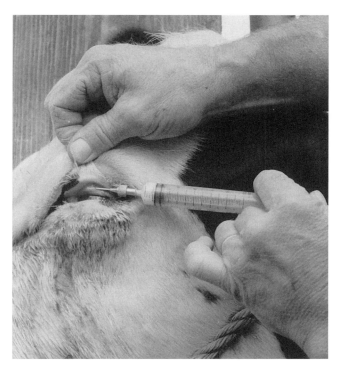

The most effective pinkeye treatment involves injecting penicillin into the lining of the upper eyelid, beneath the membrane on the inside of the lid.

repeated 48 to 72 hours later, if necessary. When the eye stops producing tears, this is a sign it is healing. In a serious case of pinkeye, the most effective treatment is a combination of systemic antibiotics, eyelid injection, and eye protection.

Nuflor (florfenicol) can be given as two injections 24 hours apart or as a single subcutaneous injection at higher dosage for longer action. Excede is a broad-spectrum antibiotic effective against gram-negative bacteria; it was designed to treat respiratory disease and is a long-acting sustained-release formulation of ceftiofur — the same drug as Naxcel. One injection of Excede, placed under the skin in the middle one-third of the back of the ear, provides high antibiotic levels in the bloodstream for 7 to 8 days.

A study at UC–Davis showed that both Nuflor and Excede are very effective as treatments for pinkeye. This is an extra-label use for these drugs, however, and you must consult your vet and obtain a prescription before giving these products. Your vet should also train you in the proper injection technique when using Excede — on the back of the ear — because if given incorrectly this drug will quickly kill the animal.

USE DISPOSABLE GLOVES

Whenever you examine, handle, or treat an eye for any reason, use disposable latex examination gloves obtained from your vet or medical-supply source. After you have examined or treated the eye or nose area, throw the gloves away, since they are likely to be contaminated with bacteria. The gloves will keep you from getting bacteria on your hands and spreading it to another animal. If you use a halter or nose tongs to restrain an animal's head, disinfect them with Nolvasan before using them on any other animal.

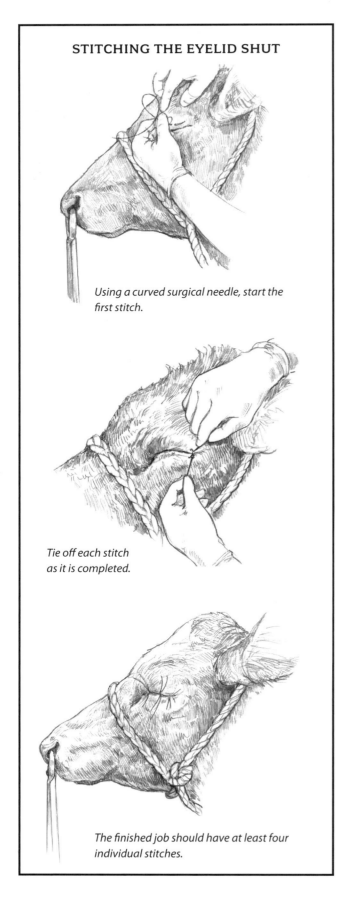

Using a curved surgical needle, start the first stitch.

Tie off each stitch as it is completed.

The finished job should have at least four individual stitches.

Eye Protection

Eyes heal faster if you combine eye protection with antibiotic treatment. The eye can be protected with a patch or by sewing the eyelids shut. A piece of denim stuck to the side of the face with rubber cement or some other nontoxic glue can be used as a patch. Commercial glue-on patches are also available for covering the eye. The disadvantage of gluing on any type of eye cover is that sometimes they don't stay on long enough; cattle often rub them off.

Stitching the eyelids shut, when done correctly, is more dependable than any patch for protecting an eye from bright light, dust, and flies, and also has the advantage of keeping the eyelids immobile. There's no blinking to rub the protruding ulcer and keep irritating the inflamed eye. With the eye continually closed, it is constantly bathed in its own tears, which has a healing effect. Stitching the eye shut for 2 or 3 weeks keeps it from drying out. Seriously affected eyes tend to bulge, prolapse, and become dried out, which delay healing.

Pinkeye cases detected and treated early are less likely to develop complications, such as deep ulceration and scarring, bubble eye, and permanent damage, but it's still important to treat eyes in the late stages of pinkeye. Not only will aggressive treatment and protection help the eye heal faster and with less permanent scarring and damage, but it also eliminates the bacteria causing the infection. This ensures that the animal won't continue to serve as a source of pinkeye for the rest of the herd.

Foreign Material in the Eye

Cattle often get pieces of hay or straw (*chaff*) or grass seeds stuck in the eye. These usually work their way over to the corner of the eye, where tears wash them out. Occasionally, though, they become trapped under the lid and cause irritation. If foreign bodies are caught in the corner of the eye or stuck in the membranes under an eyelid, they are very painful, and the eye waters profusely. A seed stuck to the underside of an eyelid may scrape the eyeball every time the animal blinks. If the surface is scratched, inflammation may create an ulcer (erosion) or a spot on the tough transparent covering of the eye (*cornea*). The lesion and tears may be mistaken for pinkeye. Large foreign particles can be found by your vet during examination of the eye and flushed free or removed with small *forceps*.

Sometimes a foreign body is easy to see because it's stuck to the eyeball, but it's not always easy to remove. Sometimes it's not visible until the eyelid is rolled back. You may need your veterinarian to help you find and remove the foreign body, since he or she has more experience at rolling back eyelids and examining eyes. The vet may apply a local anesthetic to the eye surface so the animal won't protest so much, making it easier to find and grasp the foreign body with forceps.

Particle-Removal Trick

If the chaff or seed is visible, you may be able to remove it with the animal restrained. It can be hard, however, to wipe it out of the eye since he'll close it tightly. If the particle is stuck to the eyeball itself or floating around, not embedded under an eyelid, try the following trick to snare it.

1. Restrain the suffering animal.

2. Squeeze a bit of sticky ointment out of a tube of eye medicine (obtained from your vet for treating eye infections) so that it's protruding from the end of the tube's nozzle.

3. Hold the eyelids open as best you can, and carefully, calmly approach the eye with the tube so as not to startle the animal.

4. Quickly press the little glob of ointment onto the floating foreign body.

5. As the animal pulls away, the foreign body will generally remain stuck to the ointment on the end of your tube. If you can't snag it with ointment, get help from your vet.

If the eye has been scratched or irritated by the particle, it is vulnerable to infection; the eye's protective covering has been penetrated, and opportunistic bacteria may gain entrance. After you've removed the foreign body, apply eye ointment along the inside of the lower lid or into the corner of the eye or squirt a liquid eye medication over the eye. Tears help disperse the antibiotic over the eye and help protect the scratched area from infection.

Microscopic Burr Slivers

Burdock slivers cause an eye problem often mistaken for pinkeye, except this irritation occurs during the wrong time of year to be pinkeye. If a sliver gets into an eye, it gets caught under an eyelid, where it scratches the surface of the eyeball (cornea) with every blink, creating abrasions and ulcers. The eye is sensitive to light, so the cow holds it shut. Other symptoms include excessive tears and contraction of the pupil and positive *fluorescein dye* uptake at the site of corneal damage (when a dye is put into the eye to detect any scratches on its surface). These symptoms can mislead the vet into thinking this is a corneal injury. An embedded foreign body may not be suspected until the corneal damage fails to respond to conventional treatment within a reasonable period. If an animal has an inflamed eye that is not responding to topical antibiotic treatment, suspect a burr fragment is the culprit.

Slivers from a burr are so small that the vet's usual eye examination tools — a strong light and a magnifying lens — are not powerful enough to locate them. Finding the general area of irritation may help locate the sliver, since actual viewing of it can be difficult without extensive magnification. But the inflamed and reddened tissues can easily hide the tiny sliver. The vet must narrow the search by looking at the portion of the eyelid rubbing the damaged cornea during eye movements and blinking.

To locate the culprit with a powerful magnifying lens, the veterinarian must first stain the eye with fluorescein die. Some slivers can be removed by grasping with forceps. Those that can't be grasped may be removed by scraping the surface of the inflamed conjunctiva with a scalpel blade.

When no sliver can be seen, scraping the inflamed conjunctiva to remove the sliver and following up with antibiotics typically resolves the problem. After the sliver is removed and topical antibiotics are given, the eye usually returns to normal, though an eye that's been inflamed a long time, with more scarring, takes longer to heal.

Stockmen who don't have access to a veterinary facility that has specialized equipment for eye examinations can treat the eye themselves. We treated winter eye infections the same as we would for a bad case of pinkeye, stitching the eyelid shut to reduce irritation and halt blinking, which also keeps the sliver from rubbing against the eyeball. Just like a tiny splinter in your finger that festers and comes out, the sliver eventually works out of the lid lining and is washed away by tears. The eye clears up and becomes normal again. This treatment works best if given before the eye is badly damaged and infected.

Burdock Hitchhikers

Burdock (*Arctium minus*) produces seeds that stick to fur, hair, and clothing — anything that brushes them — because they have microscopic hooks and barbs. Cocklebur is lowgrowing, with small egg-shaped brown burrs, and burdock is 6 feet [1.8 m] tall or more, with large composite leaves and round, prickly burrs.

Burdock was brought from Europe and Asia by burrs stuck to imported animals. It thrives in moist soils along fences, roads, and ditches, where ground has been disturbed, or in burned areas. It often grows in shady places. Cattle that go into the brush for shade become covered with burrs.

The plants bloom in late summer; the burrs mature by mid-August in southern regions and later in northern climates. When burrs ripen they release hundreds of microscopic barbed slivers. If a burr is shredded during attempts at removal from fur or hair, these seeds are scattered. Slivers can become embedded in human flesh, causing irritation. They are too small to see with the naked eye and are hard to remove.

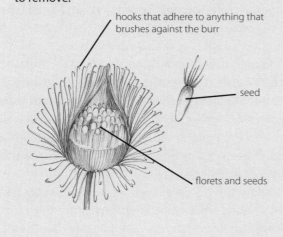

hooks that adhere to anything that brushes against the burr

seed

florets and seeds

Dried burr from a burdock plant

The Offending Plant

Fall and winter are common times for burdock eye problems. Burrs are hanging on the plant, ready to latch onto anything that passes by. They may stay all winter on the dead, dry plant that might still be standing in spring, even after new plants are growing. A horse or cow may also get a burr sliver in an eye any time of year if feed or bedding contains shredded burrs, as when burdock plants get baled with hay or straw. If the animal roots around in the hay or bedding or slings and shakes a flake of hay while eating, tiny slivers from shreds of mashed burrs may disperse in the air and could end up in an eye.

Burdock is a biennial; it comes up from the roots the next year to produce blooms and seeds. Chopping or spraying at proper times to keep it from going to seed can control burdock. Spraying for 2 years gives the best control, but if you don't want to use *herbicide*, you can eventually get rid of patches just by chopping down all plants, leaving none to go to seed. We reduced winter eye problems in our cattle by diligently chopping down patches of burdock in the brush. If you do it too early, however, plants grow back and still go to seed. You'll have better results if plants are chopped after they bud but before burrs are ripe. A few plants may grow from old seeds, so you still have to check the areas each year and chop any plants that come up, but this will help reduce the burdock problem.

Cancer Eye

Eye cancer (bovine ocular *squamous cell carcinoma*) is the most common type of cancer in cattle. Eighty percent of all *tumors* reported at slaughter involve the eye and are the leading cause of carcass condemnation at packing plants resulting in losses of more than $20 million per year in the United States. Cancer eye causes significant economic loss to cattle producers, due to the decreased salvage value of affected cows, condemnation of carcasses in advanced cases, and shortened productive life. Cows with cancer eye often must be culled during their productive years. If this condition is detected early, however, it can usually be successfully treated and cured, since the first stages are not malignant. Neglect is a common reason for lost value on an animal. It's important to recognize the early signs of cancer.

DURING THE EARLY 1980s on our ranch, we had a few cases of irritated, watering eyes every winter. Some of the affected eyes became ulcerated, blue, and temporarily blind. We had to treat several of our bulls for bad eyes when they were on winter pasture in the fields along our creek and usually treated at least two or three cows each winter.

We couldn't understand why cattle would get pinkeye so late in the year, and neither could our vet. Fly season was long past, and our cattle had been on a good IBR-BVD control program since 1976. IBR sometimes affects eyes, and BVD can impair the immune system and make animals susceptible to other diseases, including pinkeye. Not knowing what was causing the winter eye problems, we treated them like pinkeye, injecting antibiotics into the inner surface of the upper eyelid, and sewing the eyelids shut to protect the temporarily blind eyeball. They all cleared up after treatment, though it often took several weeks.

The cause of the eye inflammation eluded us. Then in 1993 we read a report from the Virginia-Maryland Regional College of Veterinary Medicine. A number of sore-eyed horses examined there had microscopic barbed "slivers" embedded in

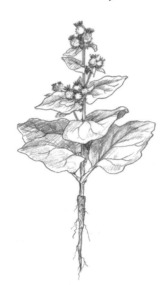

The young growing burdock plants can be controlled by chopping or spraying after they bud but before they go to seed.

the eyelid tissues — fragments from burr seed heads of the burdock plant. Veterinarians at the New York State College of Veterinary Medicine at Cornell University found the same cause for mysterious eye problems in horses and cattle.

We talked with one of the vets at Cornell, who told us the tiny slivers become entangled in folds of the eyelid lining and are very hard to locate and remove. When caught under the lid, they create a sore by scraping against the eyeball each time the animal blinks, just as a larger particle would. Soon the cornea becomes ulcerated, and the eye may turn cloudy blue, with a white spot or bulge from inflammation and infection.

When we learned about the burdock menace, our "winter pinkeye" mystery was solved. The cattle that had developed eye problems in fall and winter were in our lower fields, where they had access to creek bottoms and thickets where burdock grows. This plant had moved onto our ranch from a nearby ditch on our neighbor's place. Burrs sticking to wildlife and cattle were spreading the plant all through the brush in those pastures. It made perfect sense that the cows on our mountain pasture in late fall never had eye problems. There was no burdock up there!

Cancer eye is very rare in young animals but can occur in mature cattle of any breed. It's most common in white-faced animals, so stockmen who own cows with dark-colored faces tend to think their cows will never get this problem, and if they are not checking for it, they may not catch the early signs. White-faced or light-skinned cattle are most susceptible to cancer because the ultraviolet rays in sunlight can damage nonpigmented skin. Sunlight is also reflected into the animal's eyes, which can irritate them. Dark skin around an eye absorbs more light, and darker pigment also makes skin tougher and less susceptible to irritation. Cattle with dark skin do occasionally develop cancer eye, however.

There are two types of cancer eye: growths on the eyeball and growths on the eyelids. The latter is more serious, especially if neglected, since the tumor grows inward and can *metastasize* (spread to other tissues) sooner. It spreads to internal lymph nodes and organs, eventually killing the cow. Tumors on the eyeball, by contrast, tend to grow out from the surface rather than inward, taking longer to become malignant. Either tumor type can be successfully treated with surgery, freezing, or burning, but treatment effectiveness depends on how soon you treat it. Cattle with multiple precancerous lesions on an eye are more likely to develop cancer. It's wise to cull them.

REMOVING AN EYEBALL TUMOR

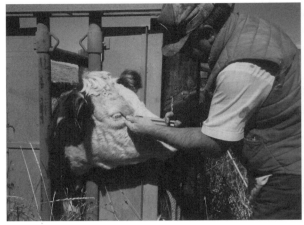

1. Small eyeball tumors can be easily removed. To begin, the veterinarian injects local anesthetic around the eye.

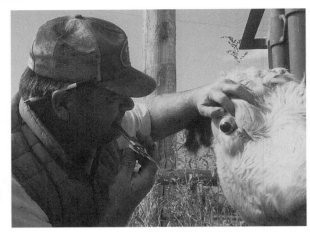

2. He or she then injects fluid behind the eye to pop the eye out of the socket so it will be easier to work on.

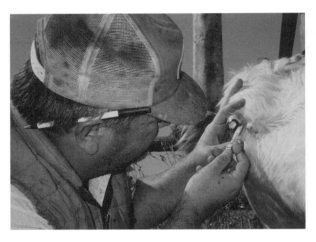

3. With the eye out of its socket, the small white growth on the side of the eyeball (where the white part meets the colored part of the eye) can be carefully sliced off with a scalpel.

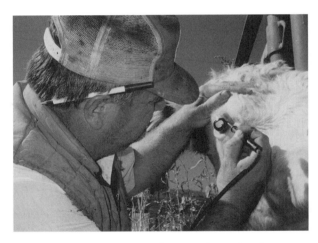

4. After removing the growth, the area is burned and cauterized to kill any stray cancer cells that might remain.

In early stages, before cancer invades deeper tissues, the eye can be saved and the tumor's growth halted with freezing or burning. If the cancer is more advanced, however, surgery is usually tried. This involves removing part of the eyelid, or removing the entire eyeball, depending on location of the cancer. By this stage, however, you may have only a 50 percent chance of saving the cow because the cancer may have already spread beyond the eye.

Eyeball Tumors
One of the most common sites for tumors is the area on the eyeball where white and dark portions meet, at the edge of the colored part of the eyeball. Few tumors originate on other parts of the eye; lesions in the center of the eye are usually due to injury or pinkeye; they are usually not cancer. The growth at the edge of the eye begins as an area that is small, white, and flat or slightly raised and pink. It is easily seen if you get close to the eye.

This type of lesion is called a *plaque* or *papilloma* and is a precursor to cancer. It grows slowly and may take months or even years before it changes into a malignant tumor. In fact, 30 percent of all plaques eventually get smaller and disappear without treatment. There's not a great deal of blood supply at the outer surface of the eye, and tumors originating on the eyeball itself are less likely to metastasize to other sites than are tumors originating in tissues around the eye. Any small white growth at the corner or edge of the eyeball should be closely watched, however. If it starts to grow, it should be removed before it becomes malignant.

Have your vet examine the eye. With the animal restrained in a chute and her head immobilized with a halter and nose lead, the vet can carefully cut the growth away with a sharp scalpel, then burn the area for 30 seconds with an electric probe to kill any stray cancer cells or freeze it. To safely cut the growth off the eye, the vet deadens the area with local anesthetic and injects a solution behind the eyeball to temporarily pop it out of its socket. That way the animal can't retract the eye and reflexively pull the *third eyelid* across it while the vet is operating.

Treating these lesions early when they are small and not yet malignant may enable a cow to have several more good productive years. Remember, however, when keeping the cow, that you should not keep a heifer (or bull) from her even if she's one of your best cows. The tendency to develop eye cancer is inherited.

Eyelid Tumors

Other common sites for cancer are the lower eyelid, third eyelid, and in the socket tissues at either corner of the eye rather than on the eyeball. These growths are not malignant in early stages but can quickly progress to a wartlike tumor that's pink or red and irregular in shape. This rough tissue can become ulcerated, bleeds easily, and may have a foul odor — all of which are signs of cancer.

The third eyelid is the most common site for malignant tumors on eyelids. In these instances, the third eyelid starts to protrude and can be seen at the inner corner of the eye as a bulge of pink tissue. These tumors readily progress to the base of the third eyelid and spread into the eye socket and surrounding bones, metastasizing more quickly than tumors on the eyeball.

On upper or lower eyelids, precursor lesions look like warty, roughened areas along the eyelash line and are called *keratomas* or wickers. Usually appearing on the lower lid, these small tumors are often

crusted over with scablike material that looks like dried eye matter. If the crust seems to be attached to the eyelashes, it probably is dried eye secretions. But if upon closer scrutiny the "scab" is really a small growth directly attached to the lid and removal causes some bleeding, then it's probably precancerous. At this stage, however, it is treatable.

These early lesions have not yet invaded deeper structures and can be completely removed by killing the superficial tissue on the surface of the eyelid. The easiest and most effective treatment for these lesions is burning them off with an electrical probe or by freezing them *(cryosurgery)* with application of intense cold; for instance, by using liquid nitrogen.

Eyelid cancer is more dangerous than tumors on the eyeball because it can get into the socket and lymph nodes much sooner. While 90 to 95 percent of early eyeball tumors can be removed successfully with heat treatment if they're not too extensive, treatment is successful in only about 60 percent of eyelid tumor cases. If cancer has already spread to lymph nodes under the ear and jaw, it will continue to spread through the body and kill the cow. A visible lump below the base of the ear is an indication that the lymph system has already been invaded; it is too late to sell the cow because her carcass will be condemned at slaughter.

Heating and Freezing Cells

Freezing cancerous lesions damages cellular structure and tends to kill surface cells quite readily. Cancer cells have a large nucleus and are more susceptible to heat than are healthy cells with a small nucleus. The electrical probe heats the cells to the point that cancer cells are destroyed, while most of the healthy cells are left intact.

Treating the lesion with heat or cold can be successful if done before the tumor has invaded the underlying surfaces and can usually save the eye. But if the tumor is already malignant, the eye and its surrounding tissues must be removed. This is not always successful, since the cancer may have already spread beyond the eye socket by then.

REMOVING AN EYELID TUMOR

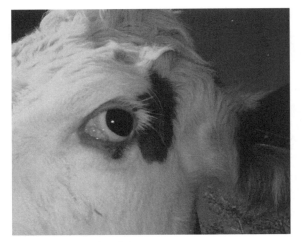

Cancer of the third eyelid

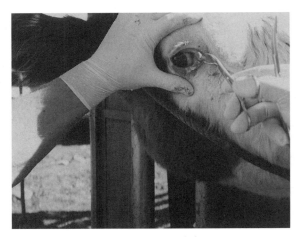

The vet pulls the tumor into view with forceps to surgically remove a cancerous tumor on the third eyelid.

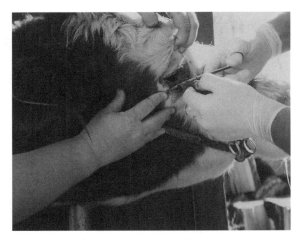

He cuts away the tumorous tissue as he removes that portion of the third eyelid.

An eyelid tumor can be treated by heat or freezing if caught soon enough, or the whole eye and socket tissues can be removed to get all the cancer before it spreads. This surgery is only successful about half the time, however. The cancer may have spread to lymph nodes under the ear and jaw before surgery.

A one-eyed cow sent to a sale for slaughter is always a cancer suspect, but you can choose to sell or butcher the cow before the disease metastasizes. A delay in slaughter to allow the cow to finish raising a calf or complete a pregnancy can be a mistake, however, since the cancer may spread explosively during that time, and you won't be able to salvage her.

Preventive Management

Check eyes closely whenever you handle cows or put them through a chute for vaccinating. Looking at them up close at least twice a year when they are in the chute will enable you to see small growths you might miss otherwise. If you discover early growths, have your vet remove them, or make a point to watch them over the next weeks to see if they grow or regress. A good rule of thumb is to remove small white eyeball plaques if they start to enlarge. Closely watch any suspicious growths on eyelids, and sell or butcher a cow if eyelid growths start to enlarge. Eyelid tumors are likely to re-grow if removed, often coming back more quickly and becoming malignant sooner, so it's often better to sell or butcher the cow rather than treat those lesions.

CHAPTER TEN

Skin Problems

THERE ARE A VARIETY OF PROBLEMS that affect the skin of cattle, everything from sunburn to allergies. Without an understanding of skin diseases, you might not be concerned about a few bald spots or some crusty skin, unless you take pride in exhibiting your beef or dairy cattle at the state fair or livestock shows. Few skin afflictions are merely matters of an animal's appearance, however, even though many of them are quite easy to see on your cows. This chapter discusses the detection, treatment, and prevention of hair loss, warts, *ringworm,* and photosensitization, among others.

Hair Loss and Bald Spots

Human hair loss is just a cosmetic concern. When cattle lose their hair, however, the consequences can be more serious, since hair provides insulation and protection against cold, wet weather, sun, and wind. Hair gives the bovine body waterproofing insulation; moisture tends to run off without soaking through to the skin, due to natural oils on the hair. Hair loss in cattle may be a problem of genetics, fever, or the animal's ever-rubbing and -scratching response to external parasites such as lice or mites (see chapter 7). Most cases of hair loss are temporary, unless the animal has a genetic defect and is born hairless.

Some types of congenital hairlessness are associated with other birth defects, many of which are fatal. In other instances a calf may be born with no hair, yet have normal skin, and may survive if kept out of the sunlight so he won't sunburn. Some of these calves may later grow a little hair, but it may not be enough to provide much protection. In other cases, such as those with the genetic defect occasionally seen in Holsteins, a calf may be born with normal hair and then gradually lose it. Herefords occasionally produce calves on which hair is scanty, but the animal does not go completely bald.

More commonly, hair loss and bald patches are a result of high fever during an illness, especially in

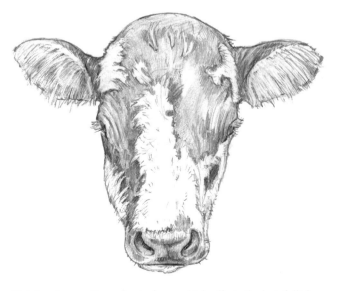

Hair loss is sometimes due to fever, which affects the hair follicles. A week or so after the fever, hair may be easily rubbed off, leaving bald spots. After the follicles recover, the hair grows back.

young calves. It is not unusual for a calf that recently recovered from scours or pneumonia to lose patches of hair. If you rub the calf, some of his hair readily comes off, but he is not itchy. By the time you notice hair loss, the calf has usually recovered from the fever and illness and is otherwise normal again.

During the stress of fever and dehydration, the hair follicles may stop producing hair temporarily. Without continual new growth, bald spots appear when the old hair falls out. It may take 3 or 4 weeks before new hair grows in on those areas. If the weather is cold, wet, or sunny during that time you should shelter the calf to keep him from getting too cold or sunburned.

Photosensitization

Photosensitization is a reaction to something the animal has eaten. Symptoms don't appear until skin is exposed to sunlight, which then creates *dermatitis* (inflammation). The harmful effects of an ingested toxin cause the animal to have sensitized skin, particularly in areas of the body where there is no skin pigment, which acts as a natural sunscreen.

When a cow ingests pasture plants (or fungi on plants) that cause *hepatitis* and liver damage, photosensitization sometimes occurs. Or photosensitization may be a result of primary liver damage and obstruction of bile ducts by tapeworm cysts, tumors, liver abscesses, or liver flukes (internal parasites; see chapter 7). Liver abscesses and damage sometimes occurs when cattle are eating high-grain diets, or if they have contracted another disease, such as leptospirosis. Anything that affects the liver's ability to *metabolize* (break down and change) or excrete harmful compounds through the bile system will predispose an animal to photosensitization.

Branding Cattle

Many states require hot iron branding as proof of ownership. Each cattle owner must have a registered brand that's always in a certain location on the animal. Brands are usually on the hip, thigh, or ribs of cattle, and identified as being on the left or right side. When selecting a brand, it must be different or on a different part of the animal than any other brand in the state. An existing brand can be purchased, however, if the former owner quits raising cattle.

If livestock are stolen, stray from the ranch, or are inadvertently sent with someone else's cattle to market, the brand identifies them and they can be returned to the proper owner. Brand inspections are required when cattle change hands or when traveling across a state line. A brand inspector looks at every animal that goes through a sale yard.

Branding, like dehorning, is stressful for cattle, and should be done with care. Don't brand during bad weather. Wet weather should always be avoided because branding a wet hide creates scalding, which is more painful and damaging to tissue (by creating a deeper, larger burn) and often results in a poor brand. Cattle should be dry when branded.

The iron should be very hot, so that it burns through the hair and top layer of hide immediately without having to be held against the animal for long. Unless the animal has short summer hair, the area to be branded should be clipped. If the iron has to burn through thick hair before it gets to the hide, it will not only take longer and be more painful but will also more severely burn the animal (burning hair keeps a larger area hot longer) and take longer to heal. The iron must be held on just long enough to sear the top layer of skin, creating a smooth surface the color of shoe leather. The top burned layer of a proper brand will later peel, creating a permanent mark on the animal where the hair either does not grow back, is shorter, or is a slightly different color, making the brand easy to see.

When selecting or creating a brand, a simple design with rounded edges rather than acute angles (an O rather than an X, for example) always results in a brand that's easier to read once healed. A brand with acute angles tends to blotch; the heat from the two edges where they come together in a sharp corner will burn the tissue in between. This results in a blob rather than crisp lines and creates a more painful brand that takes longer to heal.

When the liver malfunctions, toxins in the body build up instead of being filtered out, and some get into the bloodstream. Plant pigments aren't metabolized and excreted properly, and if some of them end up in skin tissue, they may be activated by sunlight, causing a serious reaction. Some forage plants contain *photodynamic agents,* substances that can intensify or induce a toxic reaction to sunlight if they get into the bloodstream; they cause photosensitization when they reach the skin. These chemicals are activated by light and make skin cells sensitive and vulnerable to the effects of ultraviolet radiation. The result is severe inflammation of the skin.

While dark skin is not affected, pink or very lightly pigmented skin is acutely affected because these areas are not as well protected from the sun's ultraviolet rays. The easiest way to diagnose photosensitization is to see if there's a pattern to the lesions. If the cow has a white face, white legs, or white udder, the pink skin underneath the white areas will be affected, while the dark skin will be normal. There will be an abrupt difference where the light and dark skin meet. This problem is most common in white-faced or light-colored animals (the latter often develop skin lesions along the middle of the back), but there have also been a few cases in solid red cattle and on the muzzles of cattle if the skin is lighter colored there.

Photosensitization is most apt to occur during the summer, when sunlight is more intense, ultraviolet light is stronger, and cattle are eating green plants. Some cases occur in the spring, when pasture grass is still short and cattle eat strange plants, or in the fall, if animals are moved to a new pasture. During a drought cattle may run out of pasture, need to be moved more often, and might be put into pastures not normally used until later when the toxic plants are dry and unpalatable. If the offending plants are still green, cattle may eat them and increase their risk. Some plants contain chemicals that cause photosensitization directly, and others cause the problem indirectly by damaging the liver.

Some plants such as alsike clover, cause photosensitivity in horses but not in cattle; others cause photosensitization in cattle but not in horses, perhaps because of rumen function or different methods of liver metabolism. Poisonous or toxic plants often

Plants That Cause Photosensitizaton

Plants that contain preformed photoactive compounds and cause photosensitization directly include buckwheat, giant rain lily, smartweed, and St. John's wort.

Plants that can cause liver damage and secondary photosensitization (which is much more common) include agava, alfalfa, Bermuda grass, birdsfoot trefoil, bishop's weed, bitterweed, blue thistle, bluegreen algae, bog asphodel, buttercup, cocklebur, comfrey, fiddleneck, heliotrope, horsebrush, hounds-tongue, Kochia (fireweed), lantana, mushrooms, mustard, paintbrush, panic grasses, puncture vine, rapeseed, rattlebox, sacahulste, senecio, showy crotalaria, signal grass, sneezeweed, spring parsley, tansy (ragwort, grounsel), and tarbush.

In Louisiana and other Gulf Coast states lantana is a problem because the ornamental plant has escaped from gardens and is found on most canal banks. In southern regions, ryegrass is associated with photosensitization, but scientists don't know if it is a primary cause or if it creates liver damage. At least 90 percent of photosensitization cases that occur in cattle are due to liver damage.

damage the liver, and then the by-products of plant digestion tend to accumulate in skin tissues instead of being filtered out of the body by the liver.

When a normal cow ingests green plants, one of the rumen metabolites of *chlorophyll* (the green coloring in plants that accomplishes *photosynthesis* to create energy for the plant) is a compound called *phylloerythrin,* which is a photosensitizing agent. This compound is absorbed when the blood goes through the liver of a healthy animal. If the liver is doing its job properly, it processes that material and excretes it in the bile, where it goes back into the intestine and never enters the blood circulation where it would end up in the skin.

When liver function is impaired, however, the by-products of chlorophyll digestion are not properly eliminated; they spill back into the bloodstream, reaching the small vessels in the skin and accumulating there. When too much phylloerythrin gets into the blood and moves to the skin, the animal suffers photosensitization when sunshine hits her body. Though this happens most commonly when cattle graze green pastures, it can also occur in affected animals that are fed entirely on hay. There is enough chlorophyll in hay or hay pellets to produce critical levels of phylloerythrin in the tissues of animals suffering from liver malfunction.

Symptoms

Unpigmented skin is most affected, especially if hair is short (as in the summer). Long winter hair protects skin from direct sunlight and diminishes the

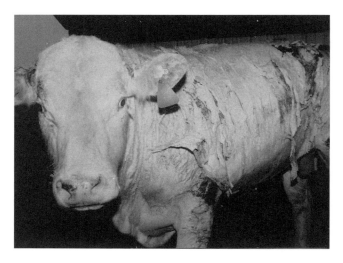

This light-skinned bull developed photosensitization and subsequent loss of hair and skin over most of his body.

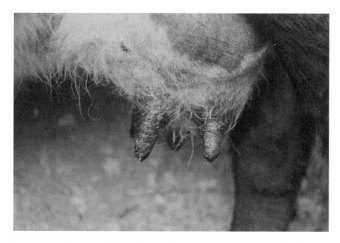

The teats of a cow affected with photosensitization may darken and become cracked and painful. Soon the skin dies and peels off.

reaction. Light-colored or pink skin is most affected if exposed to the sun; the face, back and sides, vulva, and tops of the ears are all damaged, as is the udder if the animal is lying down and sunlight falls on the udder. If the reaction is severe, you'll see photosensitization in unpigmented areas as well.

The ultraviolet rays of sunlight on sensitized tissues cause cell death, swelling, and intense itching. The animal may rub the affected areas. It may look like sunburn at first but soon grows worse. Irritated areas become red and swollen, then develop oozing blisters and cracks. The skin becomes very scaly or develops thick crusts and painful scabs. The animal is dull and depressed, goes off feed, loses weight, tries to stay in the shade (sunlight on the affected skin creates a great deal of pain), and may have a fever. Eyes may water or have a thick discharge.

Photosensitization was earlier called *"blue nose disease"* because the first signs are often a swelling of the nostrils and a slightly purple color on unpigmented, hairless areas on the muzzle close to the nostrils. The teats and vulva of cattle may darken. Teats may become cracked and painful, and an affected cow may kick off her calf or become difficult to milk. Mastitis may develop due to bacterial contamination of the cracked skin. In severe cases, cows have been known to lose some of their teats.

The animal may become quite sick, and patches of skin will start to slough off. These areas will eventually heal, however, leaving some hairless scar tissue if the deeper layers sloughed away. If the animal has a white face, the swelling and crusty skin may extend up the face, and the eyelids may swell. Eyes may become irritated and water profusely. Breathing can be impaired if there is very much swelling around the face. Some animals go off feed.

Animals can develop signs of nervousness or become overly excited if toxins from the dying skin enter the bloodstream and affect the nervous system. If skin lesions become extensive or severe, pulse rate and temperature are elevated, and in serious cases the animal may go into shock. Severe cases have been seen in cattle put into alfalfa fields in late fall after wet weather produced fungal growth on the plants; certain fungi can produce liver damage that creates photosensitization and can be fatal.

OUR ONLY CASE of photosensitization occurred in a black, white-faced Angus/Hereford cow named Prue. Other than our milk cow, she was often the only cow that stayed home from the range in summer. Prue was born with a cleft palate and raised as a pet, and she often reared extra calves with her own if we happened to have an orphan. That summer she was raising only her own calf, Prunella.

Prue and her calf, a couple of our yearlings, and our milk cow all lived in small pastures near the barnyard, including swamp pastures that were too boggy to make hay. Although we didn't realize it at the time, the marshy areas, fed by springs, were probably ideal snail habitat. Prue may have suffered liver damage from flukes, a condition that primed her for photosensitization.

About a week after moving her to new pasture where she may have sampled different plants, we noticed that she didn't feel well. She was very dull, stayed in the shade, and was not grazing. We brought her and her calf in from the pasture, took her temperature (she had a fever), and tried to figure out what was wrong. She was a black cow with a white face and a white udder. The skin of her face was red and swollen, and her teats were so sore that she didn't want her calf to nurse. After consulting with our vet we learned she was suffering from photosensitization, so we put her and her calf in our old milk barn, out of the sun, and fed her hay.

We treated her daily with medication to reduce inflammation, put salve on her teats, which were starting to crack, and supervised nursing time (putting a flank rope on Prue so she wouldn't kick her calf). The skin on her light-colored teats turned black and peeled off, along with some of the skin on the sides of her udder. The skin on her white face also sloughed away like a flap of dead hide, leaving raw spots underneath. We treated those areas with a medicated, soothing salve until they healed and hair began to grow back.

Being a pet, she trusted us, and that made it easier to treat her. We kept her and her calf in the barn during the daytime for several weeks. She recovered fully, except for some scars on her face. We never did figure out what plant she ate to trigger the skin reaction, and it never happened again. She continued raising calves until she was 14 years old.

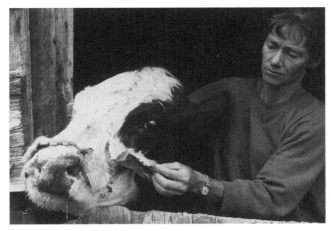

Our pet cow Prue (with a cleft palate) developed photosensitization in the summer of 1985. All unpigmented areas of skin were affected, although her black areas remained normal. We had to keep her in the barn during the hours of direct sunlight until she recovered. Here her dead face skin is sloughing off.

Risk Factors

Photosensitization typically occurs sporadically, depending on weather and growing conditions. The problem usually only affects a small number of animals in a group or maybe just one cow. It's often a springtime problem when cattle are put into new lush pasture when plants are growing rapidly. Animals that develop primary photosensitization are usually affected within 4 to 5 days of being put into a new pasture. The liver may have difficulty metabolizing all that chlorophyll at once, especially if the liver has some minor impairment from previous injury, like liver flukes.

Eating certain weeds or even alfalfa hay can cause photosensitization if molds are involved. Some dairies that feed alfalfa hay, for instance, have problems nearly every spring and summer, and the only consistent factor is the hay. Rain-damaged hay may be a risk, but researchers don't yet know which molds are the ones that cause problems. Toxicity may also vary with the growing conditions and the stage of hay maturity at harvest. Often the most problems occur in wet years or if hay is overly mature and put up in wet, humid conditions that are conducive to mold.

Cattle grazing on wheat stubble sometimes get photosensitization if they've been on hay all winter and are then put into a green field. With the sudden change, they don't seem to be able to handle the excess chlorophyll or they metabolize it poorly at first. The symptoms are similar to that of animals with liver damage. The ruminant animal needs time to adapt to the green feed. Introducing them to it slowly instead of suddenly can prevent problems.

A few cases are seen in early spring after a period of cloudy weather. If the weather suddenly clears and the sun is bright, some cows may develop photosensitization due to having eaten toxic plants and suddenly being subjected to bright sunshine. Often, risk factors must be present simultaneously in order for problems to occur: a photodynamic agent (plant) is ingested on a sunny day by an animal without enough pigment to protect the skin. And there may be a few animals that have a genetic predisposition for this problem. In some cases related animals have been the only cattle affected in their herd. They may have inherited a different type of liver metabolism.

Treatment

Any animal that develops photosensitization should be removed from the pasture or feed that caused it and put into a shelter out of the sunshine. Protecting the animal from sun will halt any further skin reaction. The barn doesn't have to be dark, just shady. The animal can be let out after sundown.

Usually by the time you see skin problems, it's been a week or more since the animal ate the offending plant, and you may not know what was eaten. Your vet can take a blood sample, however, and look for any elevation in liver enzymes. This can indicate whether it was a primary photosensitizing plant (if the enzymes are normal) or a secondary problem due to liver damage. This can help narrow your search for whatever plant might have caused it.

When treating the affected animal, steroids like dexamethasone can help reduce the inflammation, pain, and swelling but should not be given to a pregnant animal, especially in the last trimester of gestation, or it may cause abortion. Steroids also suppress the immune system and should not be given for more than a few days in a row. Other anti-inflammatory drugs, such as Banamine, can be given to ease the pain. Most vets also recommend a systemic antibiotic, such as LA-200, to combat any secondary skin or liver infections. The need for antibiotics will depend on the degree of illness.

Washing the skin lesions, maintaining clean skin, and using soothing creams or ointments on the raw areas may help reduce the pain, prevent itching and infection, and help them heal faster. Photosensitization is like a massive burn; the skin damage is similar. A severely affected animal should be treated with intravenous fluids if there are symptoms of shock. You'll want to consult your veterinarian for help. If the animal's eyes are irritated, your vet can recommend a good eyewash or eye ointment.

Just getting the animal out of the sun during the daytime until healing is well begun and using skin-tinting medication such as gentian violet on white markings can alleviate mild symptoms. Most affected animals make a complete recovery if treated promptly, though some may have residual scarring. If the problem is caused by liver damage, however, the animal may react to sunlight again in the future when eating certain plants. Care should be taken to avoid the pastures, hay, or plants that seem to cause trouble for that individual.

Allergies

Certain types of allergies affect the skin. Reaction may be triggered by sensitivity to something eaten or injected or by skin contact with the allergen. Drugs, sprays, insect bites, and weeds are among the many things that might elicit an allergic response. The reaction may take the form of skin redness, *hives* (raised lumps), or swelling of the eyelids. A severe reaction may involve the respiratory system, constriction of the airways, or the lungs filling with fluid.

The affected skin may be red, hot, swollen, and itchy, and in severe cases may ooze. You may need help from your vet to determine the allergen so it can be removed from the animal's environment or feed. Dexamethasone and *antihistamines* may be needed to reduce the inflammation and itching, along with a soothing or anesthetic salve. If the reaction is severe, the animal may need IV fluids.

Warts

Warts are unsightly skin growths caused by a virus and can thus be transmitted from one animal to another. Once they become established in a herd of cattle, they can be difficult to eliminate completely. Even though affected animals develop immunity and may never have them again, warts may be continually spread to younger animals in the herd by direct contact from infected cows.

The virus may become a continual problem in a herd, due to the long incubation period. After exposure, it can be about two months before the warts show up in a susceptible animal. This virus is host specific, meaning that it only affects cattle.

Warts may suddenly appear in several animals at once, such as a group of weanlings or yearlings that were exposed earlier. They often crop up in places where the skin has been broken, allowing the virus to enter the deeper layers of the skin. They may develop in ears after tagging, for instance, or any other area of the body where the skin has been punctured or scraped. The virus can be transmitted from one animal to another by instruments that puncture the skin (such as tagging or tattooing tools, needles) and by biting flies such as horn flies, horseflies, and stable flies that feed on first one animal and then another.

Warts are most common in calves and yearlings; young animals have not yet developed immunity to the virus. The growths often appear quickly and grow swiftly into a rough-looking or smoothly shaped mass. They may be small and rounded or become very large. A large warty mass inside the ear may make it so heavy that the ear droops down. There are several types of warts, including growths shaped like cauliflower, others like small horny bumps, and some that are more smooth and flat. Warts may appear on head, neck and shoulders, in the mouth or vagina, on the teats, or on the vulva or penis.

Warts on an affected animal often spread rapidly from the area in which they started, such as in an ear, around the mouth or neck, along the shoulders or *brisket,* or on the teats and udder. Then, almost as quickly as they appeared, the warts may seem to dry up and fall off or shrink up and disappear — once the animal's body has had time to develop antibodies against the virus and build an immune defense

---

FENCE WARTS

The virus is in highest numbers at the outer surface of the wart; this is why it can spread so readily on an animal or to other animals by direct or indirect contact. If an infected animal rubs the wart on a fence or feed bunk, the next animal that comes in contact with that object may pick up the virus.

---

against it. Thus the best treatment for warts is time. After a while they always disappear, though in some animals it may take several months to a year.

A healthy animal in good condition will build immune defenses and will generally never experience warts again. This is why warts are mainly a problem only in young animals or in the occasional adult that has not yet encountered the virus.

Prevention and Treatment

To prevent the transmission of warts to other animals in the herd, isolate the affected individual when you first notice the wart — when it is small and just starting to grow. Otherwise a number of others will develop warts, since the virus tends to affect any exposed animal that has no immunity. Isolating the infected animal is no guarantee of preventing the spread of warts, however. Due to the long incubation period, that animal may have already infected others by the time you notice the warts.

If warts appear on the teats or around the mouth or nostrils, where they interfere with milking, breathing, or eating, they can be surgically removed by your veterinarian. This usually means cutting them off with a sterilized knife or surgical scissors or tying them off with thread. If removed during their early growing stages, however, wart regrowth may be stimulated. It is safest to remove them after they are past their peak of development. Your vet can usually give a fair estimate of the wart's development, having seen numerous types of warts in various stages.

In their later stages, their disappearance can be hastened by carefully pulling, twisting, or snipping off one of the warts, crushing a small one, or removing part of a large mass of warty tissue to make it bleed a bit. Disrupting the wart in this manner puts

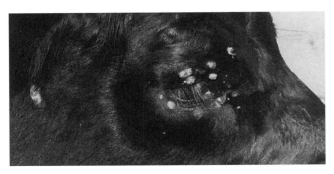
Warts around the eyes

the virus into contact with the bloodstream, and prompts the animal's immune system to create antibodies and fight the warts. Thus it's best to remove or disrupt warts only when they're starting to regress.

Commercial wart vaccines are available, but they don't always work. An autogenous vaccine (created from something within the animal's own body) is more effective. This stimulates the body to mount a strong defense against the virus and get rid of the warts more quickly and can also be used to protect susceptible animals that might come into contact with the infected one. Your veterinarian can make this vaccine from a piece of the warty tissue.

It's usually not a good idea to use iodine or any other caustic disinfectant on warts. These treatments are effective for ringworm but not for the wart virus and may be harmful to the animal. Iodine burns the skin and may create more sore areas. The simplest treatment is time. You can choose to leave the warts alone to disappear on their own, unless they must be eliminated quickly for health reasons. In that case, you should consult with your vet about removing them or trying an autogenous vaccine.

Vaccination Reactions

Some vaccines cause local reactions, such as a lump at the site of the injection. The area may be quite swollen before the reaction subsides. In some cases the reaction creates a permanent lump (called a *sterile abscess*) that remains at the site even after the initial heat and swelling subside. Animals that react to a certain vaccine may react to it again in the future and may have more severe reactions in subsequent years, due to increased sensitivity from the prior encounters with that product (see chapter 1).

Several vaccines, especially the seven- or eight-way clostridial injections for blackleg, redwater, and malignant edema, are notorious for prominent allergic reactions and often leave a lump under the skin at the injection site (see chapter 1). The animal may have heat and swelling at that site for several days. If the injection was given in the neck (as recommended by label directions), within a few hours the neck may become so sore that the animal has trouble reaching down to the ground for feed or water. Often these animals are so lame that they can hardly walk. It may take several days for the pain and swelling to subside so they can move freely again.

Ringworm

Calves and yearlings often become infected with a fungus that causes ringworm. There are several species of *Trichophyton* fungi that can cause skin lesions. The resulting crusty patches were named ringworm in earlier years because some believed their circular shape was caused by a tiny parasitic worm.

Microscopic spores spread ringworm from animal to animal. Spores may also remain viable for a period of time on any equipment used on an infected animal or on skin that was shed or rubbed off by an infected animal. Lice also may transmit the fungus spores from one animal to another.

Personalized Vaccine

If you want to make sure the rest of your young cattle don't get warts, ask your vet to create a custom wart vaccine from the infected animal's own ground-up wart tissue in which the virus is killed with formalin. Following directions from your vet for dosage, administration, and frequency, this vaccine can protect other cattle in the herd from warts.

There is no commercial vaccine against warts that is 100 percent effective, since there are many types of virus. An autogenous vaccine made from an animal on your farm is much more effective to protect your other cattle, since it will contain the specific virus that has colonized among your cattle.

The spores are hardy and can survive in the dry scabs shed by cattle for several years in shady places like barns or stalls. Sunlight tends to kill them, but winter sun is usually not strong enough in most parts of the United States and Canada to give much protection against ringworm. These fungal spores can establish new infections on the skin of a susceptible animal and then enter the hair follicles. The lesions show up two to four weeks after exposure.

Symptoms

In its early stages ringworm may go unnoticed because the affected areas are small, with slightly raised skin and rough hair. After several weeks the hair falls out or breaks off, and within 2 to 3 months the infection creates thickened patches of rough, scaly, gray material. Lesions are often on the face and neck or around the eyes, though any area of the body may be affected. The scaly area may encircle the eyes and affect the eyelids. These areas are itchy, and the animal usually rubs them. Patches on the face and neck may be small or may grow to be 3 or more inches (7.6 cm) in diameter.

Adult cattle usually have some resistance to the fungi and don't get ringworm, but if spores are present on their bodies they may pass the disease to young animals. Ringworm tends to appear in groups of young cattle that have not previously been exposed and appears most commonly during the winter months, when days are short and there's less sunlight.

Treatment

The disease generally runs its course within a few weeks or months and disappears without treatment. Sunlight and adequate vitamin A in the diet may help the animal get rid of the lesions quicker. Ringworm that goes through a group of yearlings during the winter will usually clear up by spring or summer, due to longer hours of more intense sunshine, and more vitamin A in the diet from green plants.

If you choose to treat the lesions, consult your veterinarian. There are a number of antifungal drugs that can be used, but none of them is 100 percent effective against ringworm, and they must be persistently applied (every day or every other day until lesions disappear) to make a difference.

If cattle are properly nourished — have adequate vitamin and mineral intake for optimum skin health and a strong immune system — they get rid of ringworm by themselves in a few weeks, though it may go through the whole group if they have no prior exposure to the fungus and no resistance. You may be able to prevent the spread of ringworm through a herd if you isolate the first ones that get it (in the early stages before they've passed the spores to herdmates) and treat them with a medication recommended by your veterinarian.

Sunburn

Animals with light skin can get sunburned, as can animals with very thin hair. Sunburn also affects cows with pink skin under white patches of hair. The skin turns red and may be a little cracked and blistered but does not itch. Sunburn merely affects the top layers of skin and rarely kills the deeper skin cells. It is never as severe as photosensitization. The animal may be uncomfortable, however, if large areas of skin are sunburnt, as happens sometimes when a calf has lost patches of hair following a fever. In these instances, a soothing salve can be applied over the sunburnt areas until they heal.

Ringworm Treatments

Some treatments, such as iodine or chlorine bleach, work satisfactorily only if you first wash the affected area and remove the scabby lesions by scrubbing with soap, water, and a stiff brush before applying the medication. The lesion must be scrubbed away completely, getting down to raw tissue. Simply putting medication on the lesion has little effect. Keep in mind that handling an animal with ringworm may put you at risk for getting this fungus.

Recommended treatments for ringworm include daily application of equal parts tincture of iodine and glycerin or using a mix of equal parts chlorine bleach and water. Your vet may suggest a commercial fungicide product.

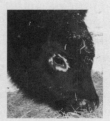

Ringworm around the eye

CHAPTER ELEVEN

Respiratory Problems

Cattle respiratory-tract infections may be as minor as human "colds" or life threatening, depending on the pathogens involved and the effect they have on the respiratory system. Respiratory disease is one of the more threatening cattle illnesses and can result in serious economic losses. The costs of treatment, slowed weight gain, weight loss, a drop in milk production, and death can be financially damaging to small farms and even larger producers. Often when an animal gets sick it's hard to know what kind of infection has invaded the herd because many diseases present similar symptoms, and multiple combinations of pathogens also may be involved.

Many infections are lumped together as "bovine respiratory disease" (BRD), since various viruses and bacteria may act alone or together. In many instances viruses are triggering agents, damaging the surfaces of air passages and giving ever-present bacteria an opportunity to invade. Other irritants that open the way for infection include dust, smoke, irritating chemicals, and *ammonia* fumes. Cattle of all ages are susceptible to respiratory infections, but stressed animals and young calves with little immunity are particularly vulnerable. Some of the most serious outbreaks of infectious respiratory diseases occur when cattle from different origins are mixed and stressed, as when sent to feedlots.

Bacteria are always present in the environment and some are normal inhabitants of the upper respiratory tract, even in healthy animals, and don't become a problem unless various factors open a way for them to enter the tissues. Viruses, by contrast, are not normally present. They are generally passed from a sick animal to susceptible animal by direct contact or via airborne droplets from coughing. Blood samples can be helpful in diagnosis. By examining the sick animal, your vet can also tell whether the infection involves only the upper respiratory tract or both the upper and lower tracts (lungs).

Upper Respiratory Challenges

Upper-respiratory-tract infections are usually mild and not life threatening unless they weaken the animal's defenses and create ideal conditions for pneumonia (see page 212). Upper respiratory infections are usually temporary and involve inflammation of the nostrils, throat *(pharynx),* and/or windpipe. The affected animal may have nasal discharge, for instance, and no other symptoms.

If infection involves the throat or windpipe or both, the animal may cough due to inflammation in the airways and may have a nasal discharge (thin and clear or thick and phlegmy) or mild fever and decreased appetite. The animal may be dull for a few days and then get better, with or without treatment. Some infections are caused by viruses rather than bacteria, and usually the only treatment that's

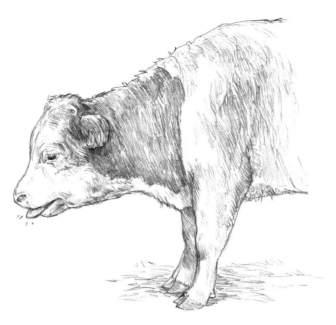

If infection involves the throat or windpipe, the animal may cough.

needed, if any, is an injection of a long-acting antibiotic to fend off any secondary bacterial infection.

Some animals have one or both ears drooping down and will seem dull but continue to eat and drink. If there's fever, it's mild. Some cases recover without treatment, but the animal should be closely watched to make sure he does not get worse, which would indicate secondary infection and a need for antibiotics. There are several things that cause the animal to have drooping ears, and some of these problems are more serious than others.

Diphtheria

When you see an animal with respiratory distress, your first thought may be pneumonia. But sometimes the problem is higher in the respiratory system and not the lungs. Infection in the mouth and throat may restrict the airways and make breathing difficult. An infection with diphtheria often involves the *larynx* at the back of the throat.

Necrotic laryngitis, more commonly known as diphtheria, is caused by a gram-negative bacterium, *Fusobacterium necrophorum,* one of the pathogens that also causes foot rot in cattle and navel ill/joint ill in newborn calves. This opportunistic bacterium is almost always present in the environment. It causes diphtheria only when conditions are right, such as when stress or injury to membranes of the mouth and throat give bacteria access to the tender tissues.

Sometimes a viral infection such as IBR or *bovine papular stomatitis* erodes the lining, causes a break in the membranes, and allows bacteria to enter. As long as the lining of the mouth and throat is intact, the animal won't get sick. But if a calf or cow eats something that scratches the larynx, or if there is IBR in the herd, the area is open to infection.

One animal cannot give diphtheria to another. It is more likely to develop if an animal's immune system is hindered but most commonly follows oral injury. The infection may settle in the larynx and pharynx (the cavity behind the nose and mouth that connects them to the esophagus) or just in the mouth, in which case the animal is not as sick.

Young cattle up to 2 years old seem most susceptible, possibly because they are shedding baby teeth, and the emerging permanent molars give entrance to bacteria if the mouth is raw. Other mouth injuries or abrasions from coarse feed or sharp seeds (such as foxtail, cheatgrass, and barley awns) can scrape the mouth and open the way for infection. If more than an occasional calf gets diphtheria, you should look at possibly vaccinating for IBR. Often after starting a vaccination program, the diphtheria, and any coinciding foot-rot problem, goes away.

Mouth Infection

If the diphtheria infection is confined to the mouth tissues, the animal may have a mild fever or be off feed. There may be swellings in the cheek area, and the animal may slobber. If you look in the mouth (with the animal restrained), you may see deep ulcers in the membrane lining the cheeks.

ONE EAR DOWN

If the animal has only one ear down, it is probably due to *Pasteurella* or *Mycoplasma* infecting the middle ear. These animals need to be treated, often for up to 10 days, or they may relapse. This infection may eventually proceed to pneumonia, but death can be avoided if you treat them. In some instances, one drooping ear can be the sign of a simple head cold, but you may need your veterinarian to examine the animal for proper diagnosis.

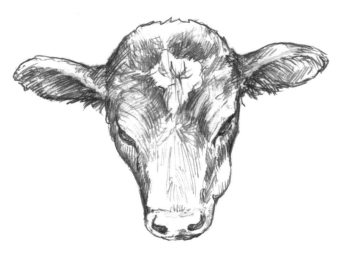

Infection in the mouth tissues may cause swelling in the cheek.

Sometimes the tongue is also ulcerated or swollen. The animal's breath may smell foul.

Ulcers in the mouth usually heal within a few days if swabbed regularly with tincture of iodine. Daily swabbing plus a course of prescribed systemic antibiotics will usually eliminate the problem. Infection in the throat, however, needs more diligent treatment, since it can be much more serious.

Throat Infection

If the larynx and pharynx in the back of the throat become infected with diphtheria, swelling in the throat tends to constrict the windpipe, making it hard for the animal to breathe. This is especially serious in calves. Adult animals have a much larger throat and windpipe and are not so apt to suffocate.

Symptoms

The animal may cough and drool if swelling makes swallowing difficult. There may be nasal discharge and foul-smelling breath. At first glance you may

---

RESPIRATION CLUE

As the larynx swells and the opening through it shrinks, breathing becomes very difficult; there's not much room for air to go through. If you watch as the animal tries to breathe, you can readily tell if it's diphtheria or pneumonia. When an animal is suffering from diphtheria, she has trouble inhaling. When she has pneumonia, she has trouble exhaling.

---

think it's pneumonia, since breathing is labored, but a closer look can help you tell the difference.

With pneumonia, the animal is quite depressed and dull, with head hanging down and ears drooping. There may be nasal discharge. *An animal with pneumonia has trouble pushing air out, due to damaged, impaired lung tissue.* She may grunt with the effort of trying to push the air out of the lungs.

With diphtheria, the head is usually extended, often parallel to the ground or higher, and the animal is usually more alert. But the most obvious clue is how the animal breathes. *Animals with diphtheria have difficulty drawing air into the lungs due to the obstruction in the throat.* You're more apt to hear wheezing from an animal with diphtheria, because of constricted airways.

Diphtheria does not affect the lungs unless the animal develops pneumonia in the later stages of a serious infection; the infection is in the larynx. As the voice box becomes inflamed, it swells, and the effect is like soaking a donut in milk. The whole thing swells, expanding the outside diameter and shrinking the hole in the center.

If the throat is infected, the animal may have a high fever. If breathing is impaired, the animal will quit eating because she is spending all her time and energy just trying to breathe. Unless treated with antibiotics to halt the infection, death may occur due to general infection in the body from bacterial toxins circulating through the bloodstream (toxemia) or from obstruction of the air passages and resultant suffocation. Complete closing of the airways is more likely to occur in a calf than in an adult.

Treatment

If a calf is very ill and not eating or drinking, she may need IV fluids. A calf dehydrates more quickly and is also more apt to be seriously affected than an adult. If you notice symptoms early, however, the infection can generally be turned around with antibiotics and medication to reduce swelling. Treatment must be aggressive and continued until the calf has a full recovery, since this condition can swiftly become life threatening. Early diagnosis and treatment can prevent complications such as pneumonia or scar tissue that makes the windpipe restriction permanent even after the infection has been eliminated. If the animal develops pneumonia in addition to diphtheria, it will be quite a challenge to save his life.

Systemic antibiotics (such as Naxcel or a combination of long-acting oxytetracycline and sulfa or some other broad-spectrum antibiotic recommended by your vet) will halt diphtheria. Antibiotic treatment should be continued as long as necessary, which may mean several weeks in a serious case. Do not quit until the animal is completely back to normal (eating, drinking, breathing easily, and with a normal temperature for at least 2 full days), or the infection may recur. A relapse can be very difficult to resolve, and the animal may die. It's best to give the antibiotic as an injection rather than a bolus; putting pills down the throat can irritate the swollen larynx and make the condition worse.

No matter what antibiotic you use, most veterinarians also recommend use of an anti-inflammatory such as dexamethasone, Banamine, or DMSO to help reduce swelling in the throat so the animal can breathe and swallow and to prevent formation of scar tissue. Dexamethasone should be given at least twice a day for the first three to five days of treatment, to help make sure the airways won't swell shut. Steroids should not be given for more than a few days, however, since they tend to suppress the immune system; long-term use can make the animal more vulnerable to other problems. Steroids can also cause recrudescence (recurrence) of the IBR virus if the animal is a latent carrier (see chapter 5). Since some cases of diphtheria may have been triggered initially by IBR (producing ulceration in the membrane that allowed the bacteria to enter), you may be putting the calf at high risk when treating with dexamethasone.

Long-term use of Banamine may not be safe either, as excessive use of Banamine or other nonsteroidal anti-inflammatory drugs can lead to gastrointestinal ulcers or, in some cases, kidney damage. Probably the safest medication, if the animal is having trouble breathing, is *DMSO (dimethyl sulfoxide)*. Mixed with a little warm water and squirted into the back of the mouth a couple times a day, this anti-inflammatory drug helps shrink the swollen tissue.

Adult cattle don't seem to get diphtheria as often as calves, and sometimes it's so mild that you don't even know they are sick, if they don't go off feed. Their throats and windpipes are so much larger that

EMERGENCY TRACHEOSTOMY

If the swelling shuts off the windpipe, the animal will die unless you or your vet can perform a *tracheostomy* so the animal can continue breathing. Air can then go in and out through this opening, bypassing the obstruction in the throat that's compressing the windpipe and closing it off. If you have to do this yourself:

1. Disinfect any available small rigid tube, such as a small (3 cc), sterile disposable syringe minus its plunger, or a ballpoint pen cover with the end cut off.

2. Take a sharp sterile knife in hand.

3. Position the knife a few inches below the jaw.

4. Slit the front of the windpipe horizontally, between two of the firm ribs of the windpipe's cartilage. Be careful to cut through just the softer tissue between the ribs of cartilage — like cutting between the ribs of a vacuum cleaner hose.

5. Gently push the tube into the slit.

6. The slit should be kept open until the vet arrives and can put a tracheal tube in place.

The tracheal tube allows the animal to breathe for a few days until the swelling in the throat can be reduced. Then the opening into the windpipe can be stitched shut again by your vet.

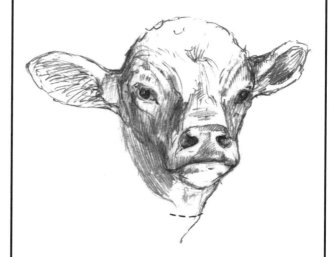

Carefully cut between the cartilage ribs, at the front of the windpipe, a few inches below the jaw, using a clean, sharp knife.

MOST CASES OF DIPHTHERIA in our herd have been calves, and some required extensive treatment and diligent care to save their lives. One challenging case, however, was a 2-year-old cow. I found her when I was riding range one day in early June. We always try to see each animal every time we ride, marking off the tag numbers in a pocket notebook. I was riding through the edge of a thicket, marking off the numbers of cows resting in the shade, when I heard an unusual sound. It was the labored, wheezing breathing of a cow in trouble.

I looked deeper into the brush and found Suzy Q, gasping for breath. I knew she'd die unless treated, so I gently herded her and her calf out of the bushes and started the long journey home. Even though home was only two miles away, it took several hours to get her there, since we had to climb over a hill. She was barely able to breathe; exertion and the hot day made it harder, so we went very, very slowly, just a couple of steps at a time.

Once we got there, I put her in a shed out of the sun. Lynn and I put a halter on her and gave her antibiotics and medication to help her breathe easier (to shrink the swelling in her throat) and carried her feed and water. She was not interested in hay, so for several days we picked armloads of tall green grass — the lushest and softest we could find — that was easier for her to eat. With extensive antibiotic treatment and tender loving care, she survived and recovered and continued to raise her calf.

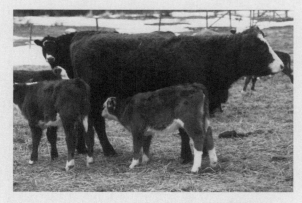

Suzy Q, a couple of years after her recovery from diphtheria, shown here with her fourth calf

a mild case won't hinder breathing. Often the main symptom is voice loss, since the infection may damage the larynx. Some cattle eventually regain their voice, but many remain almost voiceless or sound squeaky and not very loud. If an infection is serious and interferes with the ability to eat or drink or causes fever or toxemia, prompt and diligent treatment is necessary to save the animal, whether he's a calf or an adult.

Pneumonia

A lower respiratory tract infection involving the lungs rather than the upper airways is called pneumonia. Infection in the lungs is often due to a downward progression of infection in the upper tract (throat, windpipe, bronchial tubes) or to failure of mechanisms meant to protect the lungs. Viruses may damage the lining of the windpipe, allowing infection to get started. Irritation from smoke or dust can also damage the lining severely enough to invite infection. More rarely, lung infection is due to systemic infection brought to the lungs via the bloodstream. Pneumonia is usually much more serious than an upper-respiratory-tract infection and more likely to be life threatening.

Pneumonia can hit cattle at any age but is most common (and often most deadly) in calves. Stress from bad weather, extreme changes in temperature, weaning, transport, overcrowding, mixing of animals from different sources, another illness (such as scours), and nutritional deficiencies can all lower the animal's immune defenses. Most pathogens that cause pneumonia are present in the environment; many normal cattle carry one or more bacterial pathogens in their upper respiratory tract without getting sick. These pathogens may get down into the lungs but are usually expelled or inactivated by the animal's immune system. Some viral pathogens produce mild signs of illness but cause severe, sometimes fatal disease when combined with other viral or bacterial pathogens and stress.

Viruses tend to reduce the resistance of mucous membranes, allowing bacteria to invade. Viruses also destroy the tiny hairlike cilia in the bronchial tubes that help keep the lower airways free of harmful pathogens. The windpipe is lined with cilia, which are in constant motion — moving like waves on the ocean in an upward sweep. They move dirt and bacteria up and out of the windpipe into the back of the throat where this debris can be safely and easily removed from the body by coughing. But when viruses damage cilia, they can no longer defend the lungs. Damage by viral infection thus makes the respiratory system more vulnerable.

Young Calves with Pneumonia

A calf in a drafty or humid barn is a prime candidate for pneumonia. Dirty bedding saturated with urine and manure emits ammonia fumes that irritate lungs and open the way for opportunistic pathogens. Young calves gain immunity against some pathogens if they ingested adequate colostrum at birth, absorbing antibodies from the dam. Calves that don't get colostrum (or don't nurse soon enough to absorb antibodies) won't have this protection.

Calves stressed by a hard birth or chilled after birth may not get up quickly to nurse or may not be able to absorb enough antibodies even if given colostrum. Stress hastens closing of the porous intestinal lining that allows passage of antibodies through it and into the bloodstream. Calves from first-time mamas may not get as many antibodies as calves from older cows; the older cow has come in contact with more pathogens during her lifetime and has more chance to develop strong immunity, which she passes to her calf via colostrum. Calves between 2 and 10 weeks of age are most susceptible to pneumonia; that's when their temporary immunity from colostrum wanes, and they have not yet developed their own immunity. But stress can hinder immunities at any age.

Secondary Bacterial Infections

A primary viral pneumonia may be mild and run its course without treatment unless a secondary bacterial infection gets started. This can turn it into an outbreak of pneumonia that affects every calf. Secondary bacterial invaders may move into the lung tissue after it's been virally damaged. When respiratory disease is severe, bacteria (such as *Streptococcus*, *Mycoplasma*, and *Chlamydia*) are almost always involved. The most common bacteria, however, is *Pasteurella*. The two types of *Pasteurella* of concern in cattle are *P. mannheimia* and *P. multocida*.

Pasteurella mannheimia (once called *Pasteurella haemolytica*) is present in the nose and *sinuses* of normal, healthy cattle; it is readily available and can move into the lungs if the cilia in the windpipe lining are damaged by viruses. As soon as *P. mannheimia* moves into the lungs, pneumonia begins.

Bacterial pneumonia is more apt to kill the calf, but usually there's a virus there first, suppressing the immune system and damaging the airway lining. Bacterial invasion follows and creates a more severe infection. In some instances, however, BRSV (bovine respiratory syncytial virus) can cause enough problems (without any bacteria involved) to create serious lung damage or even kill the animal.

Some cases of acute viral pneumonia can be fatal in a few hours, but many cases of uncomplicated viral pneumonia recover in 4 to 7 days unless bacteria become involved. If that happens, the animal may develop toxemia; bacterial toxins get into the blood and travel throughout the body, making the animal even sicker.

Cattle of any age may develop pneumonia if weather conditions are stressful. Fall and spring are especially dangerous with hot days and cold nights. This is why most pneumonia cases occur in spring or fall. Stress-related pneumonia is often due to *Pasteurella* and may not need a viral catalyst. When temperature extremes have a differential of 40 to 50°F (4.4 to 50°C) or more (80 to 90°F [26.7 to 32.2°C] afternoons in the fall, dropping to 40 degrees at night, or 60°F [15.6°C] afternoons in the spring, dropping to 20°F [−6.7°C] at night), there are more *Pasteurella* pneumonia cases.

Symptoms

An animal with pneumonia quits eating, is dull and depressed, and may spend a lot of time lying down. If standing, the animal is usually humped up. Ears may droop, respiration may be fast or labored, there may be coughing or noisy breathing. The nose may be snotty or crusted, and there may simply be nasal and eye discharges (clear or thick). If the animal moves, she moves slowly because of pain. In severe cases, breathing is difficult. The animal may breathe with her mouth open or make a grunting sound as air is forced out of impaired lungs. In the last stages of pneumonia, before the animal is too weak to stand up, she may stay on her feet rather than lie down, since the lungs are so impaired; it's easier to breathe standing up than when lying down.

Confine the animal, and take her temperature. Cattle with pneumonia may have a fever of 104 to 108°F (40 to 42.2°C). Generally, fever up to 104 is indicative of a bacterial pneumonia, whereas fever of 106°F (41.1°C) or higher is due to a virus. A fever of 106 to 107°F (41.1 to 41.7°C) could indicate a BRSV infection, which can be quite serious.

Fever in respiratory disease indicates the animal is still fighting the infection; the body is producing an inflammatory response. If fever comes down or temperature drops into subnormal ranges and the animal is obviously still sick, this is not a good sign; immune response is waning, and the body is giving up or going into shock. Energy resources may also be depleted, which makes the body less capable of producing a higher temperature.

Cattle don't have strong lungs, and pneumonia can be an uphill battle unless you catch it early. Once the lungs are damaged and filling with fluid, the animal may be hard to save. It's very important to spot the early warning signs. If you can detect that an animal is not feeling well and diagnose the problem early, pneumonia is easier to clear up than if you delay treatment until the animal is in serious trouble. Early treatment can help prevent development of complications, such as abscesses in the lungs,

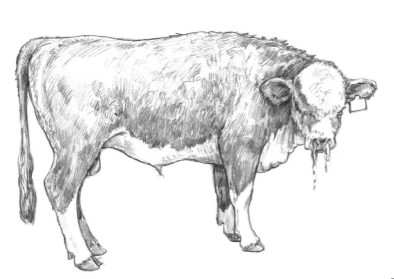

An animal with pneumonia is dull and depressed and may be humped up, with drooping ears. In severe cases, the sick animal may try to breathe with his mouth open, gasping and grunting.

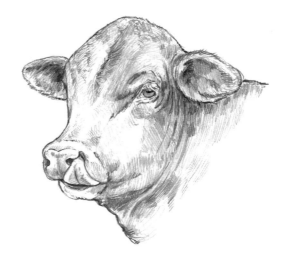

The healthy animal keeps her nose clean by licking out any discharge. A sick animal often has a "snotty" nose, partly because there's more nasal discharge but also because she doesn't feel well enough to keep her nose cleaned out.

inflammation of the lung lining, chronic dilation of the bronchial tubes, or pus-producing infection.

Endotoxemia

In some instances of bacterial pneumonia, endotoxins are produced as bacteria die and their cell walls break up. As toxins circulate through the blood, they cause damage in the lungs and adversely affect other organs of the body, creating a life-threatening situation. The heart rate may be weak and rapid, the respiratory rate fast and shallow, and a normally pink nose and gums dark, due to lack of oxygen in the tissues. Without immediate treatment to reverse this toxic condition, the animal will die.

Antibiotic Treatment

Antibiotics are usually given when an animal has respiratory disease. Although antibiotics don't halt viral progression, treatment helps prevent or combat any bacterial infection. There are several good drugs available for treating pneumonia, including Baytril, Naxcel, Nuflor, Micotil, A180, Excede, and Draxxin, that are often more effective for treating severe bacterial infections than the standard penicillins or oxytetracyclines and sulfas. The newer drugs all require proper diagnosis and a vet's prescription (see chapter 2).

Some stockmen still use oxytetracyclines or a combination of these drugs with sulfa, however, and in many instances these still work well. But keep in mind that sulfa should never be given to a dehydrated animal or it may damage the kidneys. Sulfa is broken down and eliminated through the kidneys, and there must be adequate fluid in the body or the sulfa will crystallize in urine and cause irreversible, fatal kidney damage.

Though some bacteria are now resistant to oxytetracycline or sulfa, these drugs are cheaper than newer products, and if they work on your farm, there's no reason to not use them. Some people start with LA-200, and if it doesn't work they change to another product. Some antibiotics work better in some animals than in others, and stockmen may have to discover what's best by trial and error. When dealing with a stubborn pneumonia that's not responding, don't wait too long before asking your vet for advice on changing antibiotics. If

Use Micotil with Caution

Micotil is designed for treating respiratory disease in cattle and is very effective against some of the common bacteria that cause pneumonia. This drug must always be used properly and carefully, because it is fatal to humans if accidentally injected. It can be given only subcutaneously to cattle.

Micotil is unique in that it concentrates in lung tissue once it gets into the animal's body and remains there at high levels for 3 days. This reduces stress to the animal, since you don't have to give daily treatments. One injection is often adequate, though some animals may need another injection after the third day.

no improvement is seen within 48 hours, in most instances you should change to something else.

Always read and follow label directions for dosage and timing. But your vet's advice trumps the label because, in some circumstances, he or she may prescribe a different dose or schedule. Some drugs must be given daily; others can be repeated every 48 hours and others every 3 to 4 days. Some of the newer drugs have a longer-lasting effect. Make sure you are using them properly.

Many vets use Micotil and Nuflor but don't recommend use of Nuflor in calves younger than 30 days because it can be hard on the digestive tract and cause scouring. Micotil (tilmicosin) has safety precautions (fatal if injected into a human), but if you are experienced in giving injections, many vets are comfortable prescribing it for clients to use. Baytril and A180 are similar in effectiveness, but A180 concentrates in lung tissue a little better is less expensive, and has a shorter withdrawal time.

Draxxin is relatively new and has the advantage of fewer treatments being necessary. It concentrates in the lungs and stays there 8 to 10 days. Thus, you can give one shot and may only need to handle the animal once. Excede (a newer formulation of ceftiofur, the same ingredient in Naxcel) is also good for treating respiratory infections. It is approved for use

Isolate the Sick Animal

You'll need to confine the animal for ease of treatment, and keeping him away from other animals will protect them from being exposed if the infection is contagious. To avoid stressing the animal more, a nursing calf should be kept with his mother and a flighty young cow or heifer should be confined near a gentle herdmate. Even though a severely sick animal may be too dull to try to get out of the confinement pen or stall, an insecure animal will be upset at being isolated and is much less stressed if there's a companion in the next stall or pen.

against *Pasteurella* and *Haemophilus somnus* and is injected under the skin on the back middle third of the ear. Its sustained-release formulation provides adequate blood levels for 7 to 8 days with a single injection. Your vet must show you how to give this injection, as giving it improperly can result in the immediate death of the animal.

Regardless of which antibiotic you use, the key to successful treatment is catching the infection quickly, though this can be difficult. Once abscesses form in the lungs, or there's too much damage and scarring, antibiotics may not be much use. You may not realize how sick the calf is until it's too late and there's already lung damage. Studies have shown that damage from *Pasteurella* can become permanent within less than eight hours. By that point there's scarring in the lungs even if you clear up the infection.

Once permanent damage exceeds 20 to 25 percent of the lung tissue, the animal may do poorly even if it survives. Calves that suffer permanent lung damage may not grow well and may die about the time you plan to send them to market — when they outgrow their lung capacity.

Antibiotics should always be given, even if a virus causes the pneumonia, since secondary bacterial infection could kill the calf. Be diligent with treatment, and don't stop too soon. Even if the animal is breathing easier and feeling better (eating and drinking again, with temperature back down to normal), keep the antibiotic levels high for at least 2 full days

after all symptoms are gone. If the animal relapses, it will be harder to save him the second time around. Secondary bacterial pneumonia will usually respond to antibiotic treatment, but relapses are common if viral infection is extensive, and by that time it may be difficult to save the calf even if you start treating him again.

Supportive Care

Supportive care is also important. Make sure the animal is warm and dry, protected from bad weather. If he's not eating or drinking, force-feed fluids and nutrients. A calf can be fed milk or milk replacer via stomach tube. An esophageal feeder works well for young calves; a larger calf or adult animal must be fed fluid and nutrients via nasogastric tube (into the nostril), since the esophageal probe is not long enough (see chapter 2).

Minimize stress as much as possible. Keep a sick calf with his mother even if he needs intensive care. The stress of being separated from Mama can be detrimental. If he needs to be under a heater, partition off a corner of the pen or barn stall so he can be kept warm but still have Mama nearby.

Anti-inflammatory drugs should be given to halt the cascading effect of prostaglandins that will destroy the lungs and to help reduce fever, pain, and inflammation and block the effects of *endotoxins*. It's usually wise to use a nonsteroidal anti-inflammatory that can reduce inflammation and halt prostaglandins without suppressing the immune system (as steroids do), but at the very beginning of the inflammatory process you can head it off best with dexamethasone.

SILENT PNEUMONIA

Even mild cases of pneumonia early in life may impair the lungs and result in less-functional lung tissue. Calves ill as babies may not grow well. Subclinical "silent" pneumonia may still affect growth and future health — these are calves you didn't even realize were sick or were just a little dull and off feed temporarily, and you didn't treat them. At slaughter, some of these animals have adhesions in the lungs or 10 to 15 percent of their lung tissue may be dead.

After that you can help shut it down with Banamine. Anti-inflammatory medication works well to minimize the lung damage in animals with pneumonia and can also help the animal feel better and resume eating and drinking.

Banamine reduces fever, cough, respiratory rate, discomfort, and lung congestion. It can be given by IV or intramuscularly. Don't give Banamine to a dehydrated animal or there's risk for kidney damage. If you are force-feeding fluids or giving IV fluids, however, the animal won't be dehydrated. Animals with pneumonia often recover faster if given Banamine, responding better than when given antibiotics alone.

Prevention Is Preferable to Treatment

Many cases of pneumonia can be prevented by vaccination. There are a number of vaccines available for helping prevent respiratory disease in cattle. Viral vaccines help prevent viral infections that open the way for other infections (see chapter 5). These viral vaccines won't protect calves from *Pasteurella* pneumonia, but there are some *Pasteurella* vaccines that will protect them.

There are many viral vaccines available. Some vets recommend vaccination at 4 to 6 months of age with

a booster 4 to 6 weeks later, to give adequate protection to weaning-age calves. The important thing is to make sure calves are vaccinated twice between 4 and 7 months of age with a product that will help prevent BVD, IBR, PI3, and BRSV. Calves vaccinated younger than 6 months of age usually need to be vaccinated again at that age, to boost immunity. Always follow label directions on vaccines. If two doses should be given initially, this tells you that the animal won't have much immunity until 7 to 14 days after the second dose is given.

Vaccination is something you should always discuss with your own vet, to develop a program that will be the most effective in your herd. Some vets recommend intranasal vaccines for young calves, on farms that have serious problems. Antibodies from this type of vaccine are not long lasting but may be effective more quickly. Always remember, however, that no vaccines give 100 percent protection. They work best in situations where herd management minimizes the risks and stresses that predispose animals to respiratory infections.

Calfhood pneumonia can often be prevented if calves get adequate antibodies in colostrum. This works best if cows have strong immunity during pregnancy (their own vaccinations for viral diseases kept up to date) so they pass high levels of antibodies to newborn calves via colostrum. There is no substitute for good colostrum, so make sure each calf gets an adequate amount within one hour of birth (while his ability to absorb antibodies is greatest). But this protection is waning by the time most calves are 3 to 4 weeks old, and many cows don't have strong immunity to *Pasteurella*. If you have spring and summer pneumonia in calves, talk to your vet about vaccinating calves for *Pasteurella* at about 1 month of age.

It's also important to make sure there are no underlying herd health problems. Cows may need higher nutrition levels to produce strong colostrum. If calves are getting pneumonia, check energy, protein, and mineral levels in the cows' diet. If a cow does not have a properly functioning immune system (because she's short on energy, protein, selenium, copper, or some other crucial nutrient) or if she's persistently infected with BVD (see chapter 5), her calf won't have good colostrum. If calves are getting pneumonia at less than 3 weeks of age, it's

Pneumonia Prevention: Calfhood Vaccine

To prevent young calves from contracting *Pasteurella,* some vets recommend giving a good vaccine against both types of *Pasteurella* to calves at about 1 month of age. This won't protect them clear through weaning, however; they need a booster just before weaning to give protection through their first winter.

If you give only one *Pasteurella* vaccination during calfhood, it's usually best to do it a couple of weeks before weaning. Most pneumonia vaccines are designed to give to weaning-age calves, to protect them during the stressful time of losing Mama. Our vet has used *Pasteurella* vaccine in the face of pneumonia outbreaks in weaned calves, and in his experience calves were usually able to build immunity within 7 days. In epidemics of pneumonia in weaned calves, he's vaccinated the whole group and says this can shut down the outbreak within a week.

usually the cows' fault; calves that have good colostrum and adequate nutrition are not as vulnerable.

Since stress is the biggest factor in whether cattle develop respiratory disease, try to eliminate or reduce all possible causes of stress (see chapter 1). Don't wean calves or sort, vaccinate, or ship cattle during bad weather. Avoid mixing different groups of cattle during weaning or processing, and try to control dust and mud.

Bovine Respiratory Disease ("Shipping Fever")

Shipping fever is actually a form of pneumonia and is so named because it usually occurs shortly after shipping or hauling cattle. The stress of transport (a long truck ride with no food or water), which is often simultaneous with the stress of being weaned, lowers immune resistance and makes ideal conditions for lung infection. Shipping fever is also called bovine respiratory disease (BRD), and it is caused by a number of (or combination of) pathogens. There are more than 20 bacteria and viruses that can be involved in lung infections.

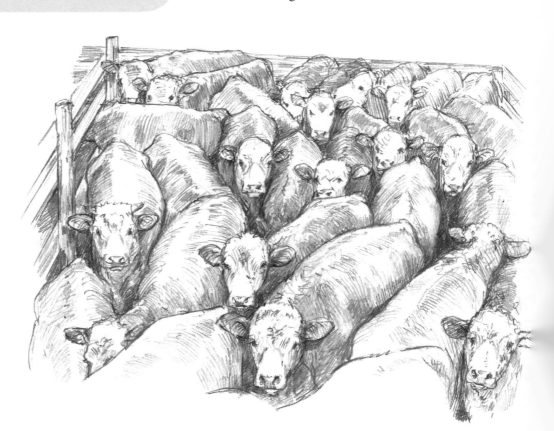

The stress of transport or enduring a sale may bring on shipping fever, which is actually a form of pneumonia.

Probably the most common culprit in shipping fever is the *Pasteurella* bacterium, which is almost always present in healthy cattle. It becomes a cause of severe illness when combined with a viral agent and stress that lowers immune resistance. Calf outbreaks of respiratory illness at weaning time can often be reduced by vaccinating calves ahead of weaning, with a *Pasteurella* vaccine recommended by your vet, and minimizing stress at weaning as much as possible (see chapter 1).

Haemophilus somnus is another bacterial pathogen sometimes involved in shipping fever. It also causes a very serious illness in feedlot cattle, often called "brain fever" or thromboembolic meningioencephalitis (TEME) (see chapter 4). There is a killed-product vaccine to help prevent this bacterial infection. It must initially be given in two doses and is most effective when administered before calves are weaned, so they'll have some immunity before the stress of weaning and being shipped to market.

Emphysema; Atypical Interstitial Pneumonia (AIP)

There are many names for this disease, including acute bovine pulmonary edema, lung fever, fog fever, and bovine asthma. It most often strikes when cattle are moved from dry pastures to green ones. The sudden change in feed quality can have disastrous results. It can also happen in feedlots, toward the last 2 or 3 weeks of their finishing period.

Affected cattle are often called *lungers* or panters. The lungs suddenly fill with fluid a few days after the change in feed. This condition is not infectious or contagious. It's like an allergic reaction, similar to human asthma, and can sometimes be successfully treated with antihistamine, epinephrine, and, for all animals but pregnant cows, cortisone.

Causes

The problem is caused by the amino acid *tryptophan*, in lush green forages. After cattle eat the forage, their rumen bacteria transform this amino acid into a poison under certain conditions. The change from dry, poor-quality pasture to verdant, rapidly growing forage results in an undesirable fermentation in the rumen, producing *3-methylindole* (3MI), which is rapidly absorbed from the rumen into the bloodstream. As blood-carrying 3MI circulates through lung tissue, a toxic intermediate compound is produced that causes lung damage and emphysema. Cattle may have trouble breathing any time between 1 and 14 days after the pasture change (most often in the first week), and death often follows within 2 to 4 days after the first symptoms appear.

Emphysema occurs frequently on certain farms yet may not affect cattle on nearby farms, for reasons not fully understood. The condition occurs worldwide. In Great Britain it's called fog fever because of its association with cattle that are grazing lush regrowth (called *foggage* in the U.K.) on green pastures. It occurs frequently in parts of Europe and Canada and throughout the United States. In the West it occurs during a dry summer or fall when cattle are moved from dry ranges to lush irrigated pastures or from any dry pasture to irrigated fields with regrowth following removal of hay.

Outbreaks of emphysema are possible whenever there are periods of active plant regrowth (as after a rainy spell following dry conditions). It can occur with any abrupt feed changes and on many types of forage, including kale, rape, alfalfa, turnip tops, small cereal grain forage, rye grass, Bermuda grass, and mixed meadow grasses. Any lush forage can apparently result

Stress and Infection

Causes of respiratory disease in cattle are many and complex but are almost always brought on by stress and a combination of viruses and bacteria. Stress factors that can lower resistance to respiratory disease include heat, cold, wet conditions, dust, fatigue, injury, anxiety, dehydration, hunger, nutritional deficiencies, and polluted air. Some of the viruses that cause respiratory disease include IBR, BVD, BRSV, PI3, adenovirus, rhinovirus, coronavirus, and herpes virus IV. Bacterial agents that cause respiratory disease include *Pasteurella*, *Haemophilus somnus*, and *Mycoplasma bovis*.

in formation of 3MI when the rumen is not adapted to the new forage. Grazing management, rather than the type of forage, is the determining factor.

The breathing problem is most common in adults that experience the feed change. The toxic reaction in the lungs results in constriction of the bronchial passages, trapping tiny bubbles of air in the lungs. This trapped air expands to form larger bubbles and some of the air sacs rupture, creating larger spaces, which further trap air. As this happens, less and less of the lung area can be utilized for oxygen exchange. The animal is also struggling to exhale, unable to get rid of the trapped air. The animal's demand for oxygen soon outgrows the available supply. The lungs become overinflated with frothy air bubbles, and the postmortem examination finds that the lungs are two to three times heavier than normal; the airways are filled with frothy fluid. Air is often trapped under the skin of the animal's back, where it accumulates after leaking from ruptured lung tissue.

Symptoms

Affected cattle show severe respiratory distress, and even slight exertion may kill them because they can't breathe. The effort of moving when you try to take them from the pasture to a corral for treatment may make the animals so short on oxygen that they collapse and suffocate. Both inhaling and exhaling are difficult because of decreased elasticity of lung tissue; the animal is slowly suffocating.

Symptoms appear suddenly. The most obvious sign is labored breathing with grunting or wheezing. The animal may try to breathe through her mouth, and froth may dribble from the mouth. The tongue is often extended and the mouth kept open. The nose may look blue due to oxygen shortage in body tissues. Yet the affected animal may seem bright and alert compared to an animal with pneumonia. There is no fever or toxemia, so the animal is not dull. In fact, she is usually anxious and restless, and may still try to eat or drink.

The cow often stands with head and neck stretched out in front of her, breathing rapidly and shallowly. Her heart rate rises due to the shortage of oxygen, and it may get as high as 150 beats per minute as she struggles to survive. If her heart rate is higher than 120, she is probably in the final stages of the disease. Death may occur within 12 hours from the beginning of the first signs, or the animal may linger for 2 or 3 days before dying.

Mild cases may recover. Some chronic cases linger for weeks or months with periods of partial recovery and relapse. Many stockmen cull any animal that suffered from emphysema because lung

A cow with emphysema breathes with her mouth open and often drools frothy saliva.

Emphysema Can Occur in Grain-Fed Cattle

Though it's less common, feedlot cattle sometimes experience emphysema, and the affected animals often die. Why they develop this acute breathing difficulty is still being debated, but research points toward a complex interplay of feed intake, feed types, individual susceptibility, and possibly environmental triggers, since some years seem to be worse than others for incidence.

Bacterial pathogens are often found in the lungs of feedlot cattle that suffer from emphysema. This is an interesting clue, suggesting that respiratory infection may be one risk factor for developing the problem. Just as in pasture cattle, it's less likely to occur when abrupt feed changes are avoided.

damage leads to increased susceptibility to other respiratory diseases.

Unless the herd is checked frequently, the first indication of trouble may be a dead cow. If the disease is acute or begins at night, cattle are often found dead, with no warning signs they were ill. The largest animals, with the highest feed-intake capacity, are most likely to succumb to this disease.

Prevention

Emphysema can often be prevented with proper management of feed and pastures. Don't put cattle into lush green pastures directly from dry pastures. A transitional period in a not-so-green pasture or feeding hay for a few days will usually prevent the condition, giving the rumen bacteria a chance to adjust gradually from the dry feed. Dry years can be especially challenging. On any pasture, cattle should be moved before they completely deplete their feed supply or else they will be very hungry by the time you move them to new pasture. When given access to lush forage, they overeat.

Research has shown that after 2 or 3 weeks of having to eat poor-quality forage with a crude-protein level that's less than 6.5 percent and with the acid detergent fiber content of plants being greater than 50 percent, rumen conditions become prime

GREEN FIELDS FOR CALVES, BUT NOT FOR COWS

Adult cattle are generally the animals affected by the change in feed when switching pastures; calves are usually not at risk. Thus, one way to avoid losses during dry years in range country is to bring cattle directly home to the corrals from summer and fall pasture instead of putting them into green fields. Calves can be weaned and put in the lush fields and the cows taken to drier pastures. This works for many ranchers — it saves the best feed for weaned calves and eliminates cow losses from emphysema.

for elevated 3MI production. Even when cows are not on overgrazed pasture, if forage has dropped in quality due to dry conditions, you can reduce the risk for emphysema by feeding hay before moving them to a greener pasture.

Preventive management when changing pasture can also include gradual adaptation to lush new forage. Feeding hay and limiting cows' access to a new pasture for the first few days help them make a safe transition. Let them graze the new pasture for only an hour or two the first day, then gradually increase

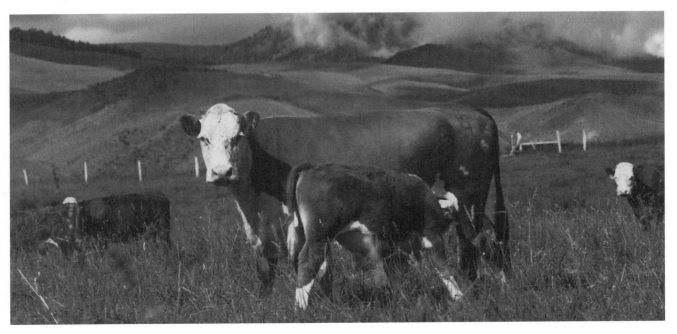

Taking cows off dry rangelands or depleted pastures and putting them into lush green pasture can put them at risk for emphysema.

their grazing time on subsequent days before you let them stay in the pasture full time.

For example, after feeding hay in the morning (so cattle are full of hay), let them graze the lush pasture for an hour in midday and then round them up again. On following days, increase grazing time by one hour over the previous day for the next 7 days, and after that you can leave them in the new pasture. This gives the rumen microbes time to adjust to the new forage and reduces the formation of 3MI. Feeding a limited amount of mechanically harvested green forage (green chop) in addition to hay is another method that can be used to help the cows' rumens adapt to the lush new forage.

Other management practices that reduce losses from emphysema include use of antibiotics (monensin) and mowing the pasture before turning in the cows. Once the mowed feed starts to dry, it is safer

TOO MUCH GREEN PASTURE

IN SEPTEMBER 1981 we brought our cows down from the range to vaccinate them and wean their calves. As was our usual practice, we kept the cows in a pasture by the corral for a few days before taking them back to our upper pasture. When we gathered them to take them back up country, we missed one.

Cow Cow was hiding in the brush along the creek. The change from dry feed to green pasture had caused emphysema, but we didn't discover this until our daughter saw the cow stagger out of the bushes two days later. We took the cow slowly to the corral. I took her temperature; it was 106°F. A phone call to our vet confirmed our suspicions about the diagnosis: the stress and lung insult from emphysema had set her up for pneumonia, so we treated her with antibiotics as well as adrenalin and antihistamine.

We put her in a barn and hoped she'd make it through the night. During the night we went to the barn and gave her more adrenalin and antihistamine and began our round-the-clock effort to save her. She would not eat or drink. The first 2 days we gave her 3 gallons of water several times a day by stomach tube, but we realized that she needed more than water to keep her alive. So we added molasses, powdered protein, and milk to her tube feedings. We'd never heard of anyone giving milk to a 2-year-old cow, but we felt it might give her energy and nutrition. We were desperate.

After the first struggle to put a stomach tube in her nose, she did not protest; she seemed to know that what we were pouring in was dinner. I added some uncooked Cream of Wheat breakfast cereal to the mix; the particles were small enough to go down the tube if I kept the concoction well stirred. Then we remembered the pig pellets we'd bought by mistake.

I soaked some of the high-protein grain pellets in warm water to soften them and ran them through the kitchen blender. We added as much of this "mush" to Cow Cow's fluid meals as we could put down the tube without plugging it up. We could probably have given her some propylene glycol for energy, but we didn't know about that option.

We weren't making progress with the pneumonia, however, and changed to a different antibiotic. She was weak, unable to stand, and struggling for every breath; her lungs were filling with fluid. On the advice of our vet we gave her daily injections of DMSO to keep her airways open and draw fluid out of her lungs. The vet suggested we change to yet another antibiotic, but she still did not improve. Several weeks had gone by, and she was a rack of bones, but she refused to give up. We gave her injections of vitamin B complex, vitamin A, and medication to help open her air passages.

Finally our vet stuck a needle between her ribs and took a sample of lung fluid to culture the bacteria and try to determine which antibiotic might work. He tried more than a dozen. There was only one that made a difference, so he prescribed it — an oral product we put into a large gelatin capsule twice daily, pushing it down her throat.

After more than a week of this, her temperature started back down, she began to take an interest in food, and we'd find her standing up when we came to the barn. We kept feeding her by tube until she began eating more hay and chewing her cud. But awe didn't take her off antibiotics until her temperature had been normal for several days; we didn't dare risk a relapse. The day she kicked at me when I gave her an injection, I knew she was going to live. We gave her fluids and food via tube for the last time 34 days after her ordeal began! We kept taking her temperature, and after several more days, we quit the antibiotics.

By this time it was November and very cold, but she'd been in the barn all this time and had no winter hair. We let for them to eat. In research trials, feeding each cow 200 mg of monensin per day (mixed with at least one pound [.45 kg] of grain) for 1 or 2 days before the pasture change and for 7 to 10 days after the change reduced 3MI formation. Monensin, an antibiotic, hinders bacterial activity. Cows fed monensin and given access to mowed, partially dried forage had lower 3MI concentrations than cows fed supplemental monensin alone. Feeding monensin is only practical if cows are already eating grain. Many beef cows are never fed grain and may not eat it; a cow that has no experience with grain will often refuse it. Even with cows that know how to eat grain, one problem with use of monensin is that some cows refuse to eat the supplement or will not eat enough of it to make a difference.

There may be a correlation in some herds between enterotoxemia and emphysema. When

her out for the first time into a small corral on a warm day. She looked like a walking skeleton but was so happy to be outside again that she gave a little buck and nearly fell down because she was so weak. She staggered when she walked. But watching her delight in being out in the sunshine warmed our hearts. We put her back in the barn each night until she'd gained some weight and grew more hair. By Christmas she was starting to look like a cow again.

The next fall when our vet saw Cow Cow, he was astonished that she was actually pregnant. We told him the only way this cow could possibly pay her way after all our efforts and the huge medical expense was to have a long life and raise lots of calves. And she did.

She was one of our favorite characters, partly because of her independent nature and partly because she beat the odds. She never had another sick day in her life, and with mischief in her eyes and a sassy kick, she made sure we knew that she would no longer tolerate any more of that "doctoring" stuff!

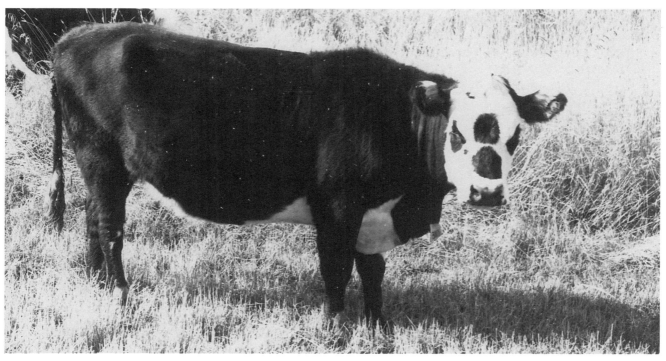

Cow Cow: fully recovered, fat, and sassy! One of the joys of working with cattle is seeing the fruits of extra efforts made while trying to save an animal and experiencing the miracle of an individual that never gave up.

cattle are routinely vaccinated with seven- or eight-way vaccines containing *C. perfringens,* there seems to be less incidence of emphysema when changing pasture.

If cattle show signs of emphysema after being moved to a green pasture, move the herd out of that pasture into a drier one (or into a corral to be fed hay), taking care to move slowly and not excite or exert them. Severely affected cows should be left where they are and treated if possible. If you must bring a cow very far for treatment, use a trailer. Forcing her to walk to a corral will kill her more quickly than leaving her alone and doing nothing.

Treatment

The most important factor in treatment is early detection. Check the herd closely at least twice a day for the first 10 days after cows are moved from dry pasture to a green one. Treatment is not always successful,

but the cow has a chance if treatment is given before her lungs become seriously compromised.

Moving the animal may result in shortage of oxygen and suffocation, so it is often difficult to bring an animal in from pasture to treat her. Sometimes the best thing to do in a serious case is to simply leave the animal alone or give injections of dexamethasone (except in pregnant cows) and antihistamine right where she is, if possible without distressing her, and then leave her alone. If the cow is not yet suffocating, you can try to save her by giving antihistamine every 8 hours to reverse the allergic condition. You may also want to use Banamine. An antibiotic like Naxcel may also be a good idea, just to head off possible pneumonia.

This treatment alone is not enough to save her if she's left in the pasture, however; she may keep eating green feed. She must be moved back to drier pasture or into a corral to be fed hay. Consult your vet.

CHAPTER TWELVE

Foot Problems

Cattle sometimes experience foot injuries and lameness. More than 90 percent of lameness cases are due to foot problems that are not related to the legs. Infectious agents, nutritional issues, or confinement often cause these ailments. Dietary deficiency can hinder healthy hoof growth. Overeating high-energy rations of grain can cause founder. Cattle are also at risk when confined in corrals or small grassy pastures, where their feet can grow too long due to lack of normal wear. Circulation in the foot may be impaired if cattle can't travel about, making the foot more vulnerable to problems. Overgrown, misshapen, and cracked hoofs can be painful.

Dairy cattle often need routine foot care and hoof trimming if they are confined in unnatural conditions and fed high-energy feed. Grass-based dairy operations provide healthier conditions for feet. Both beef and dairy cattle can suffer from foot problems, and lameness takes a toll on production. Research at Michigan State University found that lame cows were 16 times more likely to take longer than average to become pregnant after calving and 9 times more likely to return to heat when bred. According to the study, lame cows were also 8 times more likely to be culled than their healthy-footed herdmates.

Wet weather and muddy ground also create a higher incidence of foot problems. Sole injuries, infection of skin around the hoof, and foot rot are all more likely to occur when wet ground softens the tissues and makes them more vulnerable to bruising and nicks and scrapes that open the way for infection. The animal may need antibiotics, pain medication, and in some cases, foot trimming or surgery.

Foot Rot

Foot rot commonly afflicts both beef and dairy cattle. A 2004 University of Nebraska study estimated that the bacterial infection costs the beef industry millions of dollars each year. Each time an animal gets foot rot it costs the producer an estimated $120 due to weight loss, lower pregnancy rates, culling of permanently crippled individuals, reduced value or

THE FOOT

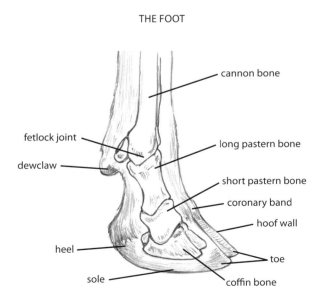

cannon bone
fetlock joint
dewclaw
long pastern bone
short pastern bone
coronary band
hoof wall
heel
toe
sole
coffin bone

condemnation of the carcass if the animal is sold, and the time and cost of treatments.

Foot rot occurs when bacteria in soil or manure invade through a break in the skin between the toes or at the heel. Usually only one foot is affected. That foot becomes hot and swollen and the skin around the hoof is red. Swelling and severe lameness appear suddenly. The animal may be fine one day, and the next day the foot is too sore to bear weight.

Causes

Several different bacteria cause foot rot, but the common culprit is *Fusobacterium necrophorum,* which can be a normal inhabitant of the digestive tract. This is the same pathogen that causes calf diphtheria, liver abscesses in feedlot cattle, and navel ill in newborn calves. *F. necrophorum* may cause foot rot by itself or in conjunction with other bacteria.

Any small cut, scratch, or puncture wound resulting from walking through such things as gravel, crop stubble, or frozen mud is all it takes to open the path for bacteria. *F. necrophorum* can live a long time in soil and persists in swampy ground, springs, and wet pastures. The skin around the feet becomes tender when wet, making foot rot a common problem in wet weather or when cattle walk through bogs. Even when weather is dry, bacteria are present in manure. Cattle may also pick up infection in shaded bedding areas that stay wet from urine and feces.

Symptoms

When bacteria enter the foot and start multiplying, they produce toxins that enable them to quickly penetrate deeper tissues. Symptoms appear 5 to 7 days after bacteria gain entrance. The resultant inflammation creates sudden swelling, especially between the toes or at the heel and around the *coronary band* just above the hoof. The most swollen area is near the site of entry. If there's a crack in the skin between the toes and that tissue is swollen, toes may be spread wide apart by the swelling.

In severe cases, the swelling extends upward as far as the fetlock joint. On first glance you might think the foot is sprained or broken because of the swelling and extreme lameness. The animal may be reluctant to put any weight on the foot, hopping

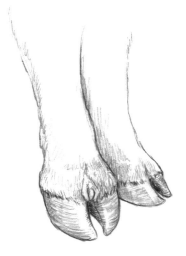

Early case of foot rot

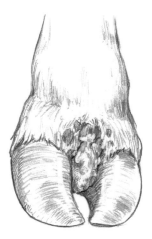

Neglected case of foot rot

on three legs when forced to move and reluctant to travel to feed or water.

The animal may have a fever and spends most of the time lying down. She loses weight because little time is spent eating or grazing. As the infection progresses, the swollen area may break open and ooze, spreading bacteria around the pen or pasture. In a long-standing case, infection may invade the joints, causing septic arthritis and permanent crippling.

Carefully examine a sore foot; not every lame animal has foot rot. A foot injury or puncture wound may produce similar symptoms. Stepping on a nail may cause severe lameness, and if infection enters the puncture, it needs aggressive treatment. Wire wrapped around the foot may also cause swelling and lameness. Look closely at the swollen foot to determine the exact cause of the problem.

Foot Rot Affects Bull Fertility

Fever between 103 and 106°F (39.4 and 41.1°C) in early stages of foot rot may hinder fertility. This temporary period of infertility starts about 60 days after the fever. Sperm formed while the animal has a fever are adversely affected; excessive heat is detrimental to sperm production. The bull is usually fertile for 60 days after suffering from foot rot because the mature sperm already in his reproductive tract may be fine unless his fever is severe. It's the immature sperm that suffer most — those that will be coming on board 60 days later. If he has foot rot early in the breeding season or a few weeks before breeding cows, you need to make sure he won't be infertile just when you need him most.

If a bull gets foot rot, take his temperature while treating him to see if he has a fever. A high fever of 104 to 107°F (40 to 41.7°C) could make him infertile later. If you know the bull had a fever during his bout with foot rot, be sure to have his semen checked a couple of months after his recovery. Otherwise, you may end up with open cows.

Treatment

Many cases of foot rot eventually clear up without treatment, but the animal is lame longer, may lose a

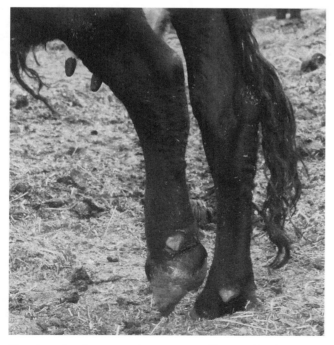

If neglected and not treated, some cases of foot rot develop septic arthritis in the joint, with permanent damage and enlargement.

lot of weight, and will spread bacteria while the foot is swollen and discharging. It's always better to treat the lame animal than to wait and see if the infection will clear up on its own. If you clear it up quickly, there is less risk for permanent damage (arthritis) to the foot. If neglected, and infection gets to a joint, the animal may develop septic arthritis. With treatment, most cases heal quickly, especially if you start treatment on the first or second day of lameness.

Antibiotics

Long-acting oxytetracycline or procaine penicillin work well for foot rot, and sulfa is also helpful in severe cases. Long-acting sulfa boluses given by mouth, in conjunction with injections of oxytetracycline (such as LA-200, which gives coverage for 3 days), repeated the third day if necessary, will usually clear it up.

In some instances your vet may prescribe a different antibiotic such as Naxcel or Micotil. If there's a chance you might want to sell or butcher the animal soon, select a drug with a short withdrawal period (see chapter 2). Topical treatments such as copper sulfate solution or an antibiotic spray may speed healing. DMSO (dimethyl sulfoxide) gel applied to swollen tissues can reduce swelling, pain, and inflammation. Disappearance of lameness is a sign of recovery. The key to successful treatment of foot rot is early and ongoing care until the animal is no longer lame. Keep the animal in a clean, dry area until healing is complete.

If no improvement is noticed after several days, you have the wrong diagnosis, you are using the wrong antibiotic, or the infection has spread into a joint. A chronic case not treated in early stages may take longer to recover. It may be necessary to clean the foot, apply local antiseptics, bandage it, and use systemic antibiotics. Sometimes it helps to glue a form-fitted block of wood under the good claw to take all the weight off the infected claw and give it time to heal. If joints or tendon sheaths are involved, prognosis for recovery is poor; surgery to remove the affected claw/toe may be necessary.

Prevention

If an animal develops foot rot, prevent additional cases by isolating him to avoid spreading the infection. Remove cattle from the causative environment (sharp stubble, boggy pasture, frozen mud with sharp protrusions), and build up their nutritional resistance. Hooves are healthiest when an animal has a proper diet that includes zinc, iodine, and manganese. If your feeds are short on these important minerals, supplement them.

There is a vaccine (Fusogard) for control and prevention of foot rot. In trails, the vaccine reduced cases by 64 percent. Label recommendations suggest vaccinating cattle at 6 months of age or older with an initial two-shot series, with each shot 60 days apart, and an annual booster thereafter. Total reliance on vaccine for control of foot rot generally doesn't work, however. It is most effective when used in conjunction with other preventive measures.

Some pens, pastures, and paddocks put cattle at risk until you drain or fence off wet areas or clean out all the manure. If any cattle had foot rot in a certain corral or pen, it should be thoroughly cleaned when cattle are taken out, and lime should be spread liberally over the ground surface (see chapter 1). If a pen is left vacant for at least a week after cleaning and liming, this will rid it of the bacteria. Help cattle in confined areas in feedlots or dairy facilities with footbaths containing 10 percent zinc sulfate or 10 percent copper sulfate.

Heel Warts

Often called hairy heel warts, strawberry warts, or digital dermatitis, wartlike lesions between the heel bulbs are caused by bacteria that infect soft tissues of the foot. This condition is found all over the world, primarily in dairy cattle. A survey of California dairy farms in the mid-1990s found that up to 75 percent of dairy herds in the state had heel wart problems.

At least five different types of *Treponema* spirochete bacteria have been found in these lesions. This infection generally occurs on the bottom of the foot between the *digits* or up the front or back of the foot. Young cattle are most susceptible; they have not yet developed immunity to these bacteria. Moist conditions can predispose cattle to heel warts if the bacteria are present. If the foot is wet, skin is softer, more tender, and more vulnerable. The best prevention is a clean, dry environment and healthy feet.

OUR FIRST EXPERIENCE WITH FOOT ROT

THE FIRST HEREFORD BULL we purchased, nicknamed Big John, was a 3-year-old. He'd been held over from the breeder's bull sale the year before because he was lame with foot rot at the time of sale. The first summer we had him he developed foot rot again and was severely lame. Our vet helped us treat him and also trimmed his feet. His hoofs were overgrown due to corral confinement before we purchased him.

Because only one digit on the lame front foot was affected, the vet glued a wooden block to the sound digit, shaping it to fit. The strong glue held it in place for several weeks, and Big John was able to travel without lameness, bearing all the weight on the good half of his foot. By the time the wooden block wore away, his foot was fully recovered, and he was able to service all his cows. He had no more problems with foot rot and turned out to be one of our best bulls, siring about 50 calves each year. He stayed sound and active until he was 10 years old.

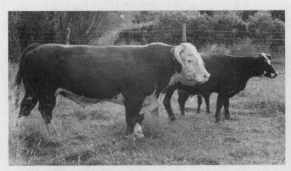

"Big John," the Hereford bull

Symptoms

Affected cattle become lame and reluctant to move; the condition may be mistaken for foot rot. In early stages the lesions are round with a red granular appearance and tiny fronds (long erect hairs) protruding from the tissue, making them look like strawberries. Most lesions are ½ to 2½ inches (1.3 to 6.4 cm) in diameter, located where skin joins the soft part of the hoof horn at the heel or midway between the claws on the bottom of the foot. The surface

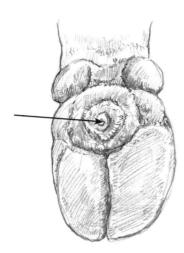

Heel warts present as a circular area at the back of the heel, with upright tufts of hair.

of the lesion is moist, bleeds readily if bumped or scraped, has a strong odor, and is painful if touched. In later stages there may be progressive separation of the hoof horn from the inner sensitive laminae, with the sole becoming *underrun* at the heel.

Hind feet are most commonly affected. The painful foot is often held off the ground, with the limb flexed and trembling, or the toe may be rested on the ground. Because of pain in the heel area, the animal tries to walk on the toes, which may become so worn that the hoof horn at the toes is worn completely away. The animal is reluctant to travel to feed or water and loses weight.

Treatment
Like foot rot, heel warts are treated with systemic antibiotics but respond best if topical antiseptics are also applied to the affected area. The foot can be sprayed daily for about 5 days with antiseptic or treated and wrapped. Use topical sprays or ointments after the lesions have been washed with water and mild disinfectant. Some dairy farms use footbaths to treat and prevent heel warts. Each cow walks through a germicidal liquid when traveling to and from the milk barn.

Prevention
Currently there is no commercial vaccine for heel warts, but ask your vet about the use of an autogenous vaccine. The high incidence of heel warts in confined dairy cows suggests that crowding and contamination help spread this disease. Clean, dry bedding and a clean environment, along with use of a foot bath once a month or once a week (depending on the incidence of this disease on your farm), can help prevent occurrence.

Sole Abscesses

Bacteria may enter the hoof itself through a crack or bruise, usually on the bottom of one of the digits (claws). A sole that's bruised from uneven weight bearing due to a misshapen foot or when an animal steps on a sharp rock may become an abscess. Damaged tissue is more likely to develop infection. Sometimes the layers of sole will separate, and a *"false sole"* develops, with pus between the layers. The abscess may break out the side of the foot or at the heel, even if the original bruise may have been at the center of the bottom of the foot. Because the infection can't break through the tough sole or hoof wall, it must travel through the foot until it reaches soft tissue in order to break out and drain.

Symptoms
Initially there is no swelling above the hoof because infection is confined inside the hoof itself. If a lame animal does not have the swollen foot that is characteristic of foot rot, suspect an abscess. The bottom of the claws should be carefully inspected. The animal may need to be confined in a chute and a rope used to help pick up the foot so you can examine it. A crack or bruise (a soft spot) on the sole should be probed with a hoof knife to find the abscess and open it up. It may need to be drained and flushed. The infection creates a foul-smelling fluid that will be obvious when the abscess is located and opened.

Treatment
If pus is present, flush out the opened abscess. Treatment generally consists of paring away all the affected horn tissue around the abscess, flushing it with an antiseptic solution like iodine and minimizing weight bearing in that area until new horn can grow and fill in the hole. Have your vet pare the affected claw so the sound one bears the weight, or glue a "shoe" or block of wood to the sound claw to

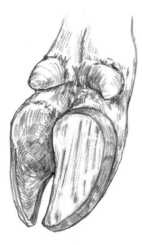

Use a block of wood to relieve sole abscesses and foot rot.

build it up so it bears all the weight. Keep the animal in a dry area so no mud, moisture, or manure can get in the hole while it heals and grows new tissue.

Puncture Wounds

Cattle have tough, hard feet unless the hoofs are constantly wet, which softens them. They rarely have hoof injuries, but occasionally an animal will suffer a puncture wound if he steps on a sharp, penetrating rock, nail, or metal piece. Cattle kept in old corrals where boards with protruding nails litter the ground or those allowed to graze around junk, dumps, or other areas where they might encounter sharp objects, are at risk for foot punctures. If the object goes into sensitive tissues, the animal will be lame and will quickly develop an infection.

Symptoms

Unless a foreign object is still embedded in the foot, the condition may be mistaken for foot rot because of the severe lameness and heat and swelling just above the hoof. Upon close inspection, however, you can generally see a dark spot left by the offending object if it penetrated into sensitive tissues. The spot, often about the size of a dime or smaller (stepping on anything with a diameter larger than a dime would probably just bruise the foot), is easy to see on a white or red foot. Even on a black foot you can often see the puncture as a darker circle, if you look closely. This is the area your vet will check.

Bull Hooves and Cow Hooves

Hoof problems in bulls are most often encountered in front feet. A bull's body is wedge shaped, wider in front, and he carries more weight on his front end where he has a hump over his neck and his wider, more muscular shoulders. His front feet grow larger to support the weight but may still be prone to bruising. If his feet become overgrown from lack of wear or from founder, usually his front feet are more severely affected.

Beef cows also have problems in their front feet, but dairy cows have about 80 percent of their foot problems in their hind feet, especially while lactating. A dairy cow may be carrying 50 to 75 pounds (22.7 to 34 kg) of milk in her udder. The extra weight stresses the hind feet, and a full udder pushing her legs and feet farther apart makes her stand differently and also contributes to the stress on the hind feet.

Treatment

If the object is still in the foot, carefully pull it out. Take note of the puncture's angle and depth of the wounds to describe to your vet so he or she can determine whether or not vital tissues were damaged inside the foot. If a nail penetrates the bone or joint capsule, the animal needs more extensive treatment, and chances for full recovery may be less. Your vet may have to pull the object out and may recommend soaking the foot, opening and flushing the puncture hole, and/or putting the animal on systemic antibiotics.

Laminitis

Lameness in cattle can be due to laminitis. This term means inflammation of the laminae — the interfacing tissues that connect the foot's sensitive bone and blood vessels to the outer, insensitive horny shell. Laminitis is often due to serious digestive problems that upset the population balance of rumen bacteria, creating bacterial toxins that enter the bloodstream and cause serious changes in the hoof (founder).

The most common cause of laminitis is grain overload. It occurs when cattle are put on grain without allowing a gradual period of adjustment to the high-grain ration or when changes in types of grain feed are too sudden. Laminitis is rare in animals that eat only forage. It is most common in feedlot cattle, young animals fed grain for faster growth, or young bulls fed grain to increase their rate of growth.

Laminitis can occur in cows fed supplemental corn in winter (for more energy during cold weather) or when pasture is short, as some stockmen do when corn is more economical than hay. Overeating corn may result in abortion or death but most often results in founder. Instances of founder dramatically increase when corn is used as a supplement, especially in mild weather when cows don't need that much energy to meet winter requirements. If they are fed more than 5 pounds (2.3 kg) of grain or corn per animal per day, there's a risk for problems, and this can easily happen if bossy individuals get more than their share. The safest feed for cattle is forage, not grain.

Just as in a horse that founders, feet become very tender from inflammation. If the laminae separate, disrupting the connection of bone to hoof horn, feet become deformed. As the attachments give way and the bone shifts downward, hoof growth patterns change. Toes become overly long and curl upward. An animal that has foundered will tend to go lame easily, due to sole bruising. If an animal has foundered once, he will be more likely to founder again.

Stress Can Cause Foot Problems

Nutrition and stress play a role in hoof diseases. Overfeeding can cause feet to grow too fast or become soft and tender. Stress or a change in feed disrupts growth and creates a change in the hoof wall, which appears as a horizontal ring or ridge growing down from the coronary band. Like tree rings, spurts of faster growth or periods of slower growth show up as changes in the appearance of the wall. The entire length of the foot from hairline to toe tip takes about 13 months to grow. A ridge or ring one-third of the way down represents a stress or change that took place 3 to 4 months earlier.

High fever from severe illness may disrupt growth and later create a visible hoof ring. Standing too long can also create stress for cattle. Unlike a horse that spends most of the time on his feet, cattle lie down to chew the cud and rest whenever they are not grazing. Cattle are not meant to stay on their feet. A horse can nap while standing; his legs are designed so the joints can lock and he can completely relax without falling down. Even though cattle may doze on their feet, they need more lie-down time than a horse.

ACUTE LAMINITIS   CHRONIC LAMINITIS, ALSO CALLED FOUNDER

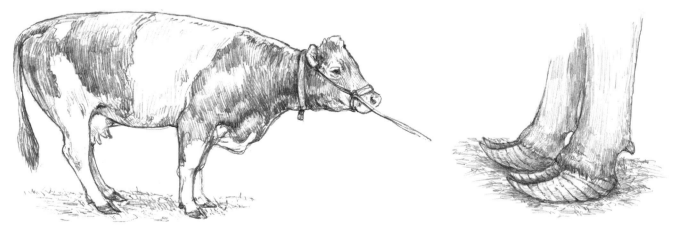

Due to severe pain in all four feet, this cow is standing with her back arched and legs bunched up under her body.

When a cow has chronic laminitis, ridges ring the hoof wall, the heels are sunken, and the toes are long and tipped upward.

Cows produce more milk, young animals grow better, and feet stay healthier if the animals can spend an appropriate amount of time lying down. Dairy cattle, for instance, lie down except when eating, drinking, or being milked. If they're standing, this generally means they don't have comfortable conditions for lying down, and this is stressful. Cattle standing in groups fighting flies (rather than lying down resting) are also stressed.

Hoof Cracks

Sometimes called *sand cracks,* hoof cracks occur most often in heavy, older animals and more commonly in feet that grow too long. Often there is a crack up the center of a toe or cracks up both toes.

A normal, healthy foot is only 3 to 4 inches (7.6 to 10.2 cm) long from the hairline to the tip of the toe, even on a large animal. A larger, heavier animal has a much broader and more massive foot, but it won't be much longer than the hoof of a smaller animal of the same age. Individual cattle have slightly different hoof angles, but toe length on healthy feet is very similar. When feet are trimmed, it's generally the toe that is overgrown and needs shortening. Only rarely do heels need trimming.

Dairy cattle need trimming more often than beef cattle, due to the unnatural conditions in which they live. If a beef animal needs trimming, genetic factors may be involved. Conscientious seed-stock producers cull animals that need their feet trimmed.

Causes

Cracks may be caused by hoof horn that becomes dry and brittle and loses its flexibility. Sometimes mineral deficiencies, especially deficiencies of selenium, copper, or zinc, can lead to loss of hoof quality and subsequent cracking. In some regions high levels of molybdenum, iron, or *sulfur* create compounds that tie up copper and keep it from being absorbed by the body (see chapter 16). This can accentuate a copper deficiency. Forage growing on alkaline ground may also be low in copper and zinc.

Excessive selenium in the diet can lead to hoof cracks, and in severe cases the animal may slough off the hoof wall. Many areas of North America are deficient in selenium, and stockmen routinely use a supplement for cattle, since adequate levels of this element are important to, among other things, normal muscle function, reproduction, healthy feet, and a strong immune system.

There are a few regions where selenium levels in soil and plants are high enough to be toxic, causing loss of tail hair, severe hoof cracks, and even death of animals eating those plants. Oversupplementing with selenium can also cause hoof cracks. The window of "healthy" levels for this trace element is very small; too much is just as harmful as too little. Find out if your region is short on selenium or not, and supplement accordingly, taking care to not double up selenium in various supplements (such as in a mineral mix and a feed product).

Cracks May Be Genetically Acquired

Some cattle have naturally strong hoofs, and others have a weaker construction, more prone to brittleness and cracking. Occasionally, the animals in a herd that develop hoof cracks are all related (mother, daughters, grandmother, sisters). Or the daughters of a certain bull will all be prone to hoof cracks. These animals may have normal feet when they have a natural diet of grass, have plenty of room to travel, and wear their feet naturally. But when subjected to unnatural conditions and stress, they tend to develop hoof problems.

Prevention and Treatment

If cattle develop hoof cracks, consult your vet and a cattle nutritionist. Mineral supplementation, especially the use of *chelated* zinc and copper (which are better utilized by the body than nonchelated) may help. Mineral supplementation is often most effective and properly rationed when given to each individual animal via bolus, drench, or injection to make sure each individual gets the proper amount.

Research studies have looked at the role of *biotin* (one of the B vitamins) in hoof health. Adding biotin to feed supplements may help cattle maintain stronger hoof horn. Biotin, like zinc, is often depleted in body tissues when the animal is under stress. Stress may include anything from weaning to seasonal dietary changes (such as going from a high-fiber diet of hay in winter to a low-fiber, high-protein diet on new spring grass). Adding biotin, zinc, copper, and other important nutrients to a supplement during stressful times of year may help the animal produce strong hoof horn and minimize hoof problems.

Hoof Wear and Tear Is Healthy

Proper hoof wear helps feet stay healthy. Many cattle don't have an opportunity to wear feet normally, if they are confined or kept on soft ground. Cattle kept on pasture where they have a normal diet of forage and enough room to travel over both rocky and soft terrain have the healthiest feet. If feet grow too long, regular trimming and removal of excess hoof horn can be very beneficial.

Hoof cracks may be more unsightly than damaging, but if they become too deep or the hoof starts to split at a toe crack, they can lead to infection of deeper tissues and cause severe lameness. Toes that

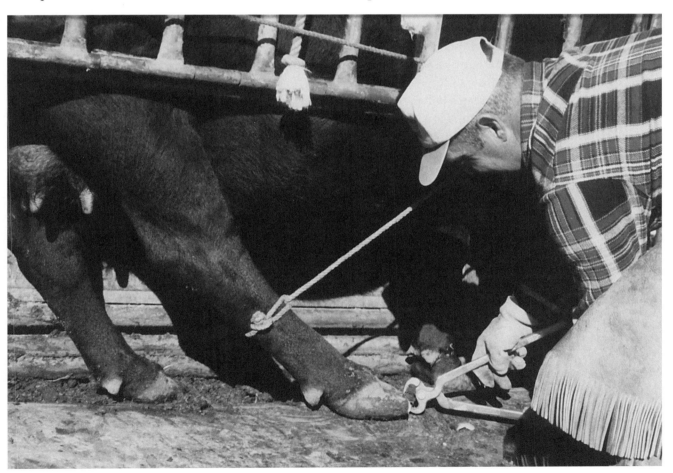

Even if you don't have access to a trimming table or a professional hoof trimmer, simply trimming off the extra-long toe with horse trimmers can help many long-footed animals.

grow too long tend to crack and split. Trimming the feet of confined animals and those of cattle on soft pasture that cannot wear their feet normally usually keeps cracks from becoming a serious problem.

In some cases hoof sealer or hoof glue can protect the outer surface of the foot and prevent cracking. There are bovine hoof products that form a bond with the hoof wall to create a tough outer surface that repels moisture and makes the hoof horn stronger. This keeps the hoof from getting soft in wet conditions and also holds in the foot's natural moisture so it won't crack in dry conditions.

If your herd or an individual animal suffers from hoof cracks, talk to your veterinarian or consult a professional hoof trimmer. In some parts of the country, especially where dairies are located, there are people who trim cattle hooves professionally.

Fescue Foot

Cattle grazing *endophyte*-infected fescue pastures may develop fescue toxicity, which causes loss of blood circulation to the extremities, especially the feet and tail. Lack of blood flow to the feet compromises the inner tissues and creates lameness, which is sometimes mistaken for foot rot. However, foot rot generally affects only one foot, and *fescue foot* may cause problems in more than one and afflict several individuals in the herd at the same time.

Lameness often appears 10 to 14 days after cattle are put into fescue pastures in cold weather. Due to the lack of blood circulation, tissues are damaged by the cold and die. Two or more weeks after lameness begins, the foot becomes gangrenous. The animal may slough off hoofs and/or lose the end of the tail. For a discussion of fescue toxicity, see chapter 17.

Preventing Foot Problems

Many foot problems can be avoided by selecting cattle with good foot and leg conformation. The ideal cattle have hooves that grow in proper alignment and balance and wear normally and evenly. Heredity plays a major role in the ability of bovine individuals to keep tough, resilient hooves. Of course, the tendency to suffer from foot problems can also be inherited. Some cattle families are genetically

---

> **CONSISTENT FOOTING IS IMPORTANT**
>
> Abrupt changes in footing can create problems, as when cattle are brought from a wet, swampy pasture (where feet have become soft) to a pen or pasture with rocky conditions or into a feed yard or auction yard with rough concrete around feed bunks (for traction). The abrasive footing, which poses no problem to hard, healthy feet, may quickly wear away soft feet and leave them vulnerable to bruising or infection, creating serious lameness. If the sole is worn away and resultant infection affects the bone, the animal may not recover.

---

predisposed to have poor feet and leg angles or have an inability to grow tough hoof horn due to soft feet or brittle feet that are easily cracked. If your herd has hoof problems such as toe cracks, check to see if the problem animals are related. You may have used a bull (or kept daughters from a particular cow) whose offspring have less-than-average hoof quality.

If cattle are kept on soft pastures and never have a chance to travel on firm, dry, or rocky ground to wear the feet, periodic hoof trimming may be necessary to keep feet from growing too long. You can schedule foot trimmings with a bovine hoof-trimming specialist, just as you'd have regular visits from a farrier for your horses.

Diet

Proper nutrition is crucial for healthy hoof growth, to avoid poor hoof horn and cracking that opens the way for infection. Nutrient imbalances and deficiencies can lead to poor hoof growth or dry, brittle feet that are prone to cracking. Trace minerals like zinc, copper, manganese, and selenium affect hoof health (see above page 232). If these are inadequate or the diet is low in vitamins A, D, or biotin, hoof horn may be adversely affected and won't grow properly.

Dietary fatty acids also play a role in growing healthy, resilient hoof horn that won't dry out or crack. Green forage plants generally contain all the elements needed for hoof health unless the soils they are grown on are mineral deficient. The healthiest feet are generally found in animals that have access to green forage plants and have room to travel, wearing the hooves at the same rate they grow.

Footing

A clean, dry environment helps prevent many foot problems. Poor footing can predispose even a healthy hoof to problems. If cattle are in wet pastures year round or spend the winter in a muddy pen, they'll often have feet problems. In different circumstances, if they must constantly travel over sharp rocks, their feet can become bruised and injured or may wear down too fast, leaving them tender-footed. Footing issues should not be ignored.

Providing mounds of dry ground in wet areas can help prevent foot rot. That way cattle can stand in dry areas instead of having their feet constantly in mud. Use of a porous, high-strength filter fabric to hold a layer of gravel near the ground surface is another way to provide drier footing in wet pens or boggy gateways. Used in highway construction, filter fabrics hold a stabilizing layer of gravel between overlaid soil and underlying dirt. The fabric allows for drainage, keeps the gravel from sinking down into the mud, and maintains a drier top layer of soil. Filter pads can prevent deep mud and improve footing in feeding areas, travel lanes, gateways, or wherever cattle tend to bog down in wet weather.

How to Construct a Drier Pen or Feed Yard

Install geotextile or grid fabric to filter water from the ground surface and to create a drier, healthier area for animals to travel and stand on.

1. Excavate the top 6 to 8 inches (15.2 to 20.3 cm) of soil in pen or roadway.
2. Place the filter pad in the hole at that level.
3. Lay in 4 to 6 inches (10.2 to 15.2 cm) of crushed rock or gravel on top of the fabric.
4. Top it with 2 to 3 inches (5 to 7.6 cm) of finely crushed rock.

This creates an effective drain for moisture, keeping the top dry and healthy for hoofs. Buildup of manure on top of the fine gravel can be scraped up and periodically removed without damaging the filter.

Tips to Prevent Foot Injury

- Keep pens clean and free of sharp stones or frozen, rough mud.
- Cover rough, frozen, hoofprint-pocked ground with straw.
- Construct concrete slabs at feed bunks, water troughs, or any other areas that tend to get boggy when cattle congregate.
- Keep pens well drained in wet weather.

Any management procedure that helps eliminate hoof damage and aids in hoof health can help prevent foot rot, sole bruising, cracks, and the invasion of bacteria in an open wound.

CHAPTER THIRTEEN

Mouth Problems

CATTLE DEPEND ON THE MOUTH AND TONGUE to eat; if any problem makes this difficult, they lose weight, experience a drop in milk production, or grow poorly. Older cows sometimes lose teeth and it becomes harder for them to eat, but cattle of any age may suffer from soft tissue injuries and infections. If the problem is severe, they may starve to death.

Lump Jaw (Soft Tissue Abscess)

Because bacteria are always present in the mouth, anything that punctures the lining of the mouth and tongue opens the way for infection. If the puncturing object stays embedded, continually irritating these sensitive tissues, the area remains infected and an abscess forms, creating the telltale "lump jaw." Sometimes it's a barley awn, foxtail, or a cheatgrass seed head that gets embedded in the inside of the cheek, but anything that can puncture the tissue and get stuck gives bacterial access and can cause infection and festering, just as a sliver in your finger will do.

Once the puncture seals over and the infection becomes encapsulated in the tissues, the abscess becomes inflamed and grows bigger as germs multiply and die, forming pus. The area can't heal until the object comes out. Nature's way to get rid of it is to create a pocket of pus around it. The infection eventually comes to a head and breaks open to drain, taking the sliver or seed with it. Sometimes, however, it's best to *lance* and drain the abscess that bulges on

the side of the animal's face, rather than waiting for it to break and drain on its own. Lancing means making a slit through the skin to enable pus to come out. The area will usually heal faster and with less scar tissue if you lance the abscess and treat it.

Causes

The infection starts with any break in the tissue surface that allows entrance, which usually occurs when the animal chews on a sharp stick or eats rough, coarse feed or grass that pokes the side of the mouth. Sometimes the offending object becomes embedded. Ulcers caused by the BVD virus create raw lesions and can also open the way for bacteria, which can enter from feed or soil.

If cattle graze a pasture short, they sometimes pull plants up by the roots and eat the dirt or sand that clings to the roots. Or cattle fed on the ground may pick up dirt or mud while eating the last wisps of feed. Dirt entering the mouth can bring with it several kinds of bacteria, and if there's a scratch or break in the tissues, infection can start the cow's inflammatory response, which may result in an abscess. A pocket of pus is walled off and surrounded by a thick wall of connective tissue, creating a lump that is often located along the lower jaw or side of the face. The lump may be hard or soft, small or large, but can be moved around if you press and push it firmly with your hand, since it is in the soft tissues and not attached to the bone.

Treatment

The best treatment for an abscess lump that has not yet broken open is to lance it, squeeze out all the pus, then flush it with strong (7 percent tincture) *iodine*.

Before you lance the abscess, restrain the animal in a chute, and tie his head around to the side so he can't move or sling his head and you can check the lump and lance it safely.

It's wise to wear clean surgical gloves to protect your hands from bacteria, especially if you have any breaks in your own skin. Make sure it's a movable soft-tissue abscess and not a bony lump (see below page 239); the latter should not be lanced.

Also check inside the mouth before you lance any lump. Sometimes the animal has a wad of feed stuck in the cheek area, making a protrusion that looks like an abscess lump. If it's just a wad of feed, pull it out with your hand (carefully, so as not to have your fingers crushed by the teeth).

If the enlargement is indeed a lump in the mouth tissues, you can go a step further to make sure it is actually an abscess rather than a tumor or some other type of swelling by poking a sterile large-diameter needle into its center. If pus comes out through the inserted needle, or the needle is covered with pus when you withdraw it, you'll know the lump is an abscess and can be lanced and drained.

If it's already broken open and draining, clean and flush the abscess with the iodine. The foreign object will drain off with the pus. You may need to make the opening larger so it can drain more completely and won't close over again before healing. The wound infection must heal from the inside out, so it must be kept open for drainage until the pus is all gone. Since the abscess is usually just a local infection, walled off from the rest of the body, it does no good to give the animal systemic antibiotics (such as an injection). Flushing out the pus with a good antiseptic solution provides the best results. One or two treatments will usually clear up the infection.

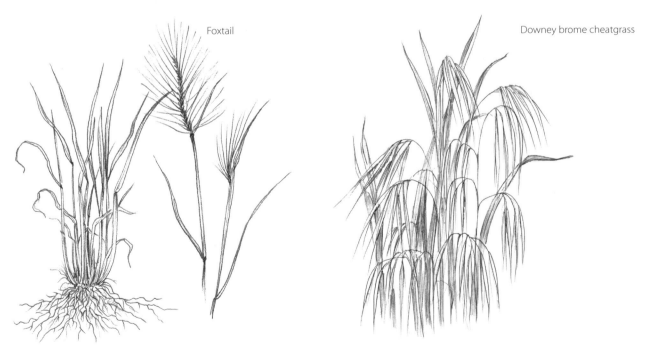

Foxtail

Downey brome cheatgrass

Sharp grass seeds from plants like foxtail or cheatgrass may puncture the mouth tissues and open the way for infection.

HOW TO LANCE AND FLUSH AN ABSCESS

1. Using a very sharp, clean knife or scalpel blade, slit the lump at the lowest edge of its softest area, if possible, for best drainage.

2. To minimize bleeding, make a vertical slit through the skin; this is less likely to cut a blood vessel than a horizontal cut (the abscess will be located between the skin and the deeper blood vessels).

3. Squeeze out all the pus you can from the lump.

4. Using a large syringe (without a needle) or a squeeze bottle, squirt an antiseptic solution of half iodine and half water into the slit several times until you are sure you've washed all the pus out and the flushing solution comes back out clean.

5. Be sure the slit is long enough to stay open for drainage, so the area can heal without more treatments. If it closes over too soon and the lump starts to enlarge again with pus, you must open it up again and flush it another time.

If an abscess keeps sealing off before it heals, keep it open and draining by soaking a strip of gauze (which comes in a roll) in iodine, wadding the gauze, and putting the gauze into the hole, leaving the end of the strip protruding through the slit. The iodine fights infection while the gauze strip keeps the slit open and serves as a "wick" to help keep pus and fluid draining out of the wound. Pull the gauze out a few days later, after the drainage has ceased, and the area will usually heal nicely.

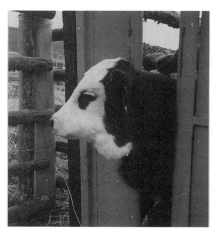

Side view of a calf with a soft-tissue abscess from a grass seed

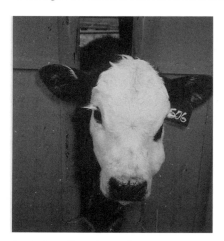

Front view of an abscess lump

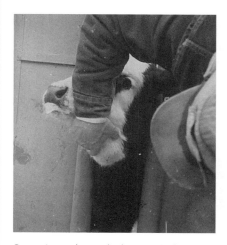

Preparing to lance the lump at its lowest spot

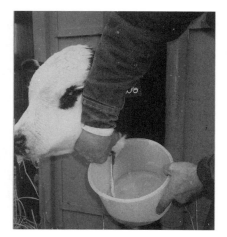

Step 3: Squeezing out all the pus

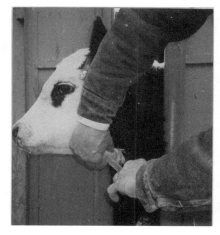

Step 4: Flushing the abscess out with antiseptic solution

Bony Lump Jaw

Less-common lump-jaw infections are bony lumps, caused by *Actinomyces bovis,* another type of gram-negative bacteria that lives in the soil. This bacterium enters a wound in the mouth the same way as bacteria in soft-tissue abscesses (from a sharp object penetrating the cheek tissue outside or inside the mouth) but can infect the bone if the puncture goes deep enough. This creates a condition called *Actinomycosis.* Since bone infection is difficult to treat and because it often recures even if it seems to get better for a while after the treatment, it usually results in having to eventually sell or butcher the animal.

Bony lump jaw occurs most often in 2- or 3-year-old cattle. Infection may be introduced by a deep puncture from an object outside or inside the cheek, but it often becomes established through the dental sockets where teeth are set into the jaw. Because young cattle are vulnerable when shedding baby teeth and their permanent teeth are coming in, they are prime candidates for the condition.

Infection gets started in the jawbone and creates a painless bony enlargement, usually at the level of the central molars. There may be multiple pockets of infection because of the reaction in the bone. The bone responds to the infection by producing more layers of new bone and sometimes a thinning of the older bone. In rare cases the infection involves the tissues of the mouth and throat, as well as the jawbone, if lacerations in those areas permit the entrance of bacteria. Bony lump jaw occurs only sporadically in affected herds but is a serious condition because of its poor response to treatment.

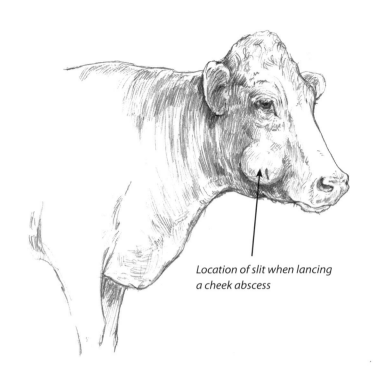

Location of slit when lancing a cheek abscess

Symptoms

Sometimes an enlargement on the lower jawbone may occur as a thickening of the lower edge of the bone with most of the enlargement appearing on the inner side of the jaw. Positioned here, the lump may not be readily observed until it becomes quite large and is already too extensive for effective treatment. More commonly, the protrusion is on the outer side of the jawbone (next to the molars) and is more easily seen. Some swellings enlarge within a few weeks, while others grow slowly over several months.

The painless bony swelling is very hard and you can't move it around with your hand, since it is part of the bone. This is the easiest way to tell the difference between bony lump jaw and a soft-tissue abscess that can be readily opened and drained (see above page 236). The bony lump is completely immobile.

There is no ill effect on the animal's health at first from a bone infection in the jaw, since it is localized and does not create systemic illness. In later stages, however, the area may become painful to the touch and will interfere with chewing. The lump may break through the skin eventually and discharge through one or more openings. A little pus or a sticky, honey-like fluid containing tiny, hard, yellow granules may ooze through the skin over the lump.

Teeth in the affected jawbone may become misaligned over time and cause pain while chewing. This makes it hard for the animal to eat, resulting in weight loss. In severe cases the infection spreads to the soft tissue and involves the muscles and lining of the throat, interfering with the animal's ability to burp up and chew her cud.

If swelling becomes extensive, it may interfere with breathing. The animal may become so thin that humane destruction is necessary, though it may take

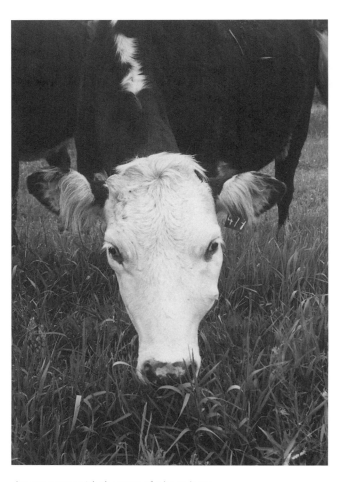

A young cow with the start of a bony lump.

a year or more for it to get this bad. If the infection spreads to the esophagus and front part of the reticulum, digestion is impaired, and the result is diarrhea (passing undigested food particles) or bloat.

Lancing the enlarged area on the jaw is pointless; unlike a soft-tissue abscess, which is comprised of pus, the bony lump is composed of infected bone and can't be drained. The oozing area may heal over only to break out again later. Trying to drain the lesion is sometimes harmful, since opening it to the outside could allow other pathogens to enter, and a secondary infection may result.

Treatment

Bony lump jaw is easy to diagnose but hard to treat. A soft-tissue abscess, by contrast, recovers quickly if opened and drained; the lump goes away. But a bony lump is always permanent. Since it is a bone infection, it must be treated from the inside out, via blood that serves the bone.

The usual treatment requires administration of a solution of 10 percent sodium iodide into the jugular vein. Dosage depends on the size and weight of the animal. This treatment may need to be repeated in

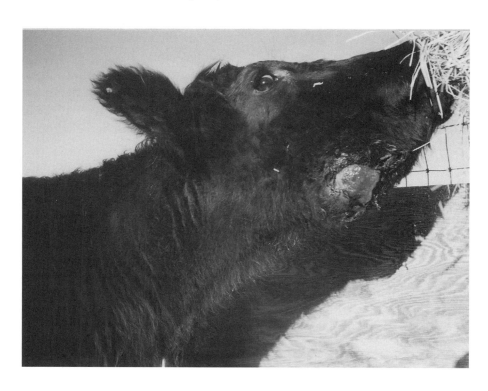

A 3-year-old cow with a bony lump that started six months earlier and has now broken through the skin.

10 days. Iodine is a poison, but *sodium iodide* is in a salt form that facilitates getting the iodine to the site of the infection through the bloodstream.

Iodides given intravenously may halt the bone infection if administered early, before the lump gets large. But many cases are stubborn and do not respond. Some lumps reduce in size once the infection is stopped but never go away completely. In other cases a lump may stop growing for a while after treatment (you might be able to get one or two more calves from the cow), but then it starts again. The cow should be culled after she relapses.

The IV administration of sodium iodide must be done slowly and carefully, or the animal may go into shock. If you are not experienced at giving IVs, your vet should do it. Even though this treatment is usually safe for pregnant cows, some abort after iodide treatment. If a cow is in late pregnancy when the bony lump is noticed, it's wise to postpone treatment until after she calves, with the hope of saving both the cow and calf. But if the cow is going downhill rapidly because she can't eat well or is not due to calve for some time, it's generally best to treat the cow and take your chances.

Wooden Tongue

Wooden tongue is called actinobacillosis by medical professionals and is caused by the bacterium *Actinobacillus lignieresii*. This pathogen is commonly found in the digestive tract of cattle and generally causes problems only when injuries to the tissues of the mouth or tongue provide an entry for it. The tissue trauma may be due to abrasions or punctures when eating coarse feed or to lacerations on the side of the tongue caused by the teeth. Local infection of the tissues causes acute inflammation, tissue death, and pus discharge. The infection may spread to nearby lymph nodes.

Symptoms
Once the infection sets in, the tongue becomes sore and stiff and interferes with chewing. The affected animal is unable to eat for a day or two and goes through chewing motions — as if trying to get rid of a foreign object in the mouth. The tongue may feel strange to the animal because it's swollen and

---

TONGUE-TIED

OUR HERD was on one of our hill pastures one December, and among them was Linda, a 10-year-old cow due to calve January 13. When we went to take the cows down to the fields for winter, we noticed that she'd lost a lot of weight. She'd probably been unable to eat for several days before we noticed her condition. She tried to eat hay but merely wadded it around in her mouth.

We brought her down to the corrals on January 1, put her on antibiotics for 7 days, and had our vet look at her. He diagnosed her with wooden tongue. Although we'd had another cow years before who responded quickly and completely to an intravenous administration of *sodium iodide*, we all agreed we couldn't risk abortion with Linda. So the vet took wads of feed out of her cheeks, rasped the sharp edges of her teeth smooth (because they could injure her tongue), and flushed her throat with iodides. We fed her water with molasses added for energy for 5 days by stomach tube, since she would not eat or drink.

Finally she started eating a little during the second week of treatment and calved on schedule. She had a healthy bull calf, even though she was very thin and weak and had a hard time getting up after her labor. We pampered her with alfalfa hay and gave her calf some extra bottles of milk for a few days until she recovered more fully and was eating better and producing adequate milk for her calf. We named him Linda's Lasses because molasses helped keep his mama alive.

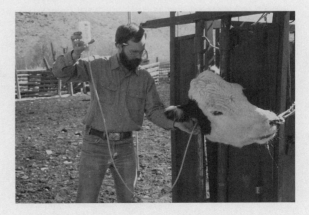

Put sodium iodide solution into the jugular vein to treat a cow with bony lump jaw or wooden tongue.

stiff. Due to constant chewing, saliva may drool from the mouth. If you open the mouth and feel the tongue, it will be enlarged and stiff, especially at the base; the tip may be normal. Handling the tongue is painful to the animal. There may be lumps and ulcerations along the side of the tongue. In later stages of infection the tongue becomes shrunken, hard and immobile; the animal continues to have trouble eating. Enlargement of infected lymph nodes may interfere with swallowing and may also cause loud snoring sounds when the animal breathes.

Treatment and Prevention

Wooden tongue responds well to iodides, which can be administered orally or intravenously. Potassium iodide can be given daily as a drench for 7 to 10 days, but this is time-consuming and labor-intensive, and the animal may develop a sensitivity to iodine, evidenced by excessive watering of the eyes, coughing, lack of appetite, and flaky skin.

It is often simpler to have your veterinarian give the animal one dose of sodium iodide (10 percent solution) intravenously, after which the symptoms of wooden tongue disappear within 24 to 48 hours. Care must be taken to administer the IV very slowly to avoid side effects such as difficult breathing and rapid heart rate. Sodium iodide may also cause abortion. Penicillin and several other broad-spectrum antibiotics are also effective, but iodides seem to give the best and most permanent results.

Isolate any animal that develops wooden tongue, and treat the infection quickly; otherwise, the affected animal may contaminate pasture and feeding areas with the pus discharges. Avoid giving your cattle coarse, sharp feed, and the incidence of oral scrapes and punctures will decrease.

Mouth and Throat Lesions

Occasionally an animal develops sores or ulcers in the oral cavity. Inflammation may be caused by trauma, such as scraping of the tissues by a stick or sharp pieces of feed, misaligned teeth, or by a balling gun or dose syringe when you are dosing the animal. An ulceration also may be caused by the animal's eating or licking something very irritating, such as certain chemicals or acid. A common cause, however, is an infection, such as diphtheria in calves (see chapter 9), wooden tongue, or lump jaw.

Ulcerations in the mouth may also be due to viral infections that erode the lining. These diseases include BVD and bluetongue (see chapter 5). Other lesions may appear as bumps inside the mouth. Bovine papular stomatitis is a mild viral disease of young cattle (2 weeks to 2 years of age) that causes small, solid, rounded elevations (papules) on the skin of the muzzle and inside the mouth and nostrils. The virus that causes this is similar to the one that causes *pseudocowpox* on teats (see chapter 15).

An animal with bovine papular stomatitis may show mild illness, but in most instances this disease goes unnoticed unless you see small bumps on the muzzle or look into the mouth. Small papules inside the mouth become dark red and develop a rough surface and may expand to the point that several lesions converge to create a large red area with a depressed center that is eventually covered with dead tissue (or a scab, on the muzzle). In the mouth the lesions may occur on all the membrane surfaces except the top of the tongue and are most common inside the lips and next to the teeth. These lesions usually heal quickly, but successive crops of lesions may appear (and keep

Observe and Check Cattle

Whenever your cattle are in close quarters for various purposes — such as putting them through a chute for vaccinations or for pregnancy checking — take advantage of the opportunity to check for any abnormalities. This is a perfect time to look closely into a cow's eyes to make sure she doesn't have the beginning of cancer eye and to do a "hands-on" examination of any lumps.

Any swellings seen on the face or jaw should be felt and pushed, to see if they are soft-tissue lumps that should possibly be lanced at that time (or flushed out if they're already broken and draining) or to see if they are bony lumps. Early treatment for a bony lump is often more successful than waiting until it is well advanced.

appearing continuously or intermittently over several months) if the animal has low resistance.

Mouth ulcers also occur with *vesicular stomatitis (VS),* or *foot and mouth disease* (see chapter 19), which is a serious foreign-animal illness. If you are uncertain as to the cause of a mouth problem or how to treat it, consult your vet. Vesicular stomatitis (see chapter 19) is a disease you must report to state health authorities (the state veterinarian) because some of the symptoms are similar to those of foot and mouth disease, a disease that authorities hope to keep out of the United States and Canada.

Symptoms and Treatment

When the mouth is sore from any type of ulceration (exposed raw tissues), the animal goes off feed or eats slowly and painfully. Chewing movements are accompanied by drooling, especially if the animal can't swallow normally. Breath may smell foul if there is bacterial infection in the lesions. In some instances the face may be swollen. The mucous membranes lining the mouth may slough away in the affected areas.

The animal should be isolated if you suspect the problem is due to infectious disease; consult your vet for proper diagnosis and treatment. The lesions can be flushed with a mild disinfectant solution. Teeth should be checked if lesions are due to trauma. The animal should be fed soft, palatable feed or fed by stomach tube or IV if unable to eat or drink.

Tooth Loss

Tooth loss is mainly a problem for older animals. A traumatic accident may knock out a tooth or teeth, but this is rare. The primary cause of tooth loss is extensive wear from eating abrasive feeds. A cow uses her incisors (the front teeth on the bottom jaw) for breaking off grass and her molars (the back teeth) for preliminary chewing and then grinding up feed more thoroughly when she chews her cud.

If cattle eat coarse forage, they wear out their teeth faster. Grass contains silica, which is abrasive and wears down teeth. A cow's teeth wear out faster in sandy soils as she takes in a little sand with some of the feed or if sand clings to the roots of easily pulled grass. Wet bottomlands with coarse swamp grasses

---

Mouth and Teeth Glossary

Broken mouthed cow. A cow that's missing some teeth. This is usually an indication of old age.

Canine teeth. The 2 outer teeth bordering the incisors in the lower jaw. In cattle, the canine teeth are smooth rather than sharp.

Cleft palate. Congenital defect creating a hole in the roof of the mouth.

Deciduous teeth. Temporary baby teeth. A calf has 8 small incisors and 12 molars, all of which are shed and replaced by larger, permanent teeth.

Dentition. The number and arrangement of teeth. Calves have 20 temporary teeth. Adults have 32 permanent teeth by the time they reach 4.5 to 5 years of age (20 on the lower jaw and 12 molars on the upper jaw). They have no front teeth; instead there is a hard dental pad. On the lower jaw the front teeth consist of 6 incisors and 2 canine teeth. The latter are not pointed; they are blunt like the incisors.

Full mouth. A solid mouth.

Incisors. The 6 largest front teeth on the lower jaw.

Mouthing a cow. Looking into the animal's mouth to examine her teeth to determine her age. The number of teeth present (or missing) and their condition can give a good estimate of her age.

Overshot jaw. An upper jaw that is longer than and protruding past the lower jaw.

Peg teeth. Small, worn-down teeth in older animals. These teeth are usually more round and cylindrical than the teeth of younger animals.

Smooth mouth cow. A cow with no teeth or whose teeth are worn down level with the gums, making it harder for her to graze and chew her cud.

Solid mouth cow. Young to middle-age cow that has all her teeth, still in good condition.

---

also wear down the teeth faster than finer grasses. Cows that pasture in the bottomlands often wear out their teeth 2 to 3 years sooner than cows grazing the finer-leafed native bunch grasses on the uplands, in regions with foothills and mountains.

Check teeth when the cow is restrained in a chute. If front teeth are worn down, the molars will be worn also. When teeth wear down too much, they may actually fall out. A cow with some of her front teeth missing is called *"broken mouthed."* An old cow may lose weight if she has lost some or all of her teeth. A 15-year-old cow with a *"full mouth"* will usually be in better body condition (and look younger) than a 10-year-old cow that's lost some of her teeth.

Choking

Blockage in the throat is probably more common than in the mouth; cattle eat so hurriedly they may try to swallow objects such as apples, or pieces of potato, that become lodged in the throat or esophagus. The obstruction is generally above the larynx, right at the back of the throat (see chapter 6).

The animal suddenly stops eating and becomes anxious and restless, frantically chewing and trying to swallow. Saliva and feed may drool from the mouth, and the animal may cough repeatedly. If the blockage is complete and the animal cannot belch, bloating begins very quickly. Many of these obstructions are temporary and resolve without treatment. The muscles of the throat or esophagus relax, and the obstruction may pass on down.

If the blockage does not quickly resolve, however, call your veterinarian. He or she may be able to reach into the throat and retrieve the object. If that fails, the animal may be given drugs to help relax the tissues so the blockage can pass on down.

Foreign Object Lesson

Cattle eat hurriedly and often get foreign material in the mouth along with their feed. Usually they sort it out with their agile tongues or spit out the mouthful when they start to chew it and find there's a rock or a stick in with the grass or hay. Calves often chew on sticks and baling twine out of curiosity or boredom, looking for something to do. On occasion an animal may get a foreign object caught or stuck in the mouth, and it may hinder eating.

Several years ago one of our 2-month-old calves was having trouble nursing his mother. He'd stand beside her and fiddle with the udder but didn't seem to take hold of the teat very effectively. He also stopped eating hay. He'd take a small mouthful but wouldn't chew it. It looked like one side of his face was a bit swollen, and we thought he might have the beginning of a cheek abscess. We caught him and felt his cheek, but it was all very hard and firm and didn't seem to have an abscess, so we looked inside his mouth and found a wad of feed stuck in the side of his mouth.

As we started digging it out, we found a stick wedged tightly in the back of his mouth, stuck between the molars on each side. The stick was effectively blocking his ability to swallow and chew. He would have starved to death if we hadn't noticed his problem. We pried the stick out and cleaned out the buildup of food in his cheek. His mouth was a little sore where the stick had poked into the tissues, but he was very, very hungry and immediately went to nurse his mama after we got his mouth cleaned out.

CHAPTER FOURTEEN

Metabolic Problems

METABOLIC DISORDERS ARE NOT INFECTIOUS or contagious but are brought on by a breakdown in normal body function, nutritional imbalances, taxing environmental conditions, and other physical circumstances. Sometimes several animals in a herd suffer the same metabolic ailment because they're all being fed the same way, experiencing the same stressful conditions, and enduring nasty weather, for example. When a number of animals become ill with the same symptoms at the same time, stockmen might think the problem is an outbreak of contagious disease. This is not always the case. Most metabolic problems are preventable if you understand the factors that trigger them and make efforts to minimize those factors.

Milk Fever

Also called *parturient paresis,* milk fever occurs mainly in dairy cows just before or after calving. It tends to affect high-producing mature cows more commonly but occasionally occurs in first calvers and in beef cows as well.

Sudden loss of calcium in the body may cause a cow to collapse at calving time. More calcium is being pulled from her body tissues for milk production than can be immediately replaced from bones and from feed in the digestive tract. Most of the time bones serve as a storage area for extra calcium; the body can pull a little calcium from these reserves during shortages. But in a cow that suddenly creates a large amount of milk, these reserves are not enough. A serious shortage has severe effects on the body because calcium is necessary for proper nerve and muscle function.

Calcium Drop

The calcium level in the blood is controlled by many factors, including the interrelationship of calcium and *phosphorus* in the feed, the amount of phosphorus in the bloodstream, vitamin D levels in the body, and the proper working of the *parathyroid* and *thyroid glands,* which play a major role in the animal's metabolism. Calcium levels in the blood may drop dramatically when the cow begins lactation, but if everything else in the body is normal, the lost calcium is generally replaced within a few hours. The parathyroid gland sends signals via certain hormones (aided by vitamin D) to release calcium stores in the bones. If the parathyroid gland is inactive, however, this signal is not sent, and stored calcium isn't mobilized into the blood to make up the shortage.

Activity of the parathyroid can be influenced by the rate of calcium intake from feed. Cows on a high-calcium diet such as alfalfa or other legumes during their *dry* period before calving again are often more susceptible to milk fever because the body is getting an excess of this mineral, and the body is lulled into a false sense of plenty. Calcium absorption from the gut alone has been adequate to maintain blood levels of calcium while the cow is dry. There is very little exchange of calcium between blood and bone, and the parathyroid gland has become dormant.

For normal function of the parathyroid gland, calcium and phosphorus intake must be in proper ratio. A dry cow on good grass pasture (or a mix of alfalfa and grass hay) will have a normal ratio of calcium to phosphorus and be less likely to develop milk fever when she starts lactating at calving.

Age plays a role in whether a cow develops milk fever because younger animals can mobilize calcium reserves more readily from the bones. As she gets older, the calcium is bound up more solidly in bones; it's less free to be drawn upon in times of shortage. As a cow ages, her ability to absorb calcium from the gut also decreases compared with a younger animal. That mature cows tend to produce more milk, hitting their peak for production flow by their third and fourth calves, is another predisposing factor. They are at greater risk for sudden calcium depletion than are first-calvers.

Symptoms

Signs of milk fever come on swiftly — over a period of 2 to 24 hours — starting with loss of appetite and slowdown of the digestive tract. The cow may stop chewing her cud and may not pass much manure.

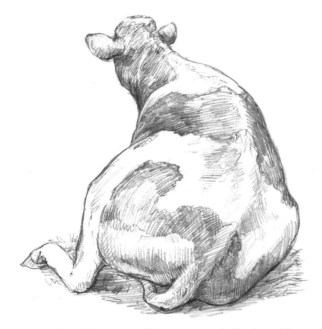

A cow with milk fever is unable to get up and often lies with an S-shaped bend in her neck as she tries to avoid lying down flat.

Her gait becomes stiff and awkward, and then she goes down and is unable to get up. After a few hours she slips into a coma and dies.

Treatment

A cow with milk fever needs an IV injection of a soluble calcium salt. The usual treatment is 400 to 800 mL of a 25 percent solution of *calcium borogluconate*. A large cow may need 1000 mL. Underdosing increases the risk of an incomplete response or a relapse, but giving too much too quickly into the vein can be toxic. In those instances, the heart rate increases dramatically (up to 160 beats per minute), the cow has trouble breathing, and may die within a few minutes. Heart rate should always be monitored while the IV is given; the rate of administration should be slowed or stopped temporarily if the heart rate rises rapidly. It's always wise to allow at least 10 minutes for giving the usual dose of IV solution.

Although intravenous administration is the preferred route because recovery is more rapid, some veterinarians split the dose and give half intravenously and the other half under the skin, to reduce the risk of toxicity. Subcutaneous administration of calcium solution is often effective if you are treating the cow yourself at the first hint of trouble, before she goes down. The dose can be put into two sites under the skin and the area massaged to help increase the rate of absorption. The cow can also be given an oral gel containing calcium chloride, to help increase her chance for recovery and to prevent a relapse.

The cow responds best if she is treated as soon as symptoms are observed, before she goes down. Even if treatment is given soon after a cow goes down, she responds rapidly. Within minutes she'll have muscle tremors and begin to show signs that her digestive tract is working again, burping and passing firm balls of feces covered with mucus. Her heart rate improves, and she'll be able to stand and usually urinates, then eats and drinks after she stands up.

But the longer she's been down, the greater the risk for muscle damage and complications, especially if she's been down for 4 hours or more. If she is lying out flat when you find her (no longer resting on her breastbone with her head up), prop her up until she can be treated to reduce the risk of choking and drawing fluid into her lungs if she regurgitates.

Prevention

Make sure cows have lower levels of calcium in their diet during late pregnancy. Requirements for calcium do not increase until after they calve and are lactating. If you overfeed calcium by offering feeds like alfalfa in late gestation, cows will become too fat and more prone to milk fever. The body gets used to a high calcium level and can't adjust quickly enough when her needs are suddenly higher after she calves. Cows do better if given feeds that are lower in calcium and higher in phosphorus until after calving.

Other methods to prevent milk fever include adding ammonium chloride salts to the feed of dairy cows during the weeks before calving or giving every cow an oral dose of calcium chloride gel at calving, followed by a diet high in calcium. For best results when using oral gel, give the first dose about 12 hours before calving (if you detect early labor signs), another dose immediately after calving, another 12 hours after calving, and a final dose 24 hours after calving. Significantly increasing the calcium content of her diet starting the day she calves can also greatly reduce the risk for milk fever.

If you have many instances of milk fever in your herd, seek advice from your vet regarding prevention and treatment. To learn how to detect stages of labor, see *Essential Guide to Calving* (Storey Publishing, 2008), the companion volume to this book.

Grass Tetany

Grass tetany primarily affects mature cattle grazing lush forage and is due to a deficiency of magnesium in the animal's bloodstream and *cerebrospinal fluid* (around the brain and spinal cord). It has been called by many names, including grass staggers, lactation tetany, milk tetany, winter tetany, transport tetany, wheat pasture poisoning, crested wheatgrass poisoning, great oat poisoning, and barley poisoning, among others.

Low blood levels of magnesium can occur in all age groups and both sexes under various management and feeding situations. However, tetany is most common in beef and dairy cows during the first 60 days of lactation, especially in older cows producing a lot of milk and grazing immature cool-season grasses. It may also occur in late pregnancy.

Milk Fever and Grass Tetany Are Similar

Milk fever is a calcium deficiency, and tetany is a magnesium deficiency, but both have similar symptoms. One way to differentiate between the two is to watch behavior: cows with milk fever are more lethargic, and cows with grass tetany are generally more violent.

Cattle may have calcium and magnesium deficiencies at the same time. For this reason supplements containing both minerals and treatment with products to restore the levels of both minerals in the body are often used.

Magnesium Drop

The problem develops when forage is low in magnesium, or when other nutrients, such as potassium and protein or nitrogen interfere with absorption and utilization of magnesium in the body. When cattle are first turned out on lush pastures in the spring, for instance, the relatively high level of potassium and protein in these grasses ties up the availability of calcium and magnesium to the body. Cereal grasses are most risky, but any high-quality lush grass tends to absorb excess potassium when growing rapidly and thus decreases the absorption of magnesium when eaten by the animal.

When to Suspect Grass Tetany

There are a number of environmental and biological conditions that invite this metabolic disorder. Suspect grass tetany:

▶ In early spring during cool, wet weather with little sunshine, when new plants that grow best in these conditions are high in potassium and soluble nitrogen

▶ In fall or winter in southern regions when rains promote lush new growth

▶ When late-gestating or lactating cows graze crested wheatgrass or immature cereal grains that have grown rapidly and are short on magnesium

- When a cow is put out on lush green grass at calving — her requirement for magnesium triples after she calves

- In winter, if cows are fed grass hay that is low in magnesium

- Whenever the mainstay of the diet is cereal greenfeed (green chop), or silage, especially if potassium in greenfeed or silage is high; high rumen levels of potassium may interfere with the absorption of both calcium and magnesium into the bloodstream

- After stormy weather or stress causes cattle to be off feed 24 hours or more, further reducing magnesium intake

- When cattle are not getting enough calcium, phosphorus, or salt in their diet

Magnesium is present in most body tissues and is crucial for normal body function, nerve impulses, and muscle contraction. About 70 percent of the magnesium is stored in bones and teeth and is not readily available if circulating blood levels drop. The body's daily requirement for magnesium must be supplied by diet. When magnesium levels in feeds are low, magnesium needed for milk production quickly depletes the levels in the blood and cerebrospinal fluid. This results in loss of normal muscle function and also affects the nervous system.

Symptoms

Signs of tetany include muscle spasms and convulsions, but the first signs may be restlessness, nervousness, or flightiness; leaving the herd; poor appetite; and excitability or aggressiveness. Upright ears, ears and face twitching, muscle twitches in the flanks and wide-eyed staring are early signs, along

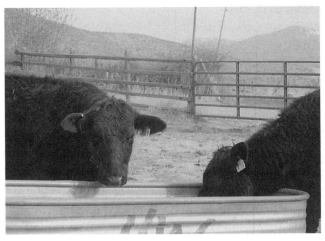

Prevent grass tetany by adding drugstore Epsom salts (magnesium sulfate) to the cows' water.

with frequent urination, getting up and down repeatedly, head and neck tremors, and high-stepping with the front legs. Muscle spasms, rapid eye movements, rapid and snapping retraction of the third eyelid, drooling, and excessive chewing are common. The affected animal is alert, easily excited, and may charge at anyone or anything that approaches. The belligerent change in attitude might be mistaken for rabies. Some symptoms may be confused with listeriosis (see chapter 4) or other conditions that affect the brain or cause sudden death.

The animal may bellow and gallop in a frenzy for no reason, often running into fences or other obstacles, or may collapse when moved or excited. Stress can bring on the *clinical signs.* The cow may be uncoordinated and staggering, then go down and be unable to get up. At this stage she may lie flat on her side with front legs paddling. She may thrash or throw her head back, drooling and breathing hard, and then lapse into a coma. Death is usually the result of respiratory failure during a seizure after the cow is down. Often the symptoms come on so suddenly, and these animals die so quickly (within 4 to 8 hours from the onset of symptoms), that you don't see them acting strangely; you simply find them dead. The ground around the dead animal is usually disturbed, due to thrashing of the animal as she dies.

Brain Fluid Diagnosis

Since cattle are often found dead, one way to determine the cause of death — and to know if other

---

RARELY BOTHERS CALVES

Mature animals are more susceptible to grass tetany because of their inability to mobilize magnesium from their bones to meet the needs of the body. They have lower magnesium stores and a reduced ability to absorb this mineral. The older the animal, the more susceptible she is.

---

cattle in the pasture are at risk — is to have your vet collect a sample of fluid from the eye or the brain. This can be analyzed for magnesium content and is more accurate than a sample of blood serum or tissue, since magnesium levels in these may return to normal at death. Blood samples of live animals are accurate for diagnosis, but putting them into a chute to collect the samples can create stress that results in life-threatening convulsions.

Treatment

Animals in early stages of tetany must be handled slowly and carefully to avoid stress. If you find an animal with tetany, immediately treat the affected individual and quietly move the rest of the herd to more mature pastures or to a location where they can be fed legume hay, which contains higher levels of calcium and magnesium than grass hay. Another option is to get supplemental magnesium into them as soon as possible via the drinking water or a concentrate feed the animals are familiar with and will definitely eat. Cattle on dry feed tend to eat more salt, which should also be provided in ample amounts.

If you find an affected cow soon enough, while she can still be moved or even if she is down and can't get up but is not yet *comatose,* the problem can be reversed within minutes by giving 200 to 500 mL of *calcium magnesium gluconate* intravenously. There are also commercial preparations of *calcium borogluconate* solution that contain 5 percent magnesium hypophosphate, which works very well.

The calcium solution can be put into the jugular vein. In a lactating cow (especially a dairy cow with big milk veins) it can be put into a vein in front of the udder, since those are easy to find. *Give the solution very slowly, and monitor the animal's heart rate closely* during IV administration; magnesium salts can be toxic if absorbed too quickly, resulting in respiratory failure. To avoid this risk, some vets recommend 200 to 300 mL injections of a *magnesium sulfate* solution (Epsom salts) under the skin rather than giving an IV injection.

Generally the cow will get up after treatment. Improvement is usually seen within 3 to 5 hours, though a few cows die in spite of treatment if they suffer another convulsion before the magnesium is fully absorbed. Relapses may occur 3 to 6 hours later.

The animal should be kept as quiet as possible. Some vets give a tranquilizer just to keep the animal from getting excited.

Another effective treatment involves dissolving 60 grams of magnesium chloride or Epsom salts (magnesium sulfate) in 200 mL of water, to give as an enema. Sometimes it is easier to deal with the cow's rear end than her head and neck if she's belligerent or having convulsions. Use a collapsible plastic bottle attached to a plastic tube inserted into the rectum, letting the fluid flow down the tube and into the rectum. The cow can absorb magnesium through the membrane lining of the rectum. Blood levels of magnesium will rise within 20 minutes.

After treatment the cow may recover quickly, but relapses are common. If you had to give an IV or an enema in a pasture, your vet may recommend a follow-up treatment orally after the cow is able to walk. Confine the cow in a chute and give 3 ounces (88.7 mL) each of magnesium oxide and dicalcium phosphate, plus 1 ounce (29.6 mL) of salt, mixed into 1 or 2 gallons (3.8 or 7.6 L) of water, via stomach tube. To play it safe, leave her in a corral for a few days where you can treat her again if necessary.

Prevention

Prevent grass tetany by using pastures that contain some mature plants. Delay turnout on pastures until grass is at least 4 to 6 inches (10.2 to 15.2 cm) tall. If that's not possible, feed a mineral supplement containing relatively high levels of magnesium (1 to 2 ounces [29.6 to 59.2 mL] of magnesium oxide or magnesium sulfate) and calcium if cattle will eat

More than One Problem

Sometimes a cow is short on both calcium and magnesium. This is why treatment is often aimed at replenishing both of these important elements. In some instances a case of milk fever will also be complicated by ketosis, in which case she responds to the calcium therapy by standing up but will continue to show signs of ketosis, which may include nervousness and circling.

enough of the supplement, or use a mineral mix containing magnesium in a palatable base. Magnesium oxide is very unpalatable, and cattle won't readily eat it. It usually must be mixed with grain or a flavoring agent if you want cattle to consume it free choice. A mineral mix should be about 6 percent magnesium, and cattle need to eat 2 to 3 ounces (59.2 to 88.7 mL) of it per day to prevent grass tetany. You can encourage salt consumption by using salt-mineral mixes containing molasses.

In many instances it's impossible to completely prevent tetany by using supplemental minerals because consumption is not consistent enough,

especially in large pastures. Always place mineral feeders where every animal will have access (such as near the water source where animals must go every day), and make sure there is adequate space in the feeders for even the timid ones to have the opportunity to eat.

It's important that each animal consume an adequate amount every day. If cattle are watered in a tank, Epsom salts can be added to the water to make sure every animal is dosed. Magnesium acetate or magnesium chloride will also work. Don't use magnesium oxide (a common source of supplemental magnesium); it is insoluble in water. After pasture grasses become more mature and/or there are more sunny days, mineral supplement or water treatment are no longer needed. Another alternative is to delay pasture turnout until grass is more mature or put less-susceptible yearlings, dry cows, or cows with calves more than 4 months old and past their peak of lactation on those pastures first.

Cows that develop tetany are more likely to do so again. They should be culled or put into a different type of feed program where risk situations are avoided.

Phosphorus Deficiency

Occasionally a dairy cow may suddenly go off feed and become extremely weak 2 to 4 weeks after calving, due to phosphorus deficiency. This may happen if cows are eating cruciferous plants like rape or turnips or large quantities of beet pulp, all of which are phosphorus poor. Soils low in phosphorus, and sometimes copper, may be a factor. High-producing dairy cows are most at risk, especially during peak production years, their third through sixth lactations. Cattle at pasture are rarely affected. Cases are more often seen in cows confined indoors for long periods, but occasionally a few animals on lush spring pasture may develop this problem.

Symptoms include blood in the urine, lack of appetite, sudden weakness, with an abrupt drop in milk production. In mild cases a cow may continue to eat, with a normal milk yield, during the first 24 hours after blood is seen in the urine. Affected cows become dehydrated, with pale mucous membranes, dry or firm feces, moderate fever, elevated heart rate,

Planning Ahead for Magnesium Intake

You can consider the risk for magnesium deficiencies in your herd and plan ahead to prevent them. One way to do this is to apply fertilizer to problem pastures and soil types. This will increase uptake of magnesium by the plants.

You can also take a pasture inventory to see what's in store for the herd by testing grasses for magnesium, calcium, and potassium content before you turn them out, especially if cool season grasses are a major part of their diet. Grass samples can be sent to any lab that does feed or forage testing.

Use the following equation to determine if a pasture may cause your cows' problems:
If the amount of potassium divided by the sum of the forage values for calcium and magnesium is greater than 2.2, the plants are likely to induce magnesium deficiency in grazing animals. Forages with less than 0.2 percent magnesium content can also be a problem.

Adding legumes like alfalfa or clover to the diet can help prevent magnesium deficiency, since legumes have higher levels of magnesium and calcium than rapidly growing grasses. If you have problems with magnesium deficiency, consult your vet or county Extension agent; one of them can help you come up with a plan to reduce the risks.

difficult breathing, and, in later stages, jaundice. Without treatment, the cow becomes weak, staggers, and finally goes down and can't get up; she may die within a few days. If she doesn't die, it may take about 3 weeks for recovery. Some cows have *ketosis* at the same time (see below).

Treatment and Prevention

Blood transfusions may be necessary in severe cases and should be given as soon as possible. A transfusion of 5 L for a large cow will usually reverse the condition, but if the cow is still weak (with pale membranes) another transfusion may be needed 48 hours later. Give IV fluids as a follow-up treatment, along with administration of phosphorus by IV and subcutaneously. Consult your veterinarian.

Cows should be fed adequate phosphorus for milk production, especially early in lactation. If any cows on your farm have this problem, you should discuss soil, crop, and feed management with your county Extension agent.

Ketosis (Acetonemia)

Ketosis most often afflicts well-fed dairy cows in good body condition during the first month of lactation. Maintenance of adequate levels of *glucose* in the blood is important for proper energy metabolism. Ketosis (ketone formation in the body) occurs when cattle have more demands for glucose and glycogen than can be met by diet and metabolism and must metabolize fat to make up the difference. The ruminant animal creates glucose in the liver from starch, fiber, and protein products of the rumen. Lowered blood levels of glucose result in lower blood insulin, which in turn results in release of long-chain fatty acids from body stores of fat and formation of *ketones*. Ketones are organic compounds, such as acetone, produced during the metabolism of fats.

In many instances ketosis occurs in high-producing fat or heavy-bodied cows being fed high-quality feed. In other instances, ketosis may result when a cow has some other disease that hinders her appetite and she does not eat enough to supply her needs for energy. It may also occur in cows that are starved and in poor body condition.

Symptoms

There are two forms of ketosis in cattle, a wasting form and a nervous form, but these are two extremes of the same condition, and some cows show varying degrees of either or both.

▸ **The wasting form** is most common. The cow has a gradual decrease in appetite and milk flow over a 2- to 4-day period. She may first refuse to eat grain, then silage, but may continue to eat hay or may want to nibble on strange things. She loses weight, more rapidly than what you'd expect from her drop in appetite, with a loss of skin elasticity due to sudden depletion of subcutaneous fat. Manure becomes firm and dry, and she may show evidence of mild abdominal pain and be reluctant to eat or move. There is the odd odor of ketones (described by some as smelling like nail polish remover; like fruit drops by others) on her breath and often in her milk.

▸ **In the nervous form,** the cow suddenly begins to act in strange ways, walking in circles, crossing her legs, pushing her head against a fence or wall, or leaning into her stanchion. She may wander aimlessly if she's out at pasture, blindly run into things, or vigorously lick herself or nearby objects. She may try to eat strange things or constantly chew and slobber. She may be hypersensitive to touch, to the point of bellowing if you stroke or pinch her. Episodes of strange behavior may last an hour or 2 and then subside, only to recur 8 to 12 hours later. The cow may injure herself during these episodes.

Treatment and Prevention

To treat the condition, give the cow an IV injection of glucose. Repeat this if necessary. In some cows response to treatment is only temporary, especially if ketosis is caused by another disease. Your vet may also recommend giving the cow propylene glycol via stomach tube, since this provides a source of quick energy. It is often beneficial in animals that are unable to eat or, in the case of ketosis, in a cow with an energy deficit or imbalance.

Prevention is difficult because many things can cause ketosis. Usually it can be prevented by making sure cows are not overly fat or starved at the time of calving and making sure that high-producing cows have adequate caloric intake during early lactation. The challenge with high-producing dairy cows is to provide enough calories while still avoiding acidosis due to a high-carbohydrate diet (see chapter 8).

Brisket Disease (High Altitude Sickness)

In mountainous areas of the West, some cattle at high elevations suffer from congestive heart failure. This condition is called brisket disease, mountain sickness, pulmonary hypertension, high mountain disease, big brisket, and dropsy. Many affected animals develop edema (swelling) in the neck and brisket due to high blood pressure forcing fluid out of the blood vessels and into surrounding tissues.

Thin Air

Above 5,000 feet (1,524 m), all mammals respond to the lower levels of oxygen by shunting more blood to the upper part of the lungs, where there's more oxygen. They do it by constricting the blood vessels and thickening the artery walls in the poorly oxygenated parts of the lung. Cattle do this at a more rapid rate than humans and other animals, and this exaggerated degree of shunting can be inherited.

If cattle suffer from too much constriction of arteries in the lungs, this results in higher blood pressure there. The muscle layer in the walls of small pulmonary arteries may thicken over time and reduce blood flow into and through the lungs. The muscle of the heart's right ventricle thickens, due to the extra effort needed to pump blood. The right side of the heart enlarges, and eventually the right ventricle loses its tone and ability to contract. As blood pressure increases and blood starts to back up into the heart, it can blow out the valves of the right ventricle.

Affected animals are short on oxygen because it's hard for them to force blood through the lungs. Cattle are more affected than sheep and other livestock because they have lungs that are small relative to the size of their bodies.

The swelling may spread up the neck to the jaws or along the underline of the belly. Sometimes, however, you never see any outward sign; you just find the animal dead from heart failure.

If cattle go to a higher elevation for summer pasture, symptoms may not become obvious in some individuals until years later or may appear as soon as 12 hours after the elevation change. Cattle living above 5,000 feet (1,524 m) are at risk for brisket disease, and the risk increases the higher the elevation. In the thinner air of high elevations, low oxygen availability triggers the problem in susceptible cattle. In these cases the heart tries too hard to supply blood to body tissues that are short on oxygen.

An Inherited Problem

Susceptibility to high altitude sickness is inherited. A few breeds are less susceptible, but brisket disease has been seen in all breeds. Cattle originating at high elevations (living at high altitudes for many generations) do not get this problem. For instance, cattle grazing at 10,000 to 14,000 feet (3,048 to 4,267 m) in Ethiopia have no hypertension; any individuals susceptible to this condition died off long ago and did not have offspring to pass on this genetic tendency.

But in breeds commonly used in North America, stockmen have selected breeding stock mainly for meat and milk production, fertility, and other marketable traits. Since most cattle live at lower elevations, in these populations there is no natural selection to eliminate the problem. There are, however, some breeds and family lines within breeds that are more naturally resistant, and there are tests to identify them (see page 253). This can help stockmen at high elevations to select resistant animals for breeding use or for purchase, and can reduce the risk of losing animals to brisket disease.

Symptoms

Cattle with brisket disease start to have problems early in life and are often lethargic. Other signs include weakness, diarrhea, bulging eyes, and difficult breathing. If you move cattle very far, those with brisket disease drop to the rear of the herd or lie down because they are short of breath. They may start to exhibit heart failure from exertion. The problem is more common in calves and yearlings.

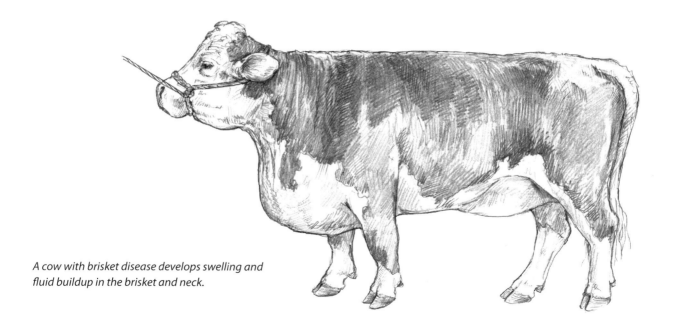

A cow with brisket disease develops swelling and fluid buildup in the brisket and neck.

Chronic cases have swelling under the jaw that may be mistaken for wooden tongue (see chapter 13). Fluid is pushed out through blood-vessel walls into the chest cavity and brisket. Sometimes there are no outward clues that the animal is ill; the animal suddenly dies for no apparent reason.

Treatment

If you see signs of brisket disease, move affected cattle to a lower elevation as soon as you can and with as little stress as possible. Some will recover, but others may die if they've suffered too much heart and lung damage. Treatment should also include administration of antibiotics to try to prevent pneumonia in the damaged lungs, and *diuretics* (drugs that draw fluid out of the tissues).

If an animal is in danger of dying before he can be moved to a lower elevation, he should be treated like a human patient with right-side congestive heart failure. Give the animal a diuretic (such as Lasix), and restrict fluid and salt intake to lower the blood pressure and fluid volume in the body. Vitamin B complex and high doses of a broad-spectrum antibiotic are also helpful.

The fluid you see on the outside of the animal (at the brisket and neck) is just a small proportion; there is more fluid inside the body. The fluid in the chest cavity is putting pressure on heart and lungs. Often veterinarians recommend draining the chest cavity of this fluid. Once you have been shown how to carry out the procedure, you can perform it yourself. To do this, you must insert a large-diameter needle through the chest wall, between the ribs. The needle must be inserted carefully, in the proper location, to avoid draining the heart cavity or poking a hole in the heart. Draining this fluid can relieve the stress on the animal, buying time until you can move him to a lower elevation.

Prevention Involves Testing

Some seed-stock producers (those who raise bulls to sell to other ranches or for artificial insemination [AI] services) test their cattle for brisket disease, using a *pulmonary arterial pressure (PAP) test*. It was developed for measuring pulmonary *artery* pressure in humans and adapted for use with cattle by Dr.

Brisket Disease Risks

Animals with respiratory disease, migrating parasitic larvae and lung worms, lung abscesses, cold-weather stress, or the stress of breathing dust, smoke, or other irritants may be more prone to developing brisket disease, but the biggest risk is genetic susceptibility. A susceptible animal may be more apt to develop the disease if any of these other factors is present.

Tim Holt at Colorado State University in the 1980s. This is a way to measure blood-flow resistance and pressure in the lungs and to predict the animal's welfare at high altitudes.

Cattle raised at lower elevations that stay at low elevation don't have problems; their lack of lung capacity may never be seen. However, if you live above 5,000 feet (1,524 m), and even more importantly above 7,000 feet (2,134 m), and buy cattle from lower altitudes, they may have problems on your farm. In cattle born and raised at high elevations, losses from brisket disease may be less than 5 percent. But when cattle are brought up from lower elevations, losses may be as high as 30 to 50 percent, depending on their genetic makeup. Cattle in Colorado, for instance, may graze at 9,000 to 12,000 feet (2,743 to 3,658 m), and brisket disease can become very costly unless new animals or bulls that produce semen selected for artificial insemination are tested to predict which ones might be at risk. PAP testing helps stockmen select genetically resistant animals.

Until recently, this genetic defect had not been recognized. Many cattle are at risk if taken to higher

Not Just an Altitude Problem

Heart failure due to brisket disease is becoming a problem in feedlots, even at low elevations. Part of the reason is that many popular bloodlines in popular breeds have this trait of susceptibility to restricted blood flow in the lungs.

Because the disease affects lung capacity (causing cattle to die of heart failure), cattle in feedlots may develop this condition when they get close to finished weight. With increased oxygen requirements for larger body bulk, the heart must work harder. Some of the cattle that have the most muscle and red meat — and who are sought after by people who want to raise calves that gain weight fast — have the most problems. There is a definite genetic correlation between fast, efficient weight gain and brisket disease in some of these cattle. Research is currently being done in feedlot cattle at 3,000-foot (914 m) elevations.

elevations. Many of the popular bulls in the Angus breed, for instance, can't be used in high country. You'd have serious problems if purchasing sons or semen (for AI breeding) from these bulls. This is why some breeders are now testing the bulls they sell, to be able to guarantee which bulls will be safe to use at high elevations.

In the 1970s, Dr. Holt studied the arterial pressure of cattle at various elevations, including those living at 15,000 feet (4,572 m), at sea level, and at all elevations in between. Now a stockman, when selecting cattle for breeding, can use PAP testing to predict early signs of congestive right-ventricle failure. PAP testing is only effective, however, when done at elevations above 5,000 feet (1,524 m), and accuracy increases at higher elevations. Most testing is done above 7,000 feet (2,134 m).

The higher the elevation you test at, the more animals you'll find with brisket disease. If breeders want their bulls tested, those bulls must live at high elevations or be taken there to stay for at least 3 to 6 weeks prior, to ensure an accurate determination of genetic susceptibility. Since most of the cattle population and AI sires in the United States reside at lower elevations and are not tested, it's a challenge for high elevation ranchers to find breeding stock that they know don't have this genetic weakness.

Researchers are currently looking at other testing methods, to find genetic markers that might show up in a blood test. This would be an easier way to determine — without having to take an animal to a high elevation — whether or not the animal is susceptible and whether offspring would inherit this susceptibility. The results of this research (a simple blood test) are still several years away, however, and in the meantime stockmen must rely on the PAP test.

Measuring Arterial Blood Pressure

The pulmonary arterial pressure (PAP) test can be done at any age, but accuracy is better if the animal is at least a year old. A calf that scores low isn't necessarily free from the risk of developing brisket disease later. His body is still growing, and his lung capacity has not yet reached its limit. A young animal with a low score should be retested later, to be absolutely sure that he will or won't be at risk for brisket disease.

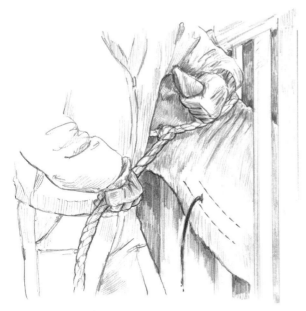

In preparation for a PAP test, the jugular vein has been located and a catheter can be inserted.

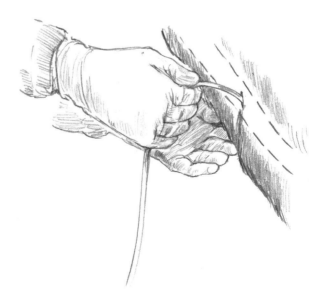

Inserting a catheter into the jugular vein in the neck and threading it through the right ventricle of the heart and out into the main pulmonary artery (between heart and lungs) to do a PAP test.

To test an animal, a catheter is inserted into the jugular vein in the neck. It is threaded through the vein into the right ventricle of the heart and out into the main pulmonary artery between heart and lungs. The pressure in this artery is measured to determine the blood pressure in the right side of the heart. The higher the blood pressure, the less capable the animal is of living at a particular elevation; the animal may already be in the process of dying due to right-heart failure

To be most accurate, the test must be done at elevations above 7000 feet (2,134 m). The PAP score goes up as the animal is taken to higher altitudes. Thus the elevation of the test site must be considered, along with the elevation of the region where the animal lives or will be living for summer pasture. Cattle raised at low elevations always have a higher probability of experiencing brisket disease when taken to higher elevations than do cattle raised at higher elevations.

PAP TEST RESULTS AND RISK SCORE

Score	Degree of Risk
30 to 35	No risk
41 to 45	Low risk for animals more than 16 months old
45 to 48	Moderate risk
49 or more	High risk; offspring are also at high risk

Any score less than 41 is acceptable for an adult animal, but yearlings should measure less than that.

Illness and stress can affect the accuracy of a PAP score because anything causing a temporary or permanent decrease in lung space can increase the PAP measurement. If there is a possibility that a high score might be due to temporary illness, the animal should be retested later.

CHAPTER FIFTEEN

Udder Problems

THERE ARE MANY AILMENTS that affect the udder. It is a complex and delicate structure that sometimes becomes injured or infected. Dairy cattle have more udder problems than beef cattle, simply because their udders are much larger, more prone to injury, and more susceptible to infection in dirty conditions. The larger udder is much more likely to get dirty when the cow is lying down, and much more easily bruised and banged by her legs if she moves faster than a walk.

Teat Injuries

Teats may be injured if a cow walks through sharp obstacles and her udder drags on something or she goes through a barbed-wire fence and snags a teat. Teats may be stepped on when a cow is lying down, or if cows are jammed together in close quarters. A bruised or ripped teat may need medical attention. Consult your vet for proper treatment, especially if a teat is cut so deeply that it needs *sutures* or if a dairy cow is injured and you don't want scarring that might interfere with use of a milking machine. Many lacerations will heal without help, however, since teat tissue has excellent blood circulation and heals rapidly. If the calf can nurse, usually no treatment is needed. You probably won't be able to use a milking machine on a dairy cow's injured teat. Carefully milk it by hand until it heals.

Chapped Teats

In cold or windy weather, a common problem is chapping and cracking. As is the case when human hands are continually in and out of water or subjected to cold, dry weather, when teats are continually wetted (as from the calf's nursing) during windy, cold weather, they can become cracked. The natural oils in the skin are depleted in dry cold and wind.

Cows with white udders and pink teats are more at risk; pigment makes skin tougher, more resistant to the effects of weather, and less prone to sunburn. Though we've had some black and red teats chap and crack, most of the chapped-teat problems in our beef herd have been in cows with unpigmented teats.

During cold, windy spring weather, a few cows get sore teats and kick at their calves. Some calves continue nursing in spite of being kicked or follow the cow around and try to nurse from behind (where the cow can't kick them so easily), but others give up. In these instances we bring the pair in from the field and put them in a small pen where the calf can easily catch up with Mama. She can't run off and may resign herself to letting her calf nurse. If that doesn't work, and she kicks him so hard he won't even try to nurse, we hobble the cow so she can't kick her calf. After a few days the teats heal, and we take the hobbles off.

Winter Teat-End Lesions

Lactating dairy cows often get teat cracks or teat-end lesions in cold weather. These can cause mastitis if they become infected, as the raw tissue opens the way for bacteria. Lesions on the ends of teats may be mistaken for frostbite (see below) or milking equipment malfunction (the vacuum is set too low or too high, creating stress to the teats), but milking equipment rarely causes winter teat-end sores. Cold weather may create lesions at the very end of the teat (around the teat opening), which can be seen if you turn up the teat and look at the end of it. Lactating dairy-cow teat ends should always be examined after a significant drop in winter temperatures.

To avoid teat-end lesions in cold, windy weather:

▸ Provide adequate windbreaks or feed dairy cows indoors during bad weather if possible

▸ Minimize teat washing in cold weather because washing and drying removes the natural oils and can be abrasive to delicate skin

▸ If you wash the teats, carefully blot them dry instead of rubbing

▸ If you dip teats after milking, blot the teat dry afterward

▸ Use a dip that not only contains an effective germicide but also a good skin conditioner

▸ Don't add extra skin conditioner to a commercial teat dip or it may inactivate the germicidal effectiveness

▸ Always use clean hands and individual towels

Frostbite

If the weather is extremely cold, or cold and windy, cows may suffer frostbite on the ends of their teats. This is generally not a problem for dry cows because their udders and teats are small, hang up closer to the body, and are less apt to be frostbitten. But a lactating or pregnant cow developing a large udder before calving is more at risk.

Sometimes after a period of cold weather the ends of a pregnant cow's teats are damaged enough to create a sore, and a scab may form. The teats may be

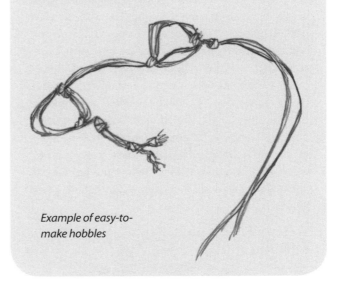
sealed over by the time she calves. In these instances, the calf is unable to draw milk from the teat; he can't suck hard enough to disturb or pull the scab or seal off the end. There may not be a visible scab but the skin is thickened, and the teat duct is sealed over. To enable the calf to nurse, you must start milking the teat for the calf. It may take a very hard squeeze to get the plug out of it.

More serious frostbite may damage the whole end of the teat, killing the skin. A few days after the cold spell, dead skin peels off the end of the teat, and it is extremely sore.

SEVERE FROSTBITE afflicted more than 50 cows in our beef herd in February 1989 after 5 days of 30-below-zero F (–34.4°C) weather, with a strong wind that had a wind chill equivalent to 100 below zero F (–73.3°C). That weather was called the Siberian Express, and it took with it the lives of many cattle in western states.

None of our young calves perished because they stayed inside the calf houses located in every field, out of the wind. They came out only to nurse their mothers and go back in again. Most of our fields had enough trees and brush to provide adequate windbreak for the cows. But in one field the wind came from the wrong direction, and all the cows in that field suffered some degree of frostbitten teats. Five days later the skin was peeling off their teats, the raw tissue was very painful, and these cows were kicking their calves. Some calves continued to nurse in spite of being kicked, but 24 calves were totally discouraged and unable to nurse. We brought those 24 pairs to the corral, put the cows through the chute, hobbled them (see box on previous page), and kept them for 3 weeks in a small pen where the hobbled cows didn't have to walk far for water. After the teats healed, we cut the hobbles off and let the cows and calves back out into the big field again.

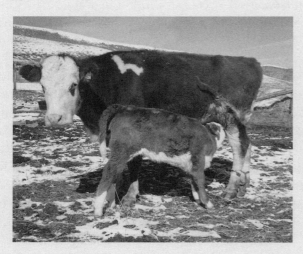

One of our cows that suffered frostbitten teats in February 1989. She and 23 others had to be hobbled until their teats healed, so they wouldn't kick their calves.

Mastitis

Inflammation of the udder (mastitis) is most common in dairy cows due to the complexity and quantity of *mammary tissue* in these high-producing animals. Their mammary tissues have many more blood vessels, are highly specialized, and more vulnerable. Mastitis can also occur in beef cows, however, and can be quite serious. If the infection does not stay localized in the udder, it may get into the bloodstream and causes septicemia. A bad case of mastitis may kill the cow.

A wide variety of bacteria may infect the udder, including several kinds of *Streptococcus*, several species of *Staphylococcus* (which can be difficult to treat), and other less-common pathogens. For instance, an occasional infection with *Klebsiella* may occur when cows are bedded on wood shavings or sawdust. This pathogen is a common inhabitant of tree bark.

Mastitis develops when a quarter becomes infected by contamination from the outside environment. When cows calve in dirty conditions or lie in mud or manure after calving, pathogens may enter the teat canal. Bacteria can be introduced to dairy-cow teats by improper or dirty milking equipment or improper handling at milking time.

Mastitis may be a sequel to bruising and trauma if the udder is bumped and bruised. The damaged tissue creates ideal conditions for infection to start even if there's no break in the skin for pathogens to enter. If a cow has infection elsewhere in her body, and germs are circulating in her bloodstream, they may find a perfect environment in bruised mammary tissue to multiply and create a serious infection.

Dairy cows' udders are more easily bruised than beef cows' udders. A pendulous, full udder is vulnerable to bruising if the cow hurries; her udder swings back and forth if she trots or gallops, and she bangs

TEAT INFECTIONS

A minor infection in the skin of the teat that evolves from scrapes, pokes, and cuts generally resolves quickly but always carries a risk for mastitis if the infection spreads into the udder. Any teat injury or infection should have immediate and proper attention.

it with her hind legs. This can also happen to a beef cow if her udder is tight and full, as at weaning time. A beef cow may still be producing a lot of milk by the time her calf is weaned, so she develops a large udder when the calf stops nursing. It may be tight and sore for several days and vulnerable to bruising if she is quite active. A tight udder signals her body to cease milk production and eventually it is reabsorbed and dries up, but for several days the udder is full, tight, and painful. It is very vulnerable to injury and bruising during this period.

Symptoms

When a cow has mastitis, milk production drops suddenly. The affected quarter is hot, swollen, tender, and sore; the cow resents having it touched. If she has a calf, she may not let him nurse that quarter. If infection stays localized, the mammary tissue in that quarter may be damaged, but the infection is not life threatening. That quarter may be permanently damaged and lose its ability to produce milk, however, unless treatment is prompt and effective. It will be small (and dry) the next time she calves or may produce some fluid right after calving and then dry up again. If the infection does not stay localized, she'll have a fever, go off feed, and may be very ill.

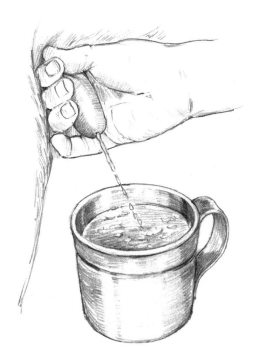

Milk that comes out stringy or clotted is a sign of mastitis.

If you suspect mastitis, inspect some milk from the affected quarter. If she has mastitis, color or consistency of the milk may be abnormal. It may be thin and watery or thick and full of clots. A few small abnormal flecks may be hard to detect unless you use a strip cup with a fine mesh to catch them.

Acute mastitis may respond to treatment or may subside on its own and then recur as a less-painful but chronic condition, flaring up again when the udder or the cow's immunity is compromised again. The aftermath of mastitis may be permanent damage and scar tissue or a lump of encapsulated pus (abscess). Some cases of chronic mastitis are not easy to detect because the udder isn't sore. The cow merely drops in milk production and has a few flakes or clots in the milk. In a dairy herd it's important to always check each cow before milking, testing the first few squirts of milk with a strip cup or a mastitis screening test to check for *somatic cells* that may be indicative of infection.

Treatment

Mastitis should always be treated as soon as you discover it. Milk the affected quarter as thoroughly as possible, then treat it with an antibiotic preparation. Mammary infusions designed for dairy cows work for beef cows also. The antibiotic preparations come in a plastic syringe with a nozzle to insert into the teat opening so you can squirt the medication into the quarter. Some infusions should be given once a day; others work better if given twice daily. Follow label directions. The main thing is to keep the quarter milked out if a calf is not nursing it.

If the animal is a beef cow with a suckling calf, it's usually okay if the calf keeps it milked out, unless the cow has a type of infection that would be dangerous to the calf. This is rare, but you can have your veterinarian check it. Often, the cow won't let the calf nurse that quarter because it is sore. And sometimes the calf doesn't like the taste of the milk or there is no milk, just watery fluid.

Beef cows can be given systemic antibiotics to help clear up mastitis even if you don't infuse the teats. Certain antibiotics that you would not give a dairy cow, because of the lengthy withdrawal time before milk can be used for human consumption, can be given to beef cattle. Your veterinarian can

WE GENERALLY KEEP the first- and second-calvers in a corral for a few days after weaning their calves, until they start to dry up and are no longer so desperate to find their babies. But a corral is dirtier than a grass pasture. Tilda, one of our young cows, developed mastitis in one rear quarter of her udder, after we weaned her calf. She may have picked up the mastitis infection in the corral, or she may have bumped and bruised that rear quarter on her 2-mile (3.2 km) trek up the mountain to the fall pasture. She'd raised a big calf because she produced a lot of milk, and she had a large udder after her calf was taken off. A couple of days after moving the cows, we rode up there to check on them and noticed Tilda had swelling in one quarter. The other quarters were beginning to dry up and shrink in size, but that one was still very large, so we brought her home for treatment.

A few years later another mama, Bella Donna, presented us with the worst case of mastitis we've ever experienced. Bella Donna had not settled when bred and came back into heat. She was "bulling," fighting other cows, riding them, and being ridden by them out on the summer range. As is often the case with an in-heat cow, constant activity and chasing around make it difficult for the calf to nurse, and the cow's udder becomes full. The calf may not be able to nurse until the cow goes out of heat, and the full and constantly jostled udder is susceptible to bruising.

While riding to check range cattle on a hot July day in 1993, I saw 8-year-old Bella Donna bulling, with a mob of cows riding her, and made a mental note to sell her in the fall. The next day when my daughter and I rode again to check the cattle, we found Bella Donna off by herself, in pain, and not eating. We found her calf, then brought them both home to the ranch. We herded them slowly, since the cow was so sick she could hardly travel. She had a high fever and a very painful udder. She would not let her calf nurse.

With diligent treatment — antibiotic injections for more than a week and twice a day squirting mastitis medication directly into the affected quarter — we saved the cow, but the infection totally destroyed her udder. One side of it eventually fell away, and our vet surgically removed the remaining tissue so the udder could heal. We treated Bella Donna with antibiotics and topical medications for 2 months to get her udder healed up and eventually sold her after she was fully recovered. Without prompt and diligent attention in the early stages of this infection, she would have died.

Odd things happen to cows, and this is one reason we check them frequently, whether they're in a pasture near the house or out on the range 5 miles (8 km) away. We ride range nearly every day in the summer, not only to check gates, fences, and water troughs, but also to make sure the cattle are healthy. Often we are able to save a cow or calf by discovering a problem and bringing the animal home for treatment.

Tiffany was one of those summertime saves. She had the strangest case of mastitis we've ever seen. We found her on the range with a swollen quarter and brought her and her calf, Rhinestone Rhonda, home to the corral to treat the infected quarter. In spite of our efforts to milk the quarter out daily and infuse antibiotic into the teat, that quarter stayed enlarged and inflamed. After several weeks it developed more swelling at the back, which eventually broke open and drained like an abscess. We flushed out the drainage hole daily with an antibiotic solution, until one day, out came a 6-inch (15 cm)- long piece of stiff grass!

We puzzled over what might cause such a bizarre situation. We guessed that her calf nursed with a bunch of grass in her mouth, and one of the grass stems must have been jammed directly into the teat canal and up into that quarter. The grass, of course, would be irritating, and carry with it enough contamination to start an infection. Our antibiotic treatments were not able to clear it up because the grass was still in there, providing constant irritation, like a sliver in a wound.

Once the grass came out, we were able to clear up the infection, though Tiffany lost the ability to produce milk in that quarter due to all the damage and scar tissue. She continued to raise calves in subsequent years, however, producing enough milk for them in her other three quarters.

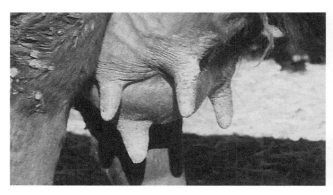

Cow with mastitis in one rear quarter; that quarter and teat are hot, swollen, and painful.

advise you on antibiotic selection, length of treatment, and dosage requirements. In some instances he or she may want to culture a milk sample to determine which bacteria are involved before recommending an antibiotic. Many vets recommend using a broad-spectrum antibiotic until the results of the milk sample culture are available.

Any beef or dairy cow that is dull, off feed, or has a fever should be given systemic antibiotics, or you may lose the cow. Mastitis can be very serious, and you'll want your vet's advice on treatment for each case. If the cow is quite ill, milk her frequently (as often as once an hour) at first, to reduce the level of bacteria and their toxins. Between milkings, use cold packs to reduce swelling and inflammation. You can improvise a cold pack using any material that will hold ice or ice water around the udder, and support it with baling twine or any type of strap over the cow's back. These measures may help save the cow, slowing the infection and inflammation until the systemic antibiotic has a chance to work.

Sometimes a dairy cow (and more rarely a beef cow) develops a case of mastitis that won't respond to standard treatments. Usually the infection is in just one quarter, and in these instances the stockman may opt to use a treatment to kill the pathogen completely and dry up that quarter, so the cow can continue to milk on the other three quarters. There are a number of products that have been used for this purpose, including infusion of chlorhexidine (Nolvasan) up into the teat. This will generally kill the pathogen, and even though the cow loses milk production from that quarter for the rest of her lactation, the quarter will usually be normal the next time she calves.

Studies of treated dairy cows show that Nolvasan residues can be detected in milk from the treated quarter for more than 42 days. Even if that quarter is not milked (and allowed to dry up), there are still residues in milk from the untreated quarters for an unacceptable period of time, so use of Nolvasan in the udder of a lactating dairy cow (whose milk is for human use) is not a legal treatment. It can, however, be used to salvage the udder of a beef cow or a cow you are going to dry up.

HOW TO APPLY ANTIBIOTICS FOR CASES OF MASTITIS

1. Milk out as much as you can.
2. Wipe the teat end with a cotton swab and alcohol or use the packaged wipe that comes with the antibiotic product to keep from pushing more bacteria up into the teat.
3. Insert the cannula and inject the medication. Milk the affected quarter at least twice a day until the infection clears up and the quarter is producing normal milk again. If the calf will nurse it, this saves you the trouble of milking it out.

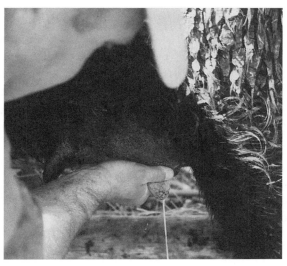

Step 1: Milk out as much of the pus and fluid as possible.

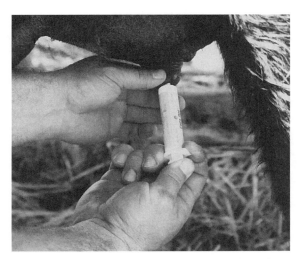

Step 3: Wipe the milked-out teat clean, insert a dose of antibiotic into the teat, and inject the mastitis medication into the quarter.

Prevention

Providing a clean environment and clean bedding goes a long way toward mastitis prevention, along with making sure you don't inadvertently spread mastitis from one cow to another in a dairy herd. Heifers are often most susceptible to mastitis because they may not have as much immunity as an older cow; it often helps to keep them separate from the older cows for at least 2 weeks before they calve.

When milking a group of cows, always milk an infected cow last, to reduce the risk of spreading the infection via your hands or the milking machine. First milk healthy first-calvers, then the healthy older cows, and then any cows or heifers that were recently purchased. Save any infected cows for last.

Always collect any milk you squirt out of the teats ahead of milking; don't just squirt it on the floor. The highest level of bacteria is in the first milk that exits the teat. Squirting it onto the floor of your milk barn will contaminate the environment when the bacteria are tracked around on human or cows' feet.

A simple and effective way to help prevent mastitis is use of a good germicidal teat dip after each cow is milked. There are some good commercial products. Ask your vet which ones to use. Diluted household chlorine bleach (four parts water and one part bleach) is also effective and kills germs for 6 hours or more. Since the teat sphincter (the muscle that opens and closes the opening) is still relaxed right after milking, the teat is vulnerable to invasion by bacteria at that time, especially if there's still a drop of milk at the end of the teat, providing an ideal habitat for bacteria. A teat dip helps prevent bacterial entrance. Be sure to rinse the teat with clean water before the next milking.

Periodic checking of equipment is equally important in a dairy where milking machines are used. If your equipment isn't functioning just right, teat injury may occur that can lead to mastitis. Minor problems are often overlooked because the equipment is still working, but if it's working too slowly or loses vacuum, this may lead to teat injury. The longer the machine is on the teats, the more chance for irritation, which can lead to infection. Proper milking procedures can reduce the incidence of mastitis.

Dairies commonly infuse a long-acting antibiotic into each teat after the final milking when a cow is to be dried up. This will generally get rid of any low-grade chronic infections and help keep the herd free of mastitis.

Udder Edema

Swelling in the udder is sometimes associated with mastitis, but generally it is simply an accumulation of fluid and occurs most often just before calving, when the udder is becoming full and distended. This is most common in heifers. Swelling may become pronounced and extend ahead of the udder along the belly. It's generally no cause for concern, disappearing a few days after the heifer calves. Lack of exercise before calving may increase the likelihood of swelling.

The udder itself may be swollen and hard (this swelling is called "cake"), and the udder may be so tender that the heifer does not want it touched. A first-calf dairy heifer may refuse to be milked after she calves, or a beef heifer may kick at her calf because the udder is sore. It can take several days of careful milking, or restraining the heifer so her calf can nurse, until the swelling resolves and the udder is no longer so sore and sensitive.

Mastitis in Baby Heifers

When raising dairy heifers, keep them separate in their early life while they are fed milk or milk replacer. Calves that nurse bottles or nipple buckets want to keep sucking after the milk is gone, so they turn to one another and suck each other's ears or udders.

In cold weather, ear sucking can lead to frozen ears, but even more damaging for a heifer is to have another calf sucking her little teats. Germs from the mouth of the sucking calf may enter the teats and cause infection, especially if calves are being fed discarded milk that can't be sold, such as milk from cows with mastitis. If a young heifer develops mastitis, you may not even know it until she grows up and has a quarter or two that are nonfunctional from early damage.

Udder edema generally needs no treatment except time and careful milking. In extreme cases, however (especially in dairy heifers, if the swollen udder makes it difficult for the heifer to walk or be milked), you can use massage and exercise to increase circulation and help the swelling resolve. Your vet may advise use of a diuretic drug to help pull fluid out of the tissues, or administration of dexamethasone to reduce the swelling on an animal that's not being milked for human consumption. Use of these drugs is not a problem for a freshly calved cow as her milk can't be used for human consumption until all the colostrum is gone, which takes several days.

Pseudocowpox

Pox viruses create small, round lesions on the teats. These raised red areas become blisterlike and rupture, then scab over and heal.

In early years, *cowpox* (also called milkmaid's disease) was common. Because the virus is related to human *smallpox,* and because people who milked cows and were exposed to cowpox did not get smallpox, the human smallpox vaccine was created from cowpox. Cowpox and smallpox have since been eradicated, but cows can still get a similar disease called pseudocowpox, which also creates lesions on the teats, but is caused by a different virus, more closely related to the virus that causes bovine papular stomatitis (see chapter 13) and is less severe than cowpox.

The pseudocowpox virus is spread from infected cows to susceptible cows by contaminated hands, washcloths, teat cups, and other equipment. Since the virus cannot penetrate the skin, there must be a scrape on the teat before it can enter the tissues. Biting flies may also spread it from cow to cow. The lesions on the teats don't have much of an adverse effect on the cow but may make milking difficult and lead to a higher incidence of mastitis.

There may be numerous lesions on one teat. The teat may first be red and swollen, then small blisters or pustules appear that may be moderately painful. These rupture within about 48 hours and then form a thick scab, after which the teat is no longer painful. The scabs fall off about 7 to 10 days after they form, leaving a horseshoe-shaped area of smaller scabs around a small, wartlike protuberance that may persist for several months. In chronic cases there may be soft yellow-gray scabs that may be rubbed off during milking, leaving the skin vulnerable to chapping.

Treat the pox by removing the scabs and applying an astringent ointment to help the area heal faster. The lesions can heal without treatment, but if scabs make milking unpleasant for the cow, an ointment applied to soften the scabs may be helpful. Be sure to burn any scabs that are removed to prevent contamination of the environment.

Prevent pseudocowpox from afflicting dairy cows by isolating infected cows and milking them last, since the virus that causes the lesions is readily

A DUTIFUL MAMA

FREDOLYN SUSTAINED one of the worst teat injuries we'd ever seen in our beef herd when, in 1967, the young, first-time Angus mama went through a barbed-wire fence and cut a front teat. It was bloody and sore for many days, but in spite of the pain, she patiently let her calf nurse it. Many cows kick their calves if a teat is sore, but not Fredolyn. She was a loyal, dutiful mama. Her ripped teat healed very well without treatment, leaving just a small scar.

transmitted from one animal to another by your hands or by milking equipment. A teat dip containing some form of iodine may be helpful. Because the virus can only invade when there is a break in the skin, care should be taken to minimize or prevent trauma to the teats.

Teat Warts

Warts can appear almost anywhere on the body (see chapter 10), but when they occur on the teats, they may interfere with milking. Warts on the teats are usually small, but the action of milking disrupts them, and they may bleed or cause discomfort. These warts may be broad and rounded or long and hanging from the teat skin by a smaller stalk. Warts may be such a problem to dairy cows that they need to be removed. Consult your veterinarian.

USE SALVE SPARINGLY ON MILKERS

Be very careful when using any type of salve on a dairy cow's teats, and be sure to clean it off your hands completely or you may spread germs from the treated cow to other cows. Salve may also result in greasy milking equipment. If you are milking a cow by hand, however, or treating a beef cow with cracked teats, you can use a greasy ointment like Bag Balm or Corona on the teats after milking or nursing to help prevent or heal cracks. The residue won't hurt a suckling calf, and on a milk cow you can wipe it off before you milk her again.

PSEUDOCOWPOX

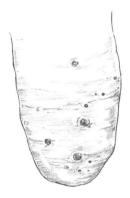

First, the teat becomes red and swollen, with small blisters or pustules appearing.

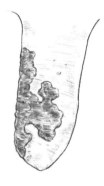

After 7 to 10 days, the small red pustular scabs that formed start falling off, leaving circular or horse-shoe-shaped lesions.

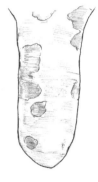

As the teats heal, the scabs slowly resolve.

PART FOUR

Other Ailments, Accidents, and Injuries

CHAPTER SIXTEEN

Mineral and Nutritional Problems

THERE ARE QUITE A FEW CATTLE AILMENTS caused by dietary problems that include deficient or excessive intake of certain minerals, vitamins, and other elements. Some of these, such as deficiencies that create metabolic problems, like milk fever and grass tetany, have been covered in previous chapters that focus on the affected body system. Other deficiencies affect reproduction and general health. For example, trace-mineral deficiencies can seriously harm cattle because certain minerals are vital for a healthy immune system.

If several animals in your herd experience health problems, poor fertility, poor response to vaccination, or lower weight gains or produce less milk than expected, your veterinarian can take blood samples or do liver biopsies on those animals or do postmortem tests on any animal that dies or is butchered, to check the mineral status of your animals. You can also have your county Extension agent help you test soils and feed samples on your farm for mineral content. Sometimes soil or forages are deficient in various important minerals.

Blood and serum samples, liver biopsies, or urine samples from live animals are generally an adequate measure of most mineral levels in the body, though disease may skew the results. Diarrhea, acidosis, stress, fever, and trauma, can all alter concentrations of certain minerals and electrolytes in body fluids and tissues. It is important to test several animals in the herd — not just a sick one or one that died — to get an accurate indication of whether your cattle have a mineral deficiency. Check the levels of about 10 animals if you're raising a small herd or 10 percent of the animals that compose a larger herd. There can be a lot of individual variation, so you need to make sure you have enough samples to get a true picture.

Mineral consumption and other measures of dietary intake should be regularly assessed when the stockman is considering the herd's health and the health of individual animals.

Selenium-Related Illness

Although many parts of the country have little selenium in the soil, a few regions have too much, creating toxicity when livestock eat certain plants that grow there. Selenium is a tricky element of diet because cattle can be unhealthy if they don't have enough and unhealthy if they ingest too much.

Selenium is vital for proper body function, but in excess it can be a deadly poison. Plants take up this trace mineral from the soil, so cattle eating pasture or hay grown in areas where selenium is adequate will not be deficient. Some plants accumulate too much selenium, however. Animals eating those plants acquire an overdose. They may suffer serious impairment or may die.

Deadly Discoveries

Long before scientists, chemists, or nutritionists knew of selenium, its effects as a poison were recognized. Marco Polo, traveling through eastern Asia in the late 1200s, referred in his journal to a "poisonous plant which, if eaten by horses, has the effect of causing hooves to drop off." Likewise, American settlers in the West discovered the deadly effects of locoweed (a selenium accumulator) when livestock were pastured in certain areas.

An army surgeon in 1857 noted loss of tails and hoofs, joint stiffness, and blindness among symptoms of selenium poisoning in horses and cattle and called it *alkali disease*. This was fitting, since selenium-accumulating plants often grow in alkaline soils. Stockmen in Wyoming and South Dakota in the late 1800s and early 1900s experienced poisoning of their livestock.

By the 1930s United States Department of Agriculture (USDA) studies identified selenium as the cause of alkali disease (or *"bob-tail disease"* as some farmers called it). Research found that poisoning could result if livestock ate feed containing more than five parts of selenium per million parts of dry matter. It was not until 1958 at Oregon State University that selenium's role as a necessary dietary element was discovered. Researchers found a connection between selenium deficiencies and *white muscle disease* in lambs, calves, and foals. The amount of selenium essential for good health and proper muscle function is so small that this important element of diet had earlier escaped notice.

Selenium, along with vitamin E, is crucial for producing an enzyme that protects muscle cells from damage during exercise and is important for muscle function. Selenium toxicity in poisonous plants is mainly a problem in certain small geographic areas. A larger problem is selenium deficiency, as a large expanse of U.S. and Canadian terrain has been found to be lacking in the element.

Finding Selenium Today

Selenium is a *metalloid* — an element intermediate in its physical and chemical properties between metals and nonmetals. It exists in the soil in several inorganic forms and in organic forms derived from

SELENIUM DISTRIBUTION ACROSS NORTH AMERICA

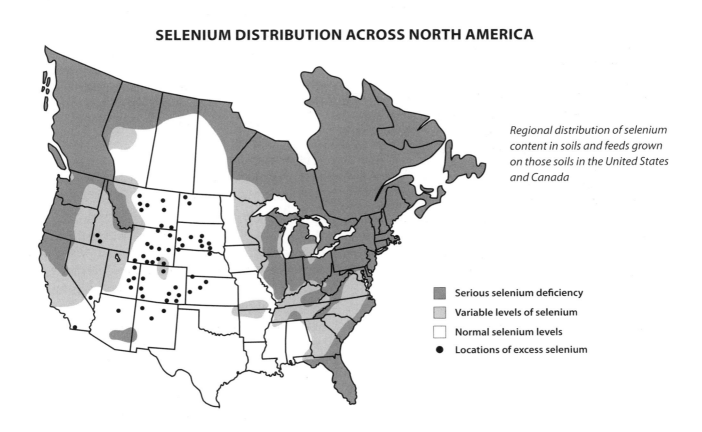

Regional distribution of selenium content in soils and feeds grown on those soils in the United States and Canada

■ Serious selenium deficiency
■ Variable levels of selenium
□ Normal selenium levels
● Locations of excess selenium

decomposed plants. There's very little selenium in soils derived from rocks of volcanic origin. Soils containing sulfur are problematic for stockmen, since sulfur can retard a plant's intake of selenium.

Natural sources for selenium in cattle diets include pasture grass, hay, and grain, if grown in soils that have adequate selenium content. Absorption by plants is greatest in regions with alkaline soils and annual rainfall of less than 20 inches (50.8 cm), such as the Great Plains and Rocky Mountain regions. In some areas where soil is highly alkaline (pH of 7 or more), selenium toxicity can occur.

Low Levels

Selenium leaches out of selenium-deficient pastures and hayfields that have been irrigated for years, making deficiency worse. Valleys with irrigation or heavy rainfall are often short on selenium, while well-drained foothills in the same region may have adequate amounts.

Selenium Accumulators

Though all plants take selenium from soil if it's there, certain plants that grow best in alkaline and seleniferous soils may contain as much as 3,000 or more parts per million of selenium. Eating these plants can produce poisoning in cattle or horses and sometimes death in just a few hours.

Common selenium accumulators are locoweed, most of the vetches, goldenweed, saltbrush, snakeweed, woody asters, and others in the aster family. If these plants grow in soils containing selenium, they accumulate it and become toxic. Some of these plants have an offensive odor and are not readily grazed, but if there's not much forage to choose from, livestock eat them. When the plants die and decay, their selenium is taken up by adjacent grass in excessive amounts. Hay and grain harvested from soils with high selenium content sometimes cause toxicity if this is the only feed an animal eats, but poisoning is more common when cattle eat selenium accumulators.

Soils in the Northwest, Southeast, Northeast, and Great Lakes states (and almost all of Canada except southern parts of Manitoba, Alberta, and Saskatchewan) are especially low because soils were derived from volcanic or coastal deposits with rainfall and leaching. Selenium deficiency is a problem in parts of 42 states, especially where soil is sandy, acid leached, or highly acidic, especially if livestock eat nothing but locally grown feeds.

Some soils are so selenium deficient that supplementation is always needed, while other areas have adequate amounts. In some regions areas with adequate levels and inadequate spots occur very close together. Small pockets with toxic concentrations exist in areas that otherwise have proper levels.

High Levels

Soils developed from cretaceous shale in Montana, Wyoming, Utah, and New Mexico often have high selenium levels. Regions that contain localized areas with too much selenium include many locations in the West and most of the Midwest and Rocky Mountain regions from the Dakotas to Texas. Feeds grown in these areas may be toxic. Common hay and pasture plants usually don't accumulate enough excess selenium to cause problems. The element is most risky when livestock eat plants that are selenium accumulators. Poisoning occurs when offending pastures are overgrazed, when animals are short on good feed and start eating unpalatable plants, or when toxic plants end up in harvested hay.

Selenium Deficiency

Small amounts of selenium are necessary for muscle growth and development and for normal functioning of the heart, liver, kidneys, pancreas, and other organs. Lack of this crucial element can lead to a wide variety of muscle diseases and weaknesses, reproductive problems, decreased fertility, increased susceptibility to disease due to a less-healthy immune system, and, in severe cases, impaired heart function. Young animals are especially at risk if their dams have inadequate selenium during pregnancy. Calves may be stillborn or die within a few days of birth or may develop muscle weakness. White muscle disease (see page 269) may occur unless the calf is given an injection of selenium at birth.

Selenium deficiency may also develop if sulfur or zinc inhibits proper utilization of selenium. These elements tie up selenium, making it unavailable to the body. Stockmen need to be careful to not overdo it when adding zinc to trace-mineral supplements.

Most plants accumulate selenium in adequate quantities for maintaining the health of grazing animals, but in some soils there just isn't enough selenium. Clover and alfalfa don't pick it up as readily as other plants. Cattle grazing legume pastures, or eating feeds grown where soil has a lot of sulfur, may develop deficiency. High crop yield, intensive irrigation (which leaches selenium out of soil), and fertilization (which stimulates plants to grow faster, with less time to accumulate minerals from the soil) contribute to selenium deficiency in some crops. The higher the yield, the smaller the concentration of selenium will be in each plant. Slower-growing plants with less yield per acre, or fewer hay cuttings per season, have time to accumulate more minerals.

Prevention

Don't buy feed grown in selenium-deficient areas. When in doubt, have feeds tested. It's always wise to know how much selenium is in the feed because there is such a narrow margin of safety. Deficiency and toxicity are separated by a fine line, so check your feeds before supplementing selenium to cattle in feed or as an injection.

White Muscle Disease

This condition is often fatal to calves born to selenium-deficient dams. Calves may be born dead or weak, dying in the first days of life.

▶ **In an acute case** a calf may suddenly become depressed, with high fever, fast respiration, and pale gums. Death may occur in 36 hours or less. In calves with respiratory distress, the problem may be mistaken for pneumonia, but they don't respond to antibiotics. Death occurs from fluid accumulation in the lungs.

▶ **In a mild case** the calf may have a stiff gait due to impairment of muscle mobility and will spend a lot of time lying down. The calf may die within a week or two unless treated. Postmortem examination shows muscle degeneration. Large

Vitamin E and Selenium

Selenium works with vitamin E to promote defense against disease. Because they're interrelated, an animal can often get by with less selenium if there's a good supply of vitamin E from green plants in her diet. Selenium and vitamin E work together to boost immunity, produce hormones, regulate carbohydrates in muscles, build and maintain bones, and protect body cells against aging and deterioration.

Both vitamin E and selenium act as antioxidants, protecting cells from damage due to natural processes that occur during metabolic function and production of energy. Tissue damage always increases during stress, trauma, or disease, weakening cell membranes. Many body cells die off daily due to damage caused by oxygen utilization in body tissues. But young, healthy cells replace these damaged cells. If more cells are destroyed than can be readily replaced, the body shows signs of damage or disease. The partnership of selenium and vitamin E works to protect cells from this kind of damage, but it functions best when both are present in the proper amounts.

areas of the normally red muscles are streaked with white, hence the name. Skeletal muscles in the legs and back and the heart muscle are often affected. The damaged muscles are largely inactive and have less *myoglobin* (the red iron-containing protein pigment of normal muscles). Calcium salts deposited in the damaged tissue add to the whiteness.

Certain internal organs are affected more than others. Scar tissue can build up in the heart, reducing its elasticity. When the calf is several weeks or months old, he may suddenly die of heart failure. Even if he survives, damage is permanent because the scarred tissue cannot be regenerated. Lack of selenium in diets of yearling and adult cattle may lead to unthriftiness, a rough hair coat, slow shedding of winter hair, lower fertility, abortion, failure to shed the placenta after calving, a compromised immune system, and, in some instances, diarrhea.

Prevention

If you know you're in a selenium-deficient area, you can prevent this problem by giving pregnant cows adequate supplementation throughout pregnancy or administering an injectable selenium product to cows. Calves can be given vitamin E and selenium injections immediately after birth. An injection gives an immediate response, but the effects are not long lasting; it may need to be repeated in 60 days. Supplementation in salt mixes or feed is more continuous, but results depend on whether the animals consume the proper amount of supplement. Selenium status can be checked with blood samples to see if your herd is deficient.

Check the labels of mineral mixes and feed supplements for selenium content. Selenium balance is tricky when cattle are fed a variety of feeds and supplements (in which the total selenium might exceed safety margins) or at the other extreme are fed only locally grown feeds that are deficient.

Unlike most minerals that have a broad range of safety, selenium has a narrow margin — only a few parts per million above the recommended levels. Read feed tags to know how much is in a commercial feed or mineral mix. Routinely adding selenium to livestock diets or supplementing with selenium in the mineral mix (or using trace-mineral salt blocks containing selenium) can add up to an overdose if you happen to live in an area that already has adequate selenium. Check your feeds (and ask your vet or county Extension agent if your area is adequate, deficient, or toxic for selenium) before using supplements.

Selenium Toxicity

Toxicity is much less common than deficiency, but the effects can be serious. Acute symptoms (as after an injection or an overdose) include diarrhea, increased heart and respiration rate, and blind staggers. When the animal ingests too much selenium in feed, similar symptoms may occur if poisoning is acute, and hooves may slough off.

Chronic poisoning comes on more slowly. Symptoms include hair loss (especially on the tail), joint stiffness and lameness, cracks or rings around the hoof just beneath the coronary band, and sometimes hoof loss. The excess selenium replaces the sulfur in proteins, causing hair loss and brittle hoofs. The animal will also have a rough hair coat and poor appetite. A cow may give birth to a deformed calf or one that shows signs of selenium poisoning.

Copper Deficiency

Copper deficiency in cattle can result in many problems. Animals suffer from a poor hair coat, reduced weight gains, impaired immune system, broken bones, or reduced reproduction rates. Often it's a subtle problem you don't suspect unless you check the copper levels in your animals. When the deficiency is corrected, they have fewer problems.

Symptoms

One of the most visible signs of copper deficiency is a change in hair color. Black animals develop a reddish or gray tint (gray is noted most around the eyes), and red animals become more bleached. The coat becomes dull instead of shiny, and cattle may be slow to shed in the spring. Copper deficiency generally has the most detrimental effect on young animals. It can result in diarrhea, poor response to vaccinations, and lameness, among other symptoms.

Without testing, it's sometimes hard to tell the difference between the signs of copper deficiency and those of internal parasites, since both can produce diarrhea, anemia, and weight loss. A positive response to copper's being added to the diet

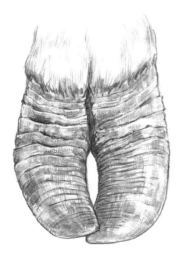

Excessive selenium in the diet can result in deformed feet (horizontal cracks that grow down from the coronary band), pain and lameness, and sometimes loss of the hoof horn.

or given as an injection or by bolus can be a sign the animals were short on this important mineral, but fecal examination for worm eggs should also be done, in case cattle are suffering from two problems at once.

One of the first signs of copper deficiency in some calves is stiffness in gait. The ends of the *cannon bones* may be enlarged and the fetlock joints painful. Pasterns may be upright, and the calf may seem to have contracted *flexor tendons,* walking on his toes. Some calves are quite lame.

When calves being weaned become severely ill, they are often found to be extremely low in copper and selenium (see page 268). Many calves that come off range pastures in the Northwest are short on copper. Some get by, but others don't.

Calves being weaned can contract pneumonia due to an unhealthy immune system, which may point to a copper deficiency. Outbreaks of pneumonia in feedlot calves are a common problem. The calves are stressed from the gathering and weaning process and from being hauled off the farm. Even if they get vaccinated immediately when they arrive at a feedlot, stressed and copper-deficient calves have a crippled immune system and may not respond very well to vaccination. This problem is avoidable, however. Try to minimize stress (see chapter 1), vaccinate ahead of weaning or shipping, make sure the calf has a healthy immune system and is not copper deficient, and he'll fare far better at the feedlot.

Copper deficiency can also impair reproduction. Heifers may be late reaching puberty. Cows may be slow to cycle after calving. Fertility in heifers may be impaired, especially when copper is tied up by molybdenum. One study showed that molybdenum in forage plants containing this element delayed puberty in beef heifers by 8 to 12 weeks. The deficiency reduced first-service conception rates in cows, lowered the rates of embryonic survival, and created a reduction in overall pregnancy rates. In situations where cows develop a severe copper deficiency due to interference by an excess of other trace elements such as molybdenum or sulfur, they may show normal estrus behavior, but ovulation does not occur. They may quit cycling. Semen quality in bulls can also be affected by copper deficiency.

Causes for Copper Shortage

A number of factors contribute to copper deficiency in cattle. A primary deficiency can happen when intake of copper is inadequate, due to a lack of copper in the soil. Secondary deficiency occurs when the dietary intake of copper is sufficient, but other factors prevent utilization of copper, which happens when there's a dietary excess of other elements that tie up copper so it can't be absorbed by the body. Elements that bind with copper include molybdenum, iron, zinc, sulfur, lead, and calcium carbonate.

Finding Copper

Many geographic regions are low in copper, while others have copper problems due to the presence of some of the binding elements. In the South and Southeast, especially in Florida, many soils are low in copper. The problem is accentuated when cattle are grazing fast-growing species of grasses that don't have time to pick up as much copper from the soil as slower-growing grasses would. Tropical grasses, for instance, may grow 8 to 10 feet (2.4 to 3 m) tall during growing season, while a western bunchgrass grows only 10 to 14 inches (25.4 to 35.6 cm), accumulating more minerals in a smaller volume of feed.

In the West, many regions have copper-deficiency problems due to the presence of molybdenum. Red clover is one plant that seems to accumulate molybdenum (and may have up to seven parts per million) and can add to the problem in certain pastures. This is most common with alkaline soils, since

Broken Bones

Molybdenum-induced copper deficiency can create weak, brittle bones in fast-growing calves. In one instance a stockman was unloading calves from a truck, where they had to jump down a few feet to the ground. Although this kind of impact would be no risk to healthy bones, several of them snapped their leg bones. The stockman had his veterinarian check the calves and perform a liver test for copper. As he suspected, the test proved that they had almost no copper in their systems.

molybdenum uptake by plants is influenced by the pH of the soil. Cattle grazing red clover pastures may show signs of copper deficiency, along with swollen feet, upright pasterns, and lameness. In the East soils are more acid. Copper-deficiency problems there are more often due to primary deficiency rather than to the presence of molybdenum.

Other soils that present a risk include peat and soils with high water tables, depending on the pH of the soil. Sulfur tends to combine with molybdenum to cause problems but can also be a problem by itself, especially in acid soils, in conjunction with lime fertilizer, or when certain regions have extra sulfur due to fossil-fuel-burning power plants.

Molybdenum is often a problem in valley bottoms or low areas; there's more molybdenum in these soils than on uplands. It is also taken up in higher concentrations in legumes than in grasses. This is why copper deficiency is more likely to occur in animals that graze the valley floor (or eat alfalfa hay) than in animals grazing high ground or range pastures where the grasses are slow growing.

Molybdenum in plants will tie up copper in a complex compound in the intestine, and this does not allow the copper to be absorbed by the body. The cattle might be getting an adequate or more than adequate amount of copper in their diet, but they can't utilize it because it is bound to the molybdenum.

Testing for Copper

If any cattle belonging to others in your region are short on copper, you should suspect your cattle might also be deficient. Even if you don't think you have a problem, it pays to check. Many people think that if they practice good management and keep cattle well fed and healthy, they won't have this problem. But copper levels in soil and forage can vary from year to year, depending on weather conditions, soil factors, and fertilization of fields.

It's difficult to figure out a copper problem just by observing your cattle because you often can't see any obvious signs like discoloration of hair coat. Your cattle may have very subtle symptoms, such as more incidence of disease due to lowered immunity. There may be an increased number of animals that develop respiratory disease or calves with diarrhea or intestinal problems. Or your calves may not grow and gain as well as you would expect. You might not even think of copper deficiency as being the cause of the other problems, but it could be the culprit.

If you suspect a copper deficiency, do some tests. Collect samples of your pasture and hay, and submit them to a lab. Your vet or county Extension agent can tell you how to collect and package them and where to send them. These tests can determine the copper and molybdenum content of feeds.

Blood tests or liver tests can show the copper status of an individual animal. Some vets hesitate to do liver biopsies because the liver bleeds profusely until the blood clots, though it doesn't hurt the animal. Other vets will perform them, feeling blood tests are not as accurate. Blood tests are not as expensive or invasive as a liver biopsy, but keep in mind that when an animal is under stress from disease or weaning, the bloodstream pulls trace minerals from the liver. This could give a false reading for copper and cause

Forage Analysis

The Cow/Calf Health and Productivity Audit of 1996 looked at forage analysis from 18 states, checking 352 samples of pasture plants. About two-thirds of 30 samples of native grass were marginal to deficient in copper. Considering the fact that some of these grasses also tend to be high in iron, which interferes with copper absorption, animals grazing these plants could have a serious copper deficiency.

Hay samples were also examined. In 109 grass-hay samples, 14 percent were deficient in copper and 50 percent were marginal. A factor that can push a marginal copper supply into the deficient category is interference by iron or molybdenum. About 10 percent of the hay samples had enough molybdenum to do that.

When evaluating a forage sample, always look at the copper-to-molybdenum ratio. When forage samples contain less than 8 to 10 parts per million of copper, they are borderline deficient. The problem is compounded when molybdenum levels are in excess of 1 to 3 parts per million or when the copper-to-molybdenum ratio falls below 3 or 4 to 1.

you to falsely believe the animal has an adequate amount. To be reasonably accurate, blood test calves during grazing season rather than when they have just been weaned and are stressed.

Another way to monitor copper levels in your herd is to take a liver sample whenever an animal dies or is butchered or from a fetus aborted in the last trimester of pregnancy. The liver can be stored in your freezer until you have a chance to send it in for testing. If the animal died from a severe infection, the liver may show low copper levels even if the copper level was normal when the animal was healthy, but in most cases an occasional sample can give good clues about your herd's copper status.

Correcting a Copper Deficiency

There are several strategies for enhancing cattle copper levels. What you do will depend on whether your problem is a primary copper deficiency (a lack of copper coming into the body) or a secondary deficiency (inadequate copper because of too much iron, molybdenum, or some other binding element). Your strategy will also depend on whether your herd is out on large pastures or close at hand where you can treat individual animals.

Supplement with a loose salt/mineral mix, injections of various copper products, oral drenching, or by giving the animals copper boluses that provide delayed release of copper. There are many ways to supplement; what you choose may depend on what's cost-effective and feasible for your situation. Work with a veterinarian or nutritionist to figure out the best way to address a herd problem and the level of supplementation. Some of the early injectable-copper products were notorious for injection-site swellings, but newer products (such as Multimin — which provides copper, selenium, zinc, and manganese) are less irritating. Trace-mineral blocks generally do not contain enough trace minerals to correct any deficiencies.

The most common way stockmen deal with copper deficiency is to put copper into a salt/mineral mix, but this is not 100 percent effective because cattle have variable salt intake. Some animals consume enough, and others won't. Some may eat too much. Cattle eat more salt when eating certain types of forage and less when eating others. It's hard to get cattle

Copper Can Be Toxic

Cattle are not as vulnerable to copper poisoning as sheep, but you need to be careful not to overdo it during long-term treatment or supplementation. A long-term supplementation program with excess copper intake can lead to chronic toxicity problems. Poisoning occurs only rarely with an injection, drench, or bolus. It's more likely to happen with long-term supplementation and more-than-adequate levels of copper in a mineral mix.

If there's too much copper going into the animal because you overestimate the amount needed, and if you are not doing occasional blood or liver sampling to assess the levels, cattle may accumulate toxic levels. Always monitor copper levels. Work with a nutritionist or vet to set up the long-term goals of your supplement program.

to eat salt when grazing forages grown on alkaline soils, for instance.

One way to ensure accurate supplementation is to use copper oxide boluses. These are tiny copper oxide needles in a gelatin capsule that you put into the rumen with a balling gun. The gelatin cover dissolves, and the needles are released, lodging in the tiny *papillae* (small protuberances) of the rumen lining. They sit there a while, then gradually pass into the abomasum, where they dissolve, making the copper available for absorption. When using these boluses, you need to know the correct dose for each individual. A bolus containing 20 to 25 grams of copper given to an adult animal at the beginning of the grazing season will usually prevent copper deficiency for about 6 months.

Getting copper into calves is sometimes a challenge. Many will eat it in a salt mix, but some of them won't. Even if their mothers are eating a mineral mix, it doesn't help the calves, since minerals are not transferred to the milk very well. Zinc levels in calves often drop dramatically after they are born, so keeping minerals in front of them is always a good idea. Use an open type of mineral feeder that calves can get into. Adult animals have learned how to use some of the covered ones that allow them to flip the rubber cover up, but calves won't do this. Before the grazing season, some stockmen give each calf an injectable product that contains copper, zinc, selenium, and manganese — all the trace minerals that are often short in cattle diets.

If you vaccinate calves (for instance, at weaning) before they've had a chance to have a deficiency corrected, their immune systems may not be able to respond to vaccine; they may get the diseases you are trying to prevent. Stockmen who bring the calves in at weaning time and immediately put them on a ration that is highly supplemented with copper may have better luck, but there's a bit of lag time before they "catch up." If you vaccinate them at the same time, they may still get sick.

Even if calves have adequate levels of copper and selenium, the stress they go through at weaning may still cause problems. If they are short of these important elements, they are doubly at risk when stressed. This is often the cause of big "wrecks" at weaning time. Even if they don't get obviously sick, many won't gain as well as they should. They may simply be "poor doers" affected by subclinical silent pneumonia (see chapter 11), which takes a toll on weight gains. Copper deficiency can be obvious, but more often it's a sneaky villain, so it pays to know the copper status of your cattle.

Iodine Deficiency

Iodine is another trace mineral that is very important yet is toxic if consumed in large amounts. Most of the iodine in the body is in the thyroid gland, where it regulates metabolism and the rate at which the body converts simple compounds (from food) into energy and building blocks for body cells, then breaks down and eliminates waste materials. Iodine-containing hormones influence metabolism, the birth process, and the ability of newborn calves to withstand cold stress.

Iodine deficiency results in an enlarged thyroid gland (goiter), seen as a lump on the underside of the neck. Iodine-deficient cows may be infertile or give birth to hairless, weak, or stillborn calves. Bulls may have lower fertility. Many areas of the United

AREAS WITH IODINE DEFICITS

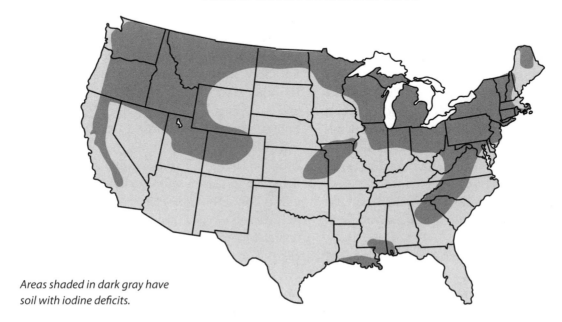

Areas shaded in dark gray have soil with iodine deficits.

States are deficient in iodine, so this important trace mineral is often added to protein supplements, salt mixes, and salt blocks.

Calcium Deficiency

Calcium is vital for bone strength and proper body function. If cattle have adequate forage in their diet, they usually are not short on calcium. Natural forage, such as pasture plants, generally contains enough of the two major minerals needed by the body, calcium and phosphorus. Grasses and most forage plants usually contain the proper ratios of calcium and phosphorus necessary for efficient and normal utilization. Legumes such as alfalfa are high in calcium and can be used to balance grain and other feeds that have low levels of calcium.

Sometimes problems create a shortage of calcium in the body. Metabolic deficiency, when a cow suddenly needs more calcium (due to heavy lactation) than feed can provide, may result in milk fever (see chapter 14). In other instances calcium deficiency may be due to long-term calcium shortage in feed, which is uncommon unless cattle are fed artificial diets containing a lot of grain and little forage. Grain is high in phosphorus, which may interfere with the body's absorption of calcium.

Symptoms of calcium deficiency include weakness, swollen joints and lameness, and broken bones. Calcium deficiency can be remedied or prevented by giving cattle access to good pasture or providing feeds (such as alfalfa hay) that are higher in calcium.

Phosphorus Deficiency

Phosphorus is important to growth and body tissues. About 80 percent of the phosphorus in the body is in the bones and teeth. Green grass and most other forage plants usually contain adequate phosphorus for the normal growth and body maintenance of cattle. Mature, dry grasses or weather-damaged hay may be short on phosphorus, however. As plants mature or become severely drought stressed and dry, their phosphorus level drops and may not be adequate for optimum growth and production. This problem is more common in geographic areas where soil is short on this important mineral or where excessive

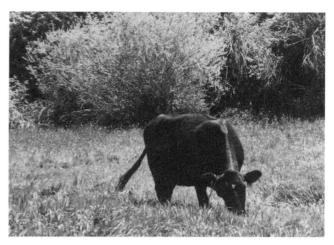

Green grass and most other green forage plants usually contain adequate amounts of both calcium and phosphorus for cattle.

amounts of other minerals bind to the phosphorus and make it less available.

Adult cattle can often get by on the lower level of phosphorus in mature forage, but young growing animals, lactating cows, or cows in late pregnancy may suffer problems. Some nutritionists say phosphorus deficiency is the most prevalent mineral deficiency in grazing cattle worldwide. By contrast, cattle that eat grain are rarely short on phosphorus because most grains contain adequate levels.

Phosphorus is crucial for growth, reproduction, and lactation. If animals are deficient, they are slow growing, have poor appetites, and weak, fragile bones. Phosphorus-deficient cows are less fertile and produce less milk. Long-term deficiency results in impaired immune function, bone abnormalities, and depraved appetite (eating strange things).

Prevention

If your forage is short on phosphorus (particularly in fall and winter pastures), it pays to supplement with this mineral. It's a good idea to check the level of phosphorus in pastures, or talk to your county Extension agent to find out if your region is low. Deficiencies can then be avoided by providing a mineral supplement while cattle are on fall/winter pasture or feeding hay that has an adequate phosphorus level. Alfalfa hay is generally higher in both calcium and phosphorus than is grass hay.

If phosphorus deficiency is a problem in your region, farm, or herd, work with your vet, your county Extension agent, or a cattle nutritionist to test your forage and plan a good feeding or supplement program to ensure that your cattle won't be short on this important mineral during fall and winter when pasture levels are low.

Vitamin A Deficiency

Although natural diets usually contain adequate amounts of most vitamins, a vitamin A shortage sometimes occurs if cattle don't have access to green forage plants or if feed is no longer green during a drought or in winter. *Carotene,* the source of vitamin A, is found in all green plants; grazing animals store vitamin A in the liver. Unless cattle haven't had access to green plants or properly cured hay for a while, they won't suffer from a shortage of vitamin A. Deficiencies are most likely to occur if animals are confined and fed artificial diets such as dried beet pulp, grain, and poor-quality hay.

Signs of deficiency include night blindness, hoof defects, poor bone growth, unhealthy skin, infertility, weight loss, and nervous-system problems. Calves born to vitamin A–deficient dams may be blind, due to constriction of the optic nerve.

The need for vitamin A increases during late pregnancy and lactation, but this can be met by adding alfalfa hay to the diet, since it has higher levels of vitamin A than most grass hay. Vitamin A can also be supplemented in feed or by injection. An overdose of vitamin A can be harmful, however, and will cause reduced growth rate, lameness, and incoordination.

Thiamine Deficiency

The most dramatic problem due to thiamine (vitamin B_1) deficiency is a nervous-system disease called polioencephalomalacia — "polio," which literally means softening of the gray matter of the brain. This problem is also called *cerebrocortical necrosis.* It is sometimes caused by eating plants, such as *horsetail (equisetum)* and several other ferns that tie up vitamin B_1 in the body. It is more often caused, however, by changes in feed that allow a specific type of rumen bacteria to multiply quickly and produce large amounts of an enzyme called *thiaminase.* Even though there may be adequate thiamine in the body or in the feed, this enzyme destroys the vitamin before the animal can utilize it. This results in blood levels that are too low, which adversely affect the brain; the ability of brain cells to control water movement in and out of the cells is impaired, and the brain tissue swells and dies.

A sudden drop in thiamine due to a feed change may occur when cattle are moved abruptly from marginal- or poor-quality pasture to lush grass or when feedlot animals are being changed to a high-concentrate ration. The problem may also occur when there are high levels of sulfur in feed or water. Sulfur can bind up thiamine.

Symptoms

Usually the first sign of thiamine deficiency is "stargazing"; the affected animals seem to be looking at the sky. Then they become blind and bump into obstacles. Soon they become disoriented and uncoordinated, staggering to try to maintain their balance, and eventually go down and can't get up. Spasms, with extreme arching of the back, stiffening of legs, and forward extension of head and neck, soon follow, and then the animal goes into convulsions. Death often occurs within a few hours after the beginning of symptoms, due to the brain damage. Symptoms may be misinterpreted as TEME (see chapter 4) or *lead poisoning* (see chapter 17).

Treatment

Even though there's no lack of thiamine in the diet, polio can be successfully treated with adequate injections of thiamine, if given before the animal goes into spasms and seizures. Injections should be given twice a day the first day and once a day thereafter unless signs are still severe. Most animals treated in early stages improve dramatically within 24 hours, and permanent brain damage is prevented.

Thiamine treatment, which can be given by IV, intramuscularly, or subcutaneously, should be continued for 3 days, even if the animal is improving. Some may take up to a week of treatment for full recovery, and some won't recover if the brain is too damaged. Some recover but remain blind. If treatment wasn't started until 8 hours or later after signs appeared, there is less chance for recovery, due to brain necrosis (tissue death) and scarring.

Prevention is achieved by avoiding pastures or hay containing toxic ferns or getting rid of those ferns and by careful feeding. Don't make feed changes suddenly. Introduce cattle to new pastures gradually, and make ration changes (to high-concentrate diets) over at least a two-week period. Some stockmen feel that supplementing a grain-based diet with thiamine or brewer's yeast (which contains vitamin B$_1$) is helpful, especially if the ration is high in concentrate without very much fiber.

Importance of Salt

One of the most important additions to cattle diets is salt, since forage contains very little *sodium chloride.* Salt blocks or loose salt should always be provided for cattle; they'll consume it as needed to balance their salt requirements. If cattle go without salt for long periods, they eat less feed, drink less water, and do poorly. If they crave salt, they often lick and chew strange things, including rocks, treated fence posts, and other objects or chemicals that may be harmful, in their attempts to eat something salty.

Salt toxicity can occur if animals have been deprived of salt for a long time and then load up

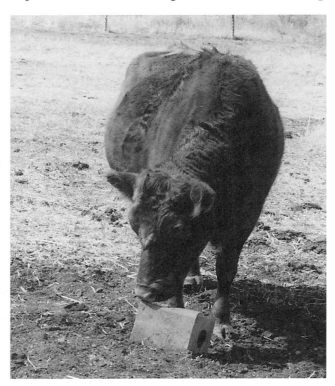

Salt should always be provided for cattle.

on it. Unless they have easy access to water and can drink enough to dilute the excessive amount of salt they consume, they may die.

Salt is also provided because mineral supplements are generally added to salt so cattle will eat the minerals. Cattle won't always eat salt, however, especially when grazing pastures on alkali soils or when moved to new pasture. If the reluctance to eat salt is not temporary, any minerals needed in these regions of alkaline soil must be provided in some other form, such as a palatable feed supplement.

Urinary Stones

Urinary stones *(calculi)* are composed of clumped-together mineral salts and tissue cells that form in the kidney or bladder or both. These stones may cause irritation and chronic inflammation that lead to bladder infection, but a more serious situation occurs if one or more stones pass out of the bladder and become lodged in the urethra (the tube between the bladder and the external opening). These stones may partially or completely block the flow of urine, and the bladder stays full.

Often called *"waterbelly,"* this condition affects steers and bulls more frequently than cows or heifers. Females have a larger urinary passage; it rarely becomes blocked. If even one animal in the herd suffers from this problem, it may mean the herd diet is out of balance and other animals are harboring bladder stones as well. Waterbelly occurs most frequently in steers between 5 and 18 months of age, usually feedlot animals, but sometimes those at pasture.

Eating feeds that contain unbalanced quantities of certain minerals cause this life-threatening problem. Minerals from feed are absorbed from the intestine into the bloodstream, where they find their way to various body parts to assist in certain functions. Iron helps create healthy red blood cells to carry oxygen, for instance. Calcium and phosphorus help build bones. Any minerals not needed by the body are filtered out by the kidneys and excreted in the urine.

If the concentration of certain minerals in the urine reaches a saturation point, however, the solution starts to crystallize. This happens more readily if the animal is short on water and the urine becomes concentrated (like saltwater evaporating, leaving salt crystals). If animals are drinking plenty of water, the urine is more dilute, and minerals rarely precipitate out of solution. If urine stays concentrated, however, mineral crystals in the bladder increase and eventually clump together to form stones.

Stones that stay in the bladder rarely cause problems and may be there for the rest of the animal's life without symptoms. Stones may readily pass out when a cow or heifer urinates. Females have short, direct, large-diameter passages from the bladder to the outside opening. But a male's urethra is much longer, makes a sharp bend, and narrows where it passes through the penis. A stone may become caught in this narrow passage and block it. Steers are most commonly affected because they have the smallest-diameter urethra, especially if castrated at a young age, since the urethra then does not enlarge very much as the animal grows. A bull's urethra is a little larger but not nearly as large as that of a female.

Animals that don't drink enough water or individuals that consume an excessive amount of minerals (especially phosphates) are more likely to develop stones because urine is more concentrated. Some people think hard water containing a high mineral level can lead to stones, but hard water generally contains calcium and magnesium, which actually help protect cattle against the formation of phosphate stones.

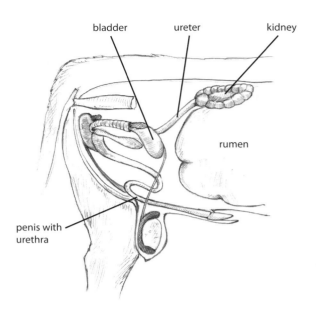

Blockage from a urinary stone is more common in males than in females because the male urethra is longer and narrower.

Two Kinds of Stones

Phosphate stones are common when steers are fed grain. The high levels of carbohydrate cause an increase of mucoproteins in urine, and grain is high in phosphorus. In urine that is slightly alkaline, these two factors result in phosphate stones, which are relatively soft. Stones made up of silicate are more common when animals are at pasture. Some plants contain high levels of silica, as do some water sources. Silicate stones, which are very hard, form when urine is slightly acidic.

Symptoms

If a stone blocks the urethra, the bladder enlarges. Urine is continually formed by the kidneys and routed to the bladder, which can no longer empty through the blocked urethra. The distended bladder puts pressure on other organs in the abdomen, causing discomfort and eventually extreme pain. The affected animal will lick or kick at his belly, stamp or tread with his hind feet, and incessantly switch his tail. Attempts to urinate may be accompanied by straining. If the stone does not completely obstruct the urethra, the steer may dribble a little bloodstained urine but is still in a lot of pain. He tries repeatedly to urinate and may grind his teeth while trying.

Pressure builds up in the distended bladder, and it eventually ruptures. This gives instant relief to the animal — the pressure is gone. He quits kicking and stops showing signs of distress, but the relief is temporary and is the start of a more serious problem. The urine from the ruptured bladder now flows into the abdominal cavity or fills the tissues around the penis. Swelling may extend under the belly skin toward the chest. In a few hours, toxins and other waste materials that were filtered out of the body via the kidneys and into the urine are absorbed back into the bloodstream and slowly poison the animal. He usually becomes dull, stops eating, and may go into shock or become weak. Death usually occurs within 48 hours after the rupture.

Treatment

At the first sign of waterbelly you can butcher the animal or have your vet try treatment or perform surgery. If you detect the problem early, often the best solution is salvage by slaughter. If this is not feasible, consult your vet for treatment or surgery. Urinary-tract relaxants may help keep the urethra as open as possible, to allow passage of stones. Giving the steer ammonium chloride may help make the urine more acid, to dissolve any phosphate stones. Surgery is probably the most effective treatment, if performed soon after the problem is discovered, but it may not save the animal if the condition has been going on for several days and the animal's health is compromised. If the bladder has already burst, there is generally no hope for recovery.

The surgical procedure is merely a temporary solution to keep the steer alive, enabling him to recover and to grow large enough to be butchered. The vet will make an incision below the rectum so the penis can be dissected out through the underlying tissues and pulled out backward through the opening. The urethra in the penis is then opened up to allow urine to drain out. This hole in the urethra is kept open by stitching it to the skin. Because the new opening is above the blockage, it creates a new exit for urine coming from the bladder.

The steer will then urinate through this hole just below the anus, similar to the route of urination in a heifer. If the surgical site heals properly and the hole stays open, the steer can continue to function, though urine will usually run down the back of his hindquarters. This emergency procedure can buy time, however, to get him over the problems caused by the stone, including tissue residues of medication and urine, and perhaps enough time to finish growing him to better butcher weight.

Prevention

For feedlot cattle a ration balanced for calcium and phosphorus (two parts calcium to one part phosphorus) will help reduce the risk for stone formation. Feeding alfalfa, which has a high level of calcium and low phosphorus, is beneficial. Adding salt and a little ammonium chloride to the feed may also help. The diet should always be well balanced, with adequate vitamin A, and plenty of clean, warm water should be supplied during cold weather so the animals will drink enough.

Pasture cattle should always have salt and plenty of water. Pastures that contain plants that are high in *silicates* and *oxalates* may be risky for steers and should only be used by cows and calves unless you can supplement with alfalfa or other legumes to reduce the intake of siliceous plants.

Water Requirements of Cattle

Water deficiency and quality are often overlooked when ranchers are trying to determine the cause of disease or illness. In reality, water is the most important "nutrient" because no animal can live very long without it. Animals can survive for many days without feed but only a few days without water. They need more water in hot weather than in cool weather, because water is lost through sweating and saliva production as the body tries to stay cool (see chapter 16). A lactating cow will need more water than a nonlactating one.

Water requirements for a nonlactating beef animal in moderate temperatures, for instance, will be about ¾ to 1½ gallons (2.8 to 5.7 L) per 100 pounds (45.4 kg) of body weight (about 6 to 15 gallons [22.7 to 56.8 L] per day for a 1,000-pound [453.6 kg] animal). Cows nursing calves may drink 18 percent of their body weight (about 24 gallons [90.8 L] per day for a 1,000-pound cow). In hot weather these amounts increase. The type of feed being eaten and the amount of salt intake are relative to how much the animal drinks. She'll drink less water when grazing lush green pasture with a high water content than when eating dry food. Similarly, the more salt she eats, the more she'll drink to balance and flush out excess salt.

In cold weather make sure water supplies are not frozen and that water is warm enough for the animals to drink an adequate amount. In hot weather or drought, water quality is often just as important as water quantity. If ponds start to dry up, the water may become more stagnant and contaminated with animal urine or feces. Pond water may also collect run-off, which contain pollutants. In some instances water may be contaminated by chemicals or nitrates and may need to be tested to see if it's healthy for livestock. Your vet or county Extension agent can advise you about how to collect and send a water sample to a diagnostic laboratory.

If water is in short supply or so unpalatable animals won't drink it, they soon become dehydrated and will also stop eating. Conscientious disease prevention includes making sure cattle always have adequate amounts of clean water.

CHAPTER SEVENTEEN

Poisoning

Poisons exist in and around every farmhouse, barn, ranch, and feedlot. They are created by humans and by nature alike. Some are plants that can be eaten by or given to an animal in small doses but can be deadly when ingested in large amounts. Others are manmade products, such as herbicides or fertilizers, that make life easier for us but can make the four-legged inhabitants of the ranch very ill if ingested or inhaled.

Poisonings can occur unwittingly, as when toxic plants end up in harvested grains and forage or curious cattle stick their noses in the wrong barrel. Certain plants cause death, illness, abortion, metabolic disorders, and other problems. It's important for anyone with cattle to be aware of the potential dangers housed in sheds and growing in the back pasture. If you understand how and when a plant or chemical is dangerous, you may be able to avoid most accidental poisoning and to treat an animal that is suffering from a toxic condition.

Poisonous Plants

Many plants are classified as poisonous, but their toxicity can vary, depending on the conditions in which they grow and other factors. Some of these plants make good feed in small amounts or in certain seasons or conditions but are poisonous in others. Toxic effects may include illness, nervous system distur-bances, damage to the fetus, sensitivity to sunlight (photosensitivity), and sometimes death.

Some plants contain substances that are directly poisonous (such as the *alkaloids* in lupine and larkspur), while others contain elements that are harmless until they become chemically changed by freezing or enzyme activity, such as the glycosides in chokecherry leaves, which can become deadly *cyanide*. Some plants absorb elements from the soil and accumulate them to toxic levels, such as selenium in locoweed and other milkvetches.

Plant poisoning of livestock depends on the palatability of the plant, its stage of development, and the growing conditions, among other factors. For example, some species of saltbush are good forage, except when grown in soils high in selenium. Moisture content can make a difference, too, as can the portion of the plant consumed. Some plants have more poison in the roots, seeds, or some other part. Plant poisoning can be suspected if sudden onset of illness or death occurs after cattle are moved to new pasture or fed different hay.

Because many poisonous plants cause death quickly, treatment may be impossible. The animal is often dead by the time you discover her. Find out what plants are growing in your fields and pastures or along the fences. Different regions have different problems; some dangerous plants may not grow in your area, and some plants may not pose a threat except under specific circumstances. Learn how to avoid situations that may lead to poisoning.

Types and quantities of poisonous plants consumed by cattle vary greatly, depending on cattle management and pasture conditions. Overgrazed pastures and ranges may have more poisonings, since cattle are forced to eat less-palatable (possibly poisonous) plants. Moving hungry cattle into pastures with high densities of poisonous plants can cause losses; cattle graze less selectively when hungry.

Turning cattle into pastures where the grasses are not mature enough to be grazed may result in poisoning because some offending plants — lupine, low larkspur, death camus, oak — are early sprouters and in their most palatable and succulent stages ahead of the grasses. Examine pastures for poisonous plants and grass readiness before moving cattle into them.

A late spring storm or early fall snow may cover shorter, more desirable plants and grasses, leaving taller ones (such as lupine or tall larkspur) more available to livestock. Storms may bring down branches or whole trees that may be nibbled by hungry cattle. Heavy rain may increase cattle losses because some plants become more toxic after a rain. Also, the ground may be softened, and toxic roots and bulbs are pulled up. In stormy weather cattle seek shelter in woods or brush and eat plants that grow in shaded soils, rather than going out to graze.

In drought areas many of the more palatable plants mature faster and dry up, while some of the poisonous ones stay green and are thus more readily eaten. In these situations cattle should be moved to safer pastures or given supplemental feed to make sure they won't consume lethal quantities.

There are hundreds of plants that can be poisonous to cattle. Some grow only in specific regions; others are widespread. Some plant varieties are always a danger, and others are only dangerous in certain conditions.

Regional Differences

Death camus and hemlock, for example, grow in many areas of Colorado, but unlike in other regions of the United States and Canada, cases of poisoning by those plants are few. Under some conditions halogeton and

> ## Alkaloids
>
> Alkaloids are organic compounds found in many plants. Many alkaloids are toxic, but some are more toxic than others. They are usually bitter in taste. Some of the common alkaloids we're familiar with are caffeine, morphine, nicotine, quinine, and strychnine. Many alkaloids can have strong, toxic effects on the body.

arrowgrass cause poisonings, but most losses in Colorado cattle are due to larkspur and locoweed.

In Nebraska the most common poisonings are a result of cattle ingesting poison hemlock, brackenfern, cocklebur (in late spring in the two-leaf growth stage or if seeds end up in harvested grain), horsetail, and Johnsongrass if grazed after a frost.

In Missouri oak and buckeye cause most of the problems. Other common poisonings in that state are a result of consumption of chokecherry (especially in spring if a late frost wilts the young leaves), cocklebur, hemlock, and pigweed. Buckeye causes poisoning in this region because it's one of the first trees to bud and is often the first green thing in the spring, making it attractive to cattle.

Poisoning in Texas is often due to milkweed, locoweed, Texas buckeye, redroot pigweed, jimsonweed, low larkspur, yellow sweetclover, and African rue (an exotic plant that spread onto rangelands in Arizona and Texas).

In the Dakotas some of the most common offenders are sweetclover, cocklebur, chokecherry, larkspur, and ponderosa pine.

In Montana and Idaho most losses are due to larkspur. Other states and climate areas have a different set of plants and problems.

There is not space for a complete list of plants that are toxic to cattle. Plants covered in this chapter are some of the common offenders and may not be the worst plants in your region. To find out which plants to look for on your farm, talk to your vet or county agent. Your vet can also advise you or help you treat an animal if poisonings occur.

Poisonous Plants

The following list may help you identify the plants on your pasture or rangeland that are poisonous to cattle and to recognize symptoms of illness so that you may treat the animal as soon as possible.

LOW LARKSPUR

Characteristics: Although various types grow to different heights, low larkspur typically grows 3 to 24 inches (7.6 to 61 cm) high. It has deep blue to purple flowers, and grows in dry to moderately moist soils on plains, foothills, and mountain pastures. It grows in grassy or sagebrush pastures on western rangeland and blooms in early spring.

Animals at risk: More deadly to sheep but causes poisoning in cattle under certain conditions

Conditions for poisoning: Most poisonous when young and growing fast in spring. Once it's bloomed, there's less risk. This plant is not as deadly as tall larkspur.

How poison impairs animal: The plants contain toxic alkaloids that affect the nervous system and muscles.

Symptoms: Weakness; trembling; constipation

Treatment: None

Prevention: Keeping cattle off heavily infested pastures until after these plants have flowered can prevent losses. On private pastures stockman have the option of spraying and getting rid of these plants.

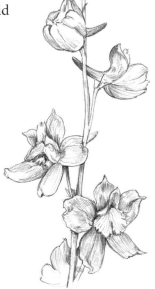

This variety of low larkspur grows 3 to 8 inches (7.6 to 20.3 cm) tall and has dark blue flowers.

TALL LARKSPUR (WILD DELPHINIUM)

Characteristics: These plants grow 3 to 7 feet (0.9 to 2.1 m) tall, with a deep, woody root. The flowers are blue and look like the delphinium that's grown in yards and gardens. It grows in thick stands in moist and shaded areas and along streams, springs, or aspen groves. It matures and blooms later than low larkspur (and the blooms are not as dark blue).

Animals at risk: All cattle

Conditions for poisoning: Poisoning is most common in summer. Most risky the first 2 weeks after cattle are moved into a new pasture containing larkspur and in late summer if weather is dry and the surrounding grass has dried out and is no longer green and palatable. If larkspur is the greenest plant, they may overeat. Larkspur growing along streams or around springs may stay green longer than upland grasses.

How poison impairs animal: The plant contains numerous toxic alkaloids and kills cattle by paralyzing the muscles. The toxic alkaloids interfere with proper functioning of the central nervous system and muscles. Death is usually a result of heart failure and respiratory distress, which may be a combination of suffocation from bloat and paralysis of the diaphragm muscles that facilitate breathing. The inability to burp up and swallow the cud may result in bloat or in spillage of rumen contents into the windpipe and lungs.

Symptoms: Beginning with mouth, ears, and tail and progressing to the diaphragm, the animal's muscles become increasingly fatigued, making it hard for the animal to breathe. Signs of poisoning develop within a few hours after the plants are eaten; the toxins cause muscle tremors and collapse. The digestive tract becomes paralyzed. Feed can't move through, and the animal can't burp, so she bloats. Any exertion worsens the effects due to muscle fatigue. Most of the affected animals die, unless the amount eaten was very small.

Treatment: No dependable or effective treatment. Poisoned cattle that are still alive should not be moved. Poisoning happens so fast you usually don't see the animal sick; you just find her dead.

Prevention: Rid your pasture of the plants by spraying, fencing off patches, not using pastures with large areas of larkspur during times when plants are most deadly, or pulling up or chopping down the plants.

Gather the chopped or pulled plants and haul them off or leave them to dry if it will be a few days before the cattle graze there. They won't eat the drying plants if there's green grass available.

Pasture Notes: The poison content of larkspur is high during early growth in the spring and then drops rapidly after the plant is mature, except in the seedpods, which still contain high levels of alkaloids. Poisoning of cattle is less likely after flowers are gone, unless a lot of plants are eaten during a short period of time.

▸ **Often cattle prefer the leaves and flowers** and may not eat much larkspur during the bud stage in spring and early summer when it is most toxic, unless other forage is sparse. They begin eating tall larkspur during its flower stage, and consumption usually peaks during the late flower stage or when pods are forming. The larkspur's toxicity is declining at that point, but cattle consumption is increasing. This results in a "toxic window" in which most cattle poisoning occurs, and cattle may be found dead. Depending on weather conditions, this toxic period may be 4 to 5 weeks long during a typical grazing season.

Tall larkspur contains up to 20 different kinds of alkaloids that vary in toxicity from very poisonous to relatively harmless. Alkaloid levels can vary greatly from one patch to another or from year to year in the same patch. These differences are part of the reason for variations in annual cattle losses. Some years it may take more pounds of larkspur to be fatal to the grazing animal.

For instance, a 1,000-pound (453.6 kg) cow would be fatally poisoned after quickly eating 3 pounds (1.4 kg) of green larkspur if the plants contain 1 percent of the most toxic alkaloid, according to studies done at the USDA Poison

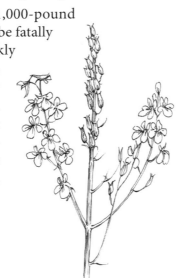

Tall larkspur (wild delphinium) grows 3 to 7 feet (.9 to 2.1 m) tall and has lighter blue flowers than low larkspur.

Plant Research Laboratory in Logan, Utah. By contrast, if the plants contain only 0.2 percent of the most toxic alkaloid, that same cow must eat more than 14 pounds (6.4 kg) of fresh larkspur within a couple of hours to be fatally poisoned. If a cow eats smaller amounts during a grazing day, she won't be adversely affected.

▸ **Cattle losses during wet years** tend to increase, perhaps due to changes in the chemistry of the plants and also their enticing luxuriant growth. In late summer, larkspur may make up as much as 25 to 30 percent of a cow's diet, especially if she spends a lot of time in the moist areas. At this stage of the plant's maturity, this amount may not be fatal, especially if cattle are eating other plants along with it and spreading their larkspur consumption throughout the entire day.

During, or just after a wet storm, larkspur consumption increases. Cattle eat much more in a short time and are more at risk. This may be because during a storm they congregate for shelter in the bottoms and brushy areas where larkspur grows, instead of spreading out to graze. Also, wet larkspur is more palatable than dry.

Annual death losses are between 4 and 5 percent of cattle grazed each summer on many Forest Service allotments, with some unfortunate ranchers experiencing more than a 15 percent loss of their herds in certain years.

▸ **Mineral supplementation** of cattle has been attempted by some stockmen to try to reduce consumption of larkspur. Effects of supplements were studied for 4 years in Utah, but the researchers found there was no level of mineral supplementation that changed the amount of larkspur eaten. In some situations it works well to graze sheep ahead of cattle since tall larkspur is not as toxic to sheep. If the sheep can be kept in the patches by herding (to eat and trample larkspur) before cattle are put in, cattle losses can be reduced.

Monitor cattle use if you have pastures with larkspur. Even if you don't actually see cattle eating the plants, take note of any evidence of plants being eaten and move cattle out of that area when they start grazing the patches. If you must use those pastures during the time of year larkspur is most deadly, your safest bet is to get rid of the larkspur.

▶ **Herbicides** are not particularly effective unless you use the proper products at the best time of year for killing the plants. You must kill the entire taproot and underground buds or the plant will come up again next year. Total eradication is sometimes impossible, but you can reduce the density of the patch and significantly lower the amount that cows will eat. But it is not safe to put cattle into a pasture where tall larkspur has been treated with herbicides, until the plants dry out and are less attractive to cattle. Although not toxic to cattle, herbicides may increase palatability, and treated plants don't lose their toxicity, so don't graze a treated pasture until the sprayed larkspur has completely dried out.

Some people worry that herbicides might kill other plants when it gets into a water source. Weed scientists at Utah State University have monitored residual herbicide levels in surface-water runoff from treated plots after larkspur was sprayed. They found that runoff contained negligible levels of herbicide; most of the residue remained in the top inch or 2 (2.5 to 5 cm) of soil, where it binds to soil particles and does not enter the groundwater.

The value of cattle saved by controlling dense patches of larkspur far outweighs the cost and labor of controlling these plants, even when using the most expensive herbicides. Your county Extension agent can advise you on which herbicides to use, when to use them, and how to use them safely. If applied properly, herbicides can greatly reduce the number of plants, and grasses

will come in to replace them. Even if a patch is not completely eradicated, if there are only a few plants left, a cow can't eat enough larkspur fast enough to kill her.

POISON HEMLOCK

Characteristics: Poison hemlock, *Conium maculatum,* is a biennial in the parsnip (wild carrot) family and is not to be confused with water hemlock. Poison hemlock grows 2 to 10 feet (0.6 to 3 m) tall, with hollow, purple-spotted stems and a solid taproot. The leaves are finely divided, like those of a carrot, and smell like parsnip when bruised. This plant is often found along roadsides, edges of fields, creeks, or ditches.

Animals at risk: Humans and livestock

Conditions for poisoning: Poisoning is most common in spring when tender, highly toxic leaves appear. It takes 10 to 16 ounces (295.7 to 473.2 mL) to poison an adult cow. All parts of the plant are dangerous, but the root is most toxic.

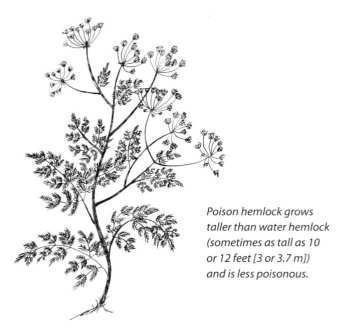

Poison hemlock grows taller than water hemlock (sometimes as tall as 10 or 12 feet [3 or 3.7 m]) and is less poisonous.

How poison impairs animal: Death is usually due to respiratory failure if the animal consumes a fatal amount.

Symptoms: Drooling, abdominal pain, and incoordination. If a nonlethal dose is eaten, pregnant animals between 30 and 70 days of gestation may later give birth to calves with skeletal defects or a *cleft palate* (similar to the defects caused by lupine).

Treatment: None

Prevention: These plants can be eradicated by digging them out, tilling the ground and replanting with a good pasture crop to crowd them out, or using herbicide before the flower buds appear.

Pasture notes: Cattle generally won't eat poison hemlock unless there's a shortage of other feed, since the leaves have a bad taste.

WATER HEMLOCK

Characteristics: Water hemlock, *Cicuta douglasii*, is a perennial in the carrot family and is even more deadly than poison hemlock. It is a wetland plant, usually grows 2 to 3 feet (0.6 to 0.9 m) tall (but can sometimes grow to double that height), often appears in small patches, and has small, white flowers that grow in umbrella-like clusters. It has thick, fleshy individual roots that grow from the bottom of the rootstalk.

Animals at risk: Any animal or human that ingests it

Conditions for poisoning: The rootstalk has many small chambers that contain a highly poisonous brown- or straw-colored liquid that is released when the stem is broken or split. Everything the liquid touches becomes a potential source of poisoning. The entire plant contains a highly poisonous alcohol with a strong, carrotlike odor. Leaves and stems tend to lose some of their toxicity as they mature, but the underground parts of the plant are always extremely poisonous.

How poison impairs animal: It only takes one bite to kill a cow. Cattle may eat the roots if they are brought to the surface by plowing or cleaning of ditches. Most affected animals die of respiratory failure. This may occur within a few minutes but more commonly happens within a few hours.

Symptoms: Muscle twitching, rapid respiration and pulse, tremors, violent convulsions, dilated pupils, slobbering, teeth grinding, bloat and coma. Signs occur one to six hours after consumption, and cattle may die 1 or 2 hours following the onset of symptoms. Occasionally a pregnant cow may eat a very small nonlethal dose that affects her fetus. She may abort or give birth to a deformed calf. The toxin tends to anesthetize the fetus, and it does not move around in the uterus as it normally would, resulting in joints that do not develop or bend properly. The cow may give birth to a "crooked" calf, similar to those with lupine deformities.

Treatment: None

Prevention: Be careful when trying to eradicate water hemlock. Herbicide increases palatability; livestock should be kept away from sprayed plants for 2 weeks. If you dig out the plants, you must get all the roots or they will regrow.

Pasture notes: Take care to not get any of the liquid from damaged plants on your hands. The thick-chambered

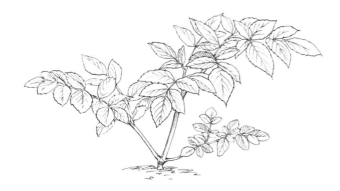

Water hemlock grows 2 to 6 feet (0.9 to 1.8 m) tall, with large divided leaves. It is often found in wet meadow or swampy areas and is very poisonous, especially the roots, which smell like parsnips.

rootstalk and bundle of fleshy roots are highly toxic even when dry, so the plants should be gathered and burned. But do not breathe the smoke; it is also toxic.

LOCOWEED

Characteristics: Locoweed is a legume (in the pea family), with pealike leaves, blossoms, and seedpods. Common in the western half of the United States, locoweed is also called crazyweed, milkvetch, or poisonvetch. It grows on arid and semiarid ranges, and there are more than 50 kinds.

Animals at risk: All cattle

Conditions for poisoning: Some types are unpalatable and are eaten only in dry years when feed is short or when grass starts late during a cold spring. Others are quite palatable, such as timber milkvetch, and can vary in toxicity, ranging from beneficial high-protein forage plants to extremely poisonous. Some types of locoweed are addictive. Once an animal starts eating it, she seeks it out and may become poisoned even if there are not a lot of locoweed plants in the pasture.

How poison impairs animal: This poison can be cumulative, building up to dangerous levels over a few days or weeks, or death may occur within a few hours of eating the plants. In fatal cases death results from heart failure or respiratory paralysis.

Symptoms: Signs of poisoning include dull, dry hair; abortion in pregnant animals or occasional birth of deformed calves; nervousness; weakness; emaciation if poisoning has been long term; depraved appetite; staring eyes; poor vision; incoordination; gait irregularity; loss of sense of direction; and difficult breathing.

Treatment: None

Prevention: Keep cattle out of pastures that contain a lot of locoweed until the grass is well grown, and remove them before the grass gets short. In pastures where locoweed is a serious problem, applying herbicide to the actively growing plants before they reach bud stages can control it.

Pasture notes: Most kinds grow on selenium-rich soils and accumulate selenium in their tissues.

LUPINE

Characteristics: Lupines are a legume, part of the pea family, and most are perennials, growing 6 inches (15.2 cm) to 3 feet (0.9 m) tall. There are several types that grow on mountain slopes, valleys or plains, grasslands, sagebrush, or forestland.

Animals at risk: More deadly to sheep than to cattle, but if pregnant cows eat toxic varieties between 40 and 70 days of pregnancy, alkaloids may affect the fetus, resulting in malformed calves.

Conditions for poisoning: Cool wet springs when growth of lupine is abundant or grazing lupine pastures during early pregnancy when the fetus might be affected.

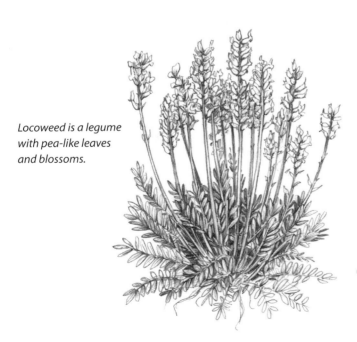

Locoweed is a legume with pea-like leaves and blossoms.

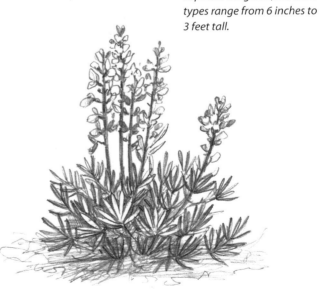

Lupine is a legume; different types range from 6 inches to 3 feet tall.

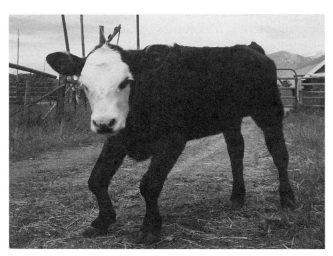

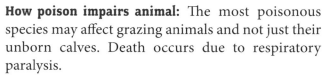

The look of a "crooked calf," caused by the dam's eating lupine during early pregnancy.

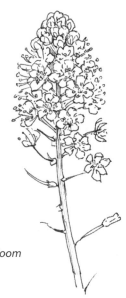

Death camus, showing the bloom and the stalk.

How poison impairs animal: The most poisonous species may affect grazing animals and not just their unborn calves. Death occurs due to respiratory paralysis.

Symptoms: Rough, dry hair coat; nervousness; depression; reluctance to move; difficult breathing; twitching leg muscles; slobbering and frothing at the mouth; convulsions and loss of muscle control; and coma. Poisoned fetuses may be born with crooked legs, twisted spine, cleft palate, or other skeletal abnormalities.

Treatment: None

Prevention: Avoid pastures containing lupine during early spring when grass may not yet be very tall, especially with cows that may be in the first trimester of pregnancy. Large patches of lupine can be controlled by use of herbicide applied before bud stage.

DEATH CAMUS

Characteristics: This perennial belongs to the lily family and has yellowish white or cream-colored flowers that grow in clusters on top of a stalk that rises taller than the leaves. The bulb is deep in the soil. The more toxic species are seldom found above 8,000 feet (2,438.4 m); they are most common in lower foothills in western pastures. The plant usually flowers in April and May, but at higher elevations the blooms may not appear until June or July.

Animals at risk: Sheep are more commonly poisoned, but it can also be fatal for cattle.

Conditions for poisoning: Cattle rarely eat death camus because it's not very palatable, but since it's one of the earliest plants to appear in spring, it may be eaten if other forage is short.

How poison impairs animal: If cattle eat death camus, toxins affect the nervous system. Death occurs within a few hours or days.

Symptoms: Rapid breathing, excessive salivation (foamy froth around the muzzle), digestive upset, weakness and staggering, then convulsions and coma.

Treatment: None

Prevention: Pasture containing a lot of death camus should not be grazed in early spring before grass is abundant. These plants can be controlled if necessary, by spraying in early spring.

BRACKENFERN

Characteristics: This large perennial herb is part of the fern family and grows in burned-over areas, woods, and shady places. It also grows on dry, sandy, or gravelly soil.

Animals at risk: Horses, sheep, and cattle

Conditions for poisoning: Cattle may eat it when other feed is short or when it is mixed in hay because plants encroach a hayfield. The leaves are poisonous whether they are green or dried. Cattle may be poisoned in late summer when other feed is scarce or when fed hay containing this fern. Cattle that have access to recently plowed fields of bracken readily eat

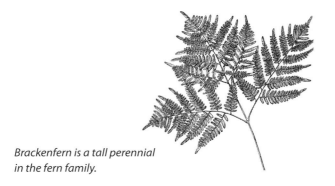

Brackenfern is a tall perennial in the fern family.

the exposed underground stems, which are 5 times more toxic than the mature leaf fronds.

How poison impairs animal: Poisoning is cumulative, and symptoms appear after cattle have eaten bracken for 2 to 4 weeks. Acute poisoning and death may occur if cattle eat a large number of immature fronds or underground stems.

Symptoms: Sudden onset of loss of appetite, high fever, difficult breathing, drooling, nasal and rectal bleeding, blood in the urine, and hemorrhage of mucous membranes. The animal is very dull. Once symptoms appear, death soon follows.

Treatment: Antibiotics and blood transfusions. This treatment is not likely to be successful in advanced cases.

Prevention: Avoid grazing woods or burned-over areas where there are large patches of ferns, and eradicate the plants where they are a problem, such as along the edges of a hayfield.

HALOGETON

Characteristics: This annual looks like Russian thistle or tumbleweed and thrives on salty soils in semiarid regions. It belongs to the goosefoot family and has a characteristic small hair on the end of each leaf. It grows along roads and trails and wherever the soil has been disturbed; dense stands are often found in burned areas, dry lakebeds, and abandoned fields.

Animals at risk: Most deadly to sheep, but cattle may also be poisoned.

Conditions for poisoning: Halogeton becomes more toxic as it grows, reaching peak toxicity at maturity. Cattle don't generally eat it if there's better feed available but may be poisoned in fall or early winter if they are hungry or after being driven where it grows along the edges of roads and trails — since they grab bites of it as they travel.

How poison impairs animal: The plant contains toxic oxalate that impairs muscle, kidney, bladder, and rumen function if eaten in large quantities.

Symptoms: If a lethal dose is eaten (less than 1 percent of the animal's body weight, or 1 to 1.2 pounds (0.45 to 0.54 kg) for a mature cow) the animal becomes dull and weak, reluctant to move. Advanced signs include drooling with white or reddish froth from the mouth and rapid, shallow breathing; then the animal collapses with a violent struggle for air, goes into a coma, and dies.

Treatment: IV or subQ administration of a solution containing calcium salts.

Prevention: Don't herd hungry animals along trails or roadways where these plants grow. Eradicate patches that have invaded disturbed soil or overgrazed areas. Make sure animals always have plenty of good, palatable feed.

PERILLA MINT

Characteristics: Sometimes called mint weed, purple mint weed, or beefsteak plant, this weed has square stems and grows 2 to 4 feet (0.6 to 1.2 m) tall, with heart-shaped leaves that have a hint of purple on the underside. The plant has a distinctive odor and grows in shady areas but may also be found in barnyards and corrals or along fences.

Animals at risk: Hungry animals that may be short on feed.

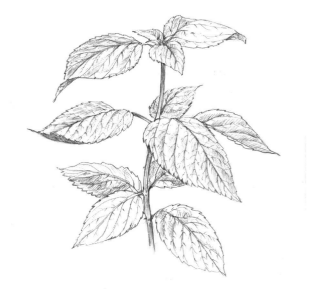

Perilla mint can cause lung damage in cattle if they graze it as it reaches seed stage.

Conditions for poisoning: Cattle may not readily eat this plant, but it is most toxic in late summer when seeding. It is toxic only after the plants have flowered. It loses toxicity following a frost that wilts it.

How poison impairs animal: Cattle eating it in late summer may suffer emphysema when plant toxins are absorbed from the digestive tract and reach the lungs via the bloodstream, where they damage the lungs. Cases show up 3 to 12 days after cattle begin eating the plants.

Symptoms: Difficult breathing may occur within 24 hours.

Treatment: None

Prevention: Eradicate the plants.

Poisonous Trees and Shrubs

Cattle are browsers as well as grazers. They like to sample a few tree leaves and nibble on shrubs while grazing, but this can get them into trouble if certain trees or bushes contain toxic substances. A number of exotic trees and shrubs are poisonous to cattle, but the most common native is wild cherry (chokecherry), which can cause *hydrocyanic acid* poisoning. The cherry laurel, often planted in yards and gardens, is also a potent source of hydrocyanic acid, as is the crab apple, but their level of toxicity varies widely between seasons and different parts of the plant.

CHOKECHERRY

Characteristics: The chokecherry grows wild in most of the United States and Canada and is found in pastures, along fencerows, and near streams or wet areas in arid regions. The chokecherry may be a tall shrub in dry areas or a full tree in places where it has plenty of water. It is easily recognized by its leaves and bark, which show its kinship with the cherry family, and by its fruit. It has clusters of tiny white blossoms and produces many small cherries that hang together in clusters, turning dark red or nearly black when ripe, depending on the variety. The pit or stone is similar to that of the pie cherry. Some people pick wild chokecherries to make jam, jelly, or syrup, but the raw fruit has a bitter, puckering taste.

Animals at risk: Sheep and cattle

Conditions for poisoning: There is always risk for poisoning if cattle eat the leaves after a frost. It's not unusual for cattle to eat leaves off the trees or off the

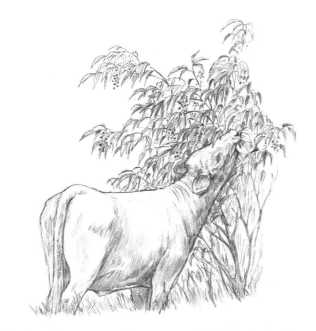

Cattle are browsers as well as grazers and often eat leaves from trees and shrubs such as chokecherry.

ground. The latter can be especially dangerous. Even though cattle may get by for many years browsing on chokecherry leaves, some years they may not be lucky if leaves are chemically changed by frost.

Poisoning is caused by toxic quantities of cyanides in certain conditions. The plant contains *cyanogenetic glycosides.* Glycosides are by-products of plant metabolism that produce sugar and other chemicals when mixed with water. Cyanogenetic glycosides are nontoxic, but hydrocyanic acid may be liberated from this organic complex by action of an enzyme (which may be present in the same plant) or by activity of rumen microbes when eaten by cattle.

The chokecherry's glycosides can produce *cyanide* in certain situations. Glycoside concentration in these plants is variable, depending on climate and other conditions affecting growth. The fruit is not poisonous, but the leaves can be toxic to cattle. Poisoning is most likely to occur when cyanide content is high, such as after a frost. If leaves wilt or freeze, the enzyme system that normally prevents release of cyanide breaks down.

How poison impairs animal: Cyanide is a fast-acting poison. In spy movies, secret agents use cyanide capsules for instant death if they get caught. Because chokecherry poisoning often occurs in a fatal dose (it takes less than 3 pounds [1.4 kg] of leaves to kill a cow), the sick animal is rarely discovered soon enough for treatment.

The poison is absorbed from the gut and circulates through the body via the bloodstream, where it is picked up by body cells. In the cells the cyanide interferes with an enzyme that is crucial to cell metabolism. This causes oxygen starvation within the cell. Every cell in the body is suffocated, and the body tissues cannot continue to function normally. Oxygen exchange no longer takes place; the oxygen is retained within the blood and can't get to the cells. The blood in early stages of chokecherry poisoning is very bright red. After a time it turns very dark, since the animal soon has trouble breathing and oxygen intake diminishes.

Symptoms: Hydrocyanic acid poisoning is almost always acute, and affected animals rarely survive more than 1 or 2 hours. Some may be affected within 10 to 15 minutes of eating the leaves. The poisoned animal is in extreme distress, becoming anxious and agitated due to the inability to get oxygen to the body. Breathing becomes difficult. The animal becomes weak from the oxygen deficiency, staggers, and falls down. There may be convulsions and muscle tremors before the animal lapses into a terminal coma. Cattle that consume large amounts of the leaves may die within minutes.

In less acute cases (if only a small amount of leaves was eaten or if they did not contain a high level of glycoside), the animal is depressed and staggering, with muscle tremors and difficult breathing. The eyes may water, and skin may become supersensitive. Muscle tremors start at the head and neck and spread to the rest of the body. Pulse is shallow, weak, and rapid. Pupils may dilate. If the animal is discovered soon enough and hasn't eaten much toxic material (and does not die before the vet arrives), you have a chance to save her.

Treatment: The animal is given a combination of sodium nitrite and sodium thiosulfate intravenously, to counteract the poison. Treatment may have to be repeated because of further liberation of hydrocyanic acid within the animal's body not neutralized by the first treatment. The sodium nitrite produces *methemoglobin,* which combines with the hydrocyanic acid to produce a compound that is not toxic. The acid is then released gradually from this compound and taken up by the sodium thiosulfate (the other ingredient in the IV solution) to form thiocyanate, which is also nontoxic and which is readily excreted from the body.

Prevention: In late fall move cattle out of pastures that contain chokecherry trees or shrubs or get rid of the chokecherry trees and shrubs.

Pasture notes: Cattle may live with chokecherries for a long time without being poisoned; we've only had one fatal case in 42 years. Since chokecherry poisoning is so acute and deadly, however, it is better to prevent it than to try to treat it.

PONDEROSA (YELLOW) PINE

Characteristics: Yellow pine grows below 4500 feet elevation in regions where there is usually more than 20 inches of annual precipitation.

Animals at risk: Pregnant cows and heifers

Conditions for poisoning: Access to ponderosa pine trees, fallen needles, or downed limbs or trees. Cattle often browse these trees or needles if snow covers the grass.

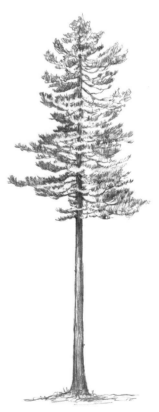

Ponderosa pine (also called yellow pine) has long needles in clusters of three.

How poison impairs animal: Ponderosa causes abortion if cattle eat the bark, tips, needles, and buds. In many cases the cow dies from a secondary infection and complications unless she is given immediate treatment and supportive care. Some cows suffer liver damage from this type of poisoning.

Symptoms: Abortion usually occurs about 2 weeks after the cow begins eating needles. She may seem normal until she aborts and then may have very weak uterine contractions and incomplete dilation of the cervix, uterine hemorrhage, and retained placenta. It's often a difficult birth and the cow needs assistance from you.

Treatment: Antibiotics to combat infection; hormone treatment to aid in shedding the placenta; fluid therapy

Prevention: Limit access to ponderosa pine trees, especially in winter or when cows are in the second half of gestation.

OAK

Characteristics: There are many types of oak trees and shrubs, but all can be toxic to cattle. Oak poisoning is common in cattle in the Southwest. Many varieties in North American regions can be browsed and cause no illness if they make up only a small part of the diet. Toxicity is highest in leaves and sprouts that contain a poisonous *tannic acid*. The acorns can also be toxic.

Animals at risk: All cattle

Conditions for poisoning: Oak poisoning occurs in spring (when cattle eat the leaves) and sometimes fall if acorns are eaten. Most cattle like the taste of acorns and seek them out, eating them off the tree or as windfalls after a storm.

How poison impairs animal: Oak contains tannic acid and phenols that cause kidney damage, abdominal pain, and constipation.

Symptoms: Often within a week after cattle start sampling the leaves or acorns of oak trees, they suffer from rumen shutdown and constipation and stop eating. Signs include abdominal pain, thirst, and frequent urination. Small amounts of hard, brownish-black pellets of manure are passed; then the bowel movements change to diarrhea if the animal survives longer.

If cattle consume too many acorns, they go off feed; develop diarrhea; may pass blood in the manure; become dehydrated, then constipated and emaciated; and sometimes die. Symptoms occur 8 to 14 days after they start eating acorns or leaves. After 3 to 7 days of clinical signs, the affected animals may go down and can't get up.

Treatment: Treatment is of little value.

Prevention: Supplemental protein may minimize instances of poisoning if cattle must graze pastures containing oak trees and acorns. Only allow oak-laden pastures to be grazed during late fall or winter after acorns have aged, turned brown, and become less toxic.

YEW

Characteristics: This ornamental evergreen (Japanese yew, English yew, *ground hemlock*) is a shrub or small tree often used in hedges or landscaping around houses and yards and along fence lines, driveways, and show barns. English yew (*Taxus baccata*) may grow up to 80 feet (24.4 m) high. Japanese yew (*Taxus cuspidata*) is a low-growing shrub. There are many varieties that have been developed for landscaping and are simply called yew or ground hemlock. The leaves of all varieties are about 1 inch (2.5 cm) long, stiff and needlelike (somewhat broad and flattened), and glossy. They are dark green on the upper side and yellow-green underneath. Seeds are produced in a small, cuplike, bright red cone. The waxy cones each contain a single seed. The wood is reddish, fine, and strong — an elastic wood used in earlier times for archer's bows.

Animals at risk: All animals, including humans

Conditions for poisoning: Deaths occur when animals have access to trees or discarded trimmings. Usually they're not planted in pastures, but cattle or horses may reach through or over a fence or have access to shrubs in a yard or barnyard. Neighbors trimming shrubs may not realize the danger and leave clippings next to your pasture fence. The plant is highly toxic whether green or dried; trimmed branches may remain deadly for a long time. Even needles from ornamental shrubs, raked up in lawn clippings and fed to animals, can cause death.

Yew is not very palatable, but animals may sample it even if they are not underfed. Often the younger, more curious ones sample it first, and this may attract some of their buddies to try it. Cattle are notorious for copying one another. The ones that ingest the most are usually the first to show symptoms and die.

How poison impairs animal: All parts of the yew plant contain a highly poisonous alkaloid called *taxine,* which has a strong depressive effect on the heart. It only takes 12 to 16 ounces (354.9 to 473.2 mL) to kill a cow and 4 ounces (118.3 mL) to kill a horse. Sudden death is due to heart failure. Often you don't see the animal ill; you just find her dead. A cow or calf may nibble on the shrub or branch trimmings and die suddenly, often with pieces of the branch still in his mouth. Yew can cause sudden death to any animal that nibbles a few bites.

Symptoms: If animals linger long enough to show symptoms, they exhibit shortness of breath, muscle tremors, difficult breathing, weakness and collapse, convulsions, and then death. A few animals have been known to survive but only because they did not get a fatal dose, simply a taste of the plant.

The animal will usually be down on the ground, cold and dull, with fast heartbeat and labored breathing and may seem blind. The pupils of the eyes may react to light, but the animal does not seem to respond or be able to see.

Treatment: There is no reliable treatment or *antidote* for this poisoning, though *atropine* has been tried, and if the animal is found in time, this may help counteract the heart-depressing effect of the poison. If the animal is still alive when found, efforts can be made to help keep the body functioning. Treatments that have been tried include large doses of mineral

oil to soothe and lubricate the irritated gut and help move toxins on through. IV administration of fluid and electrolytes may help combat shock and prevent circulatory failure. Steroids and anti-inflammatory drugs may help reduce tissue swelling in the lungs and brain and combat shock.

If the animal survives the first day or two, there is a chance for recovery. But most victims of yew poisoning don't live long enough to give you a chance to call your veterinarian. Most animals die within 4 hours of ingestion (or much sooner) and usually within minutes of the first abnormal signs. Some will appear normal and then just drop dead.

Prevention: Find out what kind of evergreens are on or near your place, especially next to your pastures or corrals. A book on poisonous plants, your county Extension agent, or someone from a plant nursery can help you identify a shrub or plant.

Miscellaneous Plants

Other common plants that can affect cattle include arrowgrass, which is readily eaten by salt-hungry cattle. It's not a true grass but grows in marshy pastures and hay meadows. Toxicity varies at different times of the year. Meadow hay containing arrowgrass may have enough cyanide in it to kill livestock, but if stored for several months, the hay gradually loses its toxicity.

Forage plants that sometimes cause problems include **birdsfoot trefoil** (a legume that is usually good cattle forage), **sudangrass, johnsongrass,** and **reed canarygrass.** All of these can cause problems if they've been stunted by lack of moisture or wilted by frost, since they all contain the same toxin as chokecherry (see above page 290).

Cocklebur can be poisonous if eaten in early spring at its two-leaf stage. **Pigweed, jimsonweed, yellow star thistle, tansy ragwort, buckeye** (horsechestnut), **greasewood,** and **prince's plume** are some of the many plants that can cause problems for cattle. Some types of **nightshade** contain a poisonous alkaloid, with unripe berries being most poisonous. **False hellebore** (called wild corn, cow cabbage, or veratrum) has large, broad leaves and is a member of the lily family. It contains alkaloids that affect the heart and cause general weakness, slobbering, irregular gait, and paralysis. Cattle may die after

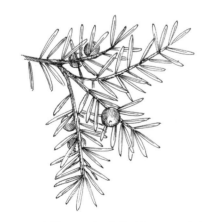

Yew is an ornamental tree or shrub that is very toxic to livestock.

eating the young shoots and roots. **Rocky mountain iris** is poisonous (native Americans used juice from iris tubers to poison their arrow tips) but rarely eaten because of bad flavor.

Greasewood, a rangeland shrub, can often be safely eaten in moderate amounts but may kill cattle if they eat too much in a short time. **Hemp dogbane** is a poisonous herb that grows 2 to 5 feet (0.6 to 1.5 m) tall and causes occasional livestock losses. **Sneezeweed** causes chronic vomiting; the poison is cumulative, and animals may die if they consume small amounts over a long period of time.

If you suspect plant poisoning, call your vet immediately; you may be able to save the animal with prompt treatment. Also consult your county Extension agent to try to identify the plant. Prevent further poisonings by eliminating that plant from your pastures, restricting cattle access to areas where the plant grows, or changing grazing management to minimize its effects.

Molds, Fungi, and Bacteria

Excessive moisture is the main reason for mold growth on plants. Some molds are harmless, while others produce dangerous toxins *(mycotoxins).* There are about 100 different fungi that grow on crops or stored feed and produce toxins. The presence or absence of visible mold (or its color) does not necessarily mean the plant or harvested feed will be toxic. Whether or not mold causes problems may also depend on moisture and temperature.

Most mycotoxin poisonings are associated with stored grains and other concentrated rations such as corn, silage, and cottonseed, but a few occur in hay and straw. Physical damage to the corn or grain, coupled with moisture, can readily lead to invasion by mold. The main effects of *aflatoxins* in grain are related to liver damage.

Some forage molds (in hay, silage, straw) may cause pregnant cows to abort. Moldy straw baled while damp or rained on after baling and eaten by pregnant cows has been implicated in births of weak and deformed calves. Calves may have congenital *spinal stenosis* (pressure on the spinal cord from narrowing of the vertebral column) with hind-leg paralysis. Some calves have shortened legs, laxity in the joints, and deformed front legs. Cows eating moldy straw may lose weight and hair and in some instances may die.

If cattle are grazing sweet potato crop aftermath (the plant parts left on the field after harvest), mold-damaged plants may cause emphysema and difficult breathing (see chapter 11). Any crop ruined by excessive moisture tends to harbor molds, some of which are toxic to grazing animals.

Some types of pasture forage, including clover and Bermuda grass, may cause photosensitization (see chapter 10) if they develop molds that contain liver-damaging toxins. Extended wet periods that lead to mold growth, followed by hot sunny days, may leave the plants toxic to livestock, and plants may retain their toxicity even after being cut as hay.

Moldy Sweetclover Hay

Sweetclover, a forage legume, is not a problem to cattle while green and growing but can become toxic when damaged or spoiled in hay or silage. When the plant molds, a toxin is produced that interferes with blood clotting. Eating large amounts of moldy sweetclover may cause swellings on the body, and the animal walks with a stiff gait. Poisoning generally occurs after the animal has been eating toxic silage or hay for at least 2 weeks. Pulse becomes fast and weak, and death is due to internal bleeding. Animals suffering from mild sweetclover poisoning may bleed to death from small wounds, dehorning, or castrating.

Fescue

Tall fescue *(Festuca arundinacea),* a nutritious cool-season perennial grass, is the most widely grown forage grass in the United States, covering more than 35 million acres (14,163,997.5 hectares). Although the plant itself is not poisonous, 90 percent of the fescue crops in the United States are infected with an endophyte fungus that can create health problems for animals that graze it.

Fescue Toxicosis

Fescue toxicosis is the term for all problems associated with ingestion of this fungus. Toxic effects include severe heat stress in hot weather (see chapter 3), reduced weight gains *(summer slump),* lower milk production and fertility, and a rough hair coat. Heifers and young bulls that consume infected fescue are slow to reach puberty. Fescue toxicosis inhibits the development of ovaries in heifers, delays release of hormones important to the start of puberty, and hinders development of testicles and the secretion of testosterone in young bulls. Problems related to fescue consumption in cold weather include impaired circulation and loss of feet, ears, or tails.

You rarely see signs of fescue toxicity when cattle are comfortable, but if the weather is too hot or too cold, they have problems due to decreased blood circulation.

▶ **In hot weather** afflicted cattle can't get rid of body heat because blood flow is part of the body's cooling mechanism and they are suffering from

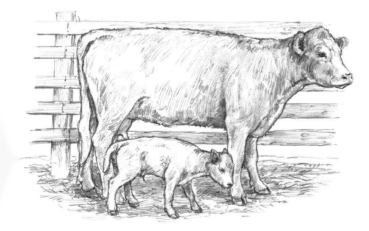

After eating moldy straw, cows may lose large patches of hair, and their calves, if not aborted, may be dwarfed.

decreased blood circulation to the skin. Normally, the circulatory system brings overheated blood from the body's core and internal organs to the body surface, where heat is dissipated into the environment if air temperature is lower than body temperature. If there's a breeze to help with sweat evaporation, this has a cooling effect as well. Cattle don't have as many sweat glands as horses do, though they still sweat enough to help cool themselves in hot weather. But if blood circulation to the skin is impaired, this cooling mechanism doesn't work; body temperature rises, respiration rate increases, and the animal salivates and drools excessively trying to cool herself by slinging saliva over her body.

Some people confuse fescue toxicosis with fever, but it is not the same. When an animal has a fever, there's an increase in metabolism caused by the body's trying to fight an infection or some other condition. Cattle with fescue toxicosis are not creating extra heat; they just can't get rid of it. They spend a lot of time in the shade or standing in water, trying to stay cool.

▶ **In cold weather** there is increased risk for frostbite. Blood flow to extremities is reduced in cold weather in a normal animal (concentrating the heat internally and attempting to minimize heat loss), but with fescue toxicosis, it is reduced even more. Nutrients such as oxygen and glucose don't get to the extremities, so the tissue dies. Normally you might expect an animal to lose ear tips or a tail tip at 30 below zero F (−34.4°C), especially if there's wind, but when cattle graze fungus-infected fescue or eat fescue hay in winter, this can happen at milder temperatures. Because of the impaired skin circulation, affected animals suffer necrosis (death) of tissues in the extremities, and if that tissue death is extensive and becomes gangrenous, the animal may lose ears, tail, or feet. The first sign may be lameness ("fescue foot"— see chapter 12). When an animal is suffering from frostbite, and it looks like she will lose a foot or feet, the stockman often must sell or butcher her.

▶ **The offending fungus,** *Acremonium coenophialum,* contains the toxin *ergovaline,* one of a number of toxins classified as ergot alkaloids that infect grasses and grain plants. This particular fungus has a symbiotic relationship with the fescue plant, making it hardier and more resistant to insects and drought. Because it grows within the cells of the plant, the fungus cannot be seen, and can only be detected by laboratory analysis. It is most concentrated in the seed head and thus most abundant on mature plants. Animals grazing fescue in early spring before the plants are mature are not as adversely affected.

It is the relationship between the fescue and the fungus that harms cattle, not the fungus alone. When plant and fungus interact, the result is release of these toxins, which are part of what makes the plant so hardy, long lasting, and resistant to parasites, heat

Fescue's Origins

Fescue is a European grass brought to this country in the 1800s. It was not used extensively until a scientist at the University of Kentucky tried planting it in various locations. It proved to be very hardy and productive, easy to establish, and able to withstand heavy grazing and trampling.

Fescue became commercially available in 1943 and was known as Kentucky 13. At that time there were very few high-producing forage grasses that did well in the central United States, so it became very popular — and also invaded many surrounding areas because of its aggressive and hardy nature. But stockmen soon noticed problems in broodmares and cattle. The cause of these problems eluded researchers until 1976, when USDA scientists discovered that the fescue plants were infected with an endophyte fungus. The term endophyte simply means a plant that lives within another plant — in this case a fungus.

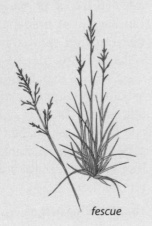

fescue

and drought, overgrazing, poor soils, and worms and insects, among other things. The alkaloid in the fungus makes infected grasses more resistant to these pests. In a stand of fungus-free fescue and a stand of infected fescue side by side, the infected fescue is almost always more lush and green and doing much better.

Fungus-free fescue is not as hardy and is more difficult to establish and maintain, especially in hot southern regions. Many insects prefer feeding on this variety of fescue and are able to develop more rapidly on the less-toxic plants. *Nematodes* (rootworms that can destroy the grass) are also more prolific on fungus-free plants. In northern climates some farmers are replacing infected stands with fungus-free varieties, but farther south this is not always an option. Even if you get a stand of fungus-free fescue planted, it may not last; infected fescue may move into the pasture from surrounding areas. The fungus-free fescue is less likely to survive and also costs more to maintain. It's often easier to try to live with the fungus and find ways to minimize the problems of fescue toxicosis.

Only seed can spread the fungus, so it can't be transmitted from one plant to another; if a stand of uninfected fescue is established, it will remain uninfected. There is fungus-free fescue seed available, but even if you establish a stand of uninfected grass, it is less hardy and may be taken over by more aggressive infected plants that come up from seed (if there were infected plants in that pasture before) or encroach from neighboring pastures. If hay is fed on the new pasture, make sure it doesn't contain infected fescue that might have seeds.

Reducing Toxic Effects and Poisoning Risk
To minimize livestock problems, keep the plants from going to seed. Fescue fields should be continually grazed and kept short or any tall patches clipped or harvested for hay before seed heads form. If cattle eat the seed heads, they get a much larger dose of the toxin. If plants get too tall before you put cattle in a pasture, mow the pasture first. If some pastures on your place are higher risk than others (pure stands of fescue without other forage plants to dilute them), it may be safest to take cattle out during summer. Fescue pastures are often safest to graze from about mid-February to mid-April in a warm climate.

The greatest negative effects for cattle occur from June through September — the hottest months of summer. Some stockmen switch to fall calving, breeding the cows in November and December after the weather cools off, since cows often have poor conception rates on fescue during hot weather. For spring calving, cows should calve early enough to breed before mid-June, when conception rates drop as temperatures increase. Some stockmen reduce breeding problems by using rotational grazing to keep fescue very short and fast growing and clip the pastures if seed heads start to form.

Legume dilution is another way to reduce fescue-related health problems. A pasture containing clover or alfalfa is less toxic and improves cattle's rate of gain. Having 20 to 30 percent legumes in the grass mix can increase weaning weights and reproductive efficiency. Extension beef specialists at the University of Georgia advise that cattle can only be expected to gain 1 pound (0.45 kg) per day on infected fescue. This can be increased to l.5 to 2 pounds (0.68 to 0.91 kg) per day if there are legumes in the pasture mix. Adding clover can significantly reduce problems.

Mixed pasture requires more management, however. The taller the grass gets, the less likely the legume will do well. Grasses must be kept short — ideally, no more than 4 inches (10.2 cm) tall — so they won't inhibit legumes. If a pasture needs to be fertilized, use lime, phosphorus, and potassium to encourage legume growth rather than grass growth. Do not add nitrogen to fescue; this may substantially increase toxicity and also boosts the grass. Some producers are able to get clover back into their pastures just by halting nitrogen fertilization.

▸ **A protein supplement** for cattle on fescue pastures may help minimize toxicity, since this has the same benefit as legumes in the diet. Adding an ionophore such as Rumensin to the protein supplement also increases feed efficiency while reducing the toxic effects of the fungus. Another type of supplement (called Tasco, marketed by Acadian Agritech in Nova Scotia) is made from sun-dried Atlantic brown seaweed and used by some stockmen ever since researchers at Texas Tech and Virginia Tech discovered that it reduced the detrimental effects in cattle grazing endophyte-infected fescue. Why and how it does this is still a mystery, but something in the seaweed increases heat tolerance and improves reproductive performance in these cattle.

There are many research efforts aimed at resolving fescue problems. Some researchers are trying to formulate a vaccine against the toxin. Some are looking at products that might be fed to cattle or administered in bolus form (to stay in the animal and be released over a 4-month period during summer) to help reduce the fungus's effects. Other researchers are trying to find cattle with genetic traits that make them more resistant. Some animals seem to be more sensitive to the toxins. On some farms stockmen don't have as many problems as they did in the past, simply because they got rid of the animals that were most sensitive to the fungus.

Studies looking at genetics of the fungus are trying to remove the toxic element without hindering plant hardiness. There is now a fescue variety (developed by plant scientists at the University of Arkansas) that's infected with a less-toxic fungus, but only time will tell whether this grass will be as hardy.

Heat Tolerance Breeds Fescue Tolerance, Too

Brahman cattle (and any other heat-tolerant breed, such as Senepol) do better than British or European breeds on fungus-infected fescue. Studies have shown that Brahman do much better than Angus, for instance, in the same pastures. This is simply because Brahman are not as stressed at the same temperature, being more adapted to hot weather. You don't see the problem of fescue toxicosis at a comfortable temperature, and if Brahman cattle are comfortable at that heat, they won't be affected.

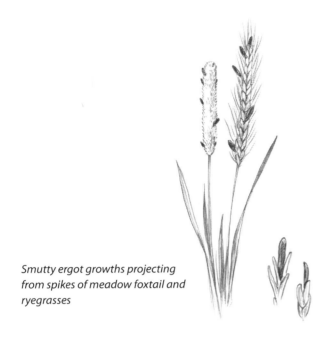

Smutty ergot growths projecting from spikes of meadow foxtail and ryegrasses

Ergot

Claviceps purpura is a fungus, commonly called ergot, that can grow on grasses and grain plants when moisture conditions are conducive. Ergot problems are rare in dry seasons. The fungus replaces the seed head with a dark brown or black mass and produces toxic alkaloids that elicit one of two kinds of responses; The animal has either a convulsive or a circulatory response. The convulsive form produces vertigo, loss of balance, muscle spasms of the hind legs, and sometimes a temporary paralysis. The circulatory form hinders blood circulation to the extremities, causing lameness and *gangrene*. Cattle may lose their ears, tail, or feet. Ergot poisoning also causes a drop in milk production, reproductive problems, and abortion.

Ergot is most common in grains but can also infect wheatgrass, brome, wild rye, bluegrass, quack grass, and a number of other wild grasses. An ergot fungus that grows on rye produces a condition called *ryegrass staggers* in cattle; this is common in countries that grow a lot of rye. There's also a type of ergot fungus that infects barley and creates another class of toxins. Often the symptoms are similar to fescue toxicosis (see above page 295), with a rise in body temperature, reduced milk and growth, and reduced circulation to the extremities.

Botulism

Botulism is an occasional risk when hay contains dead animals or when silage is improperly fermented, allowing growth of certain bacteria (see chapter 4).

Weeds in Harvested Hay

Some poisonous plants are more of a problem in hay than when they are growing in a pasture because cattle are more apt to eat them in hay. When allowed to select their food while grazing, they may not choose to eat a poisonous plant, but when it's mixed with hay, they may not sort it out. Some plants lose their odor or bad taste when cut and dried, and cattle may be less fussy about eating them.

Weeds in hay that cause nitrate toxicity in certain conditions include kochia, pigweed, carelessweed, Russian thistle, and lamb's-quarter. Whorled milkweed contains toxic glycosides and poisonous resins that are partly retained even after the plant is dry, which makes milkweed poisonous at all stages of growth and even when put up in hay.

Another weed that occasionally ends up in hay, spreading into a hayfield from where it grows along ditch banks and fences, is hound's-tongue. Cattle generally won't graze it but will eat it in harvested hay. The toxin in this weed is a *pyrrolizidine alkaloid* that causes liver damage, and toxic effects are cumulative if the animal continues to eat contaminated hay. Signs of liver damage may not appear until several months after the contaminated forage is eaten. The animal suddenly dies a few months later when stressed by illness or calving.

Blister Beetles in Hay

Blister beetles are small flying insects, ¼ to 1½ inches (0.64 to 3.8 cm) long, with a broad head and narrow neck, that feed on blooms of alfalfa, soybeans, tomatoes, and potatoes in most of the United States and Canada. The larvae feed on grasshopper eggs in soil. Some species of beetle are more toxic than others, but their bodies all contain a lethal toxin, *cantharidin*. When feeding in swarms on alfalfa blooms, they may be injured or killed by haying equipment and end up in hay. The hay may be toxic even if dead beetles are no longer in it; if they were squashed during haymaking, their poison may leak out into the hay. Cantharidin is a stable compound, and the hay can be toxic for a long time. Horses are especially vulnerable to this poison, but cattle can also be affected.

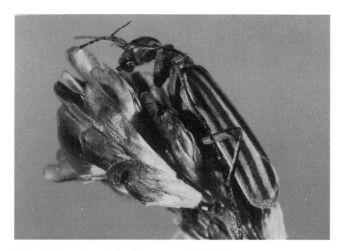
Striped blister beetle feeding on an alfalfa bloom

The beetles' toxin causes blistering of skin. If a beetle walks across your hand, it leaves a string of tiny blisters that burn painfully if broken. When an animal eats blister beetles in hay, the digestive-tract lining is blistered. Digestive action ruptures the blisters, causing sores and ulcers. The animal goes off feed and in severe cases may die. You may not ever figure out the cause of death unless you find the telltale beetles in the hay.

To avoid poisoning, use hay that was cut before blooming, since beetles are only attracted to blooming hay. If harvesting the hay yourself, monitor the fields for beetles arriving in large swarms. If even one beetle is found in a bale of hay, there's a good chance there will be more; thousands may get trapped in just the few bales that came from the portion of the field where these insects were feeding at the time the hay was cut. The hay in these bales can be extremely poisonous.

Hydrocyanic Acid (Prussic Acid)

Cattle may be poisoned when eating certain plants that contain cyanogenetic glycosides. Some otherwise beneficial forage plants, such as Sudan grass (sorghum), johnsongrass, sorghum hybrids, and others, can become toxic under certain conditions and cause heavy mortalities. Some plants and shrubs (such as chokecherry, see above page 290) that grow in pastures or along fences or ditches may also contain enough cyanogenetic glycosides to be toxic.

Linseed meal or cake may be highly toxic if eaten in large quantities.

Concentration of toxic material in plants varies. Poisoning is most likely to occur when cyanide content is high and eaten very quickly. The plants are most toxic when they grow rapidly after a period of stunting. This can occur when fall rains cause rapid growth after a summer drought or when a crop like johnsongrass or sorghum is eaten down by livestock or grasshoppers and then has rapid regrowth. These plants are also very toxic after they've wilted or been frozen. The most dangerous time is between the first light frost that merely wilts the plant and a complete freeze-down that kills the plant. The compound in the wilted plant that converts to cyanide does so because cells have been crushed or have ruptured.

The plants may also be more toxic than usual during drought or when grown in soil with a high nitrogen content, especially when phosphorus content is low. The risk for poisoning is also high when hungry animals suddenly eat a large amount of this forage, as when breaking through a fence out of a dry summer pasture and into a field of lush, immature Sudan grass or sorghum.

Symptoms

Affected animals usually die quickly, rarely surviving more than an hour or 2, and sometimes die 10 to 15 minutes after eating the toxic plants, 2 to 3 minutes after starting to show signs of poisoning. Symptoms include difficult breathing, restlessness and anxiety, stumbling and incoordination, collapse, and convulsions.

Treatment and Prevention

Treatment may be effective if given quickly and consists of intravenous administration of sodium nitrite mixed with sodium thiosulfate. Treatment may have to be repeated. The problem with this type of poisoning is that time is crucial, and you may not be able to treat the animals quickly enough to save them. Other animals in the herd that have been exposed to the toxic plants (but are not yet showing signs) should also be treated with an oral dose of sodium thiosulfate.

Poisoning potential is highest after a light frost, so don't let cattle graze these pastures at night if temperatures will drop below freezing. It's best to keep them out of that pasture for 2 weeks after a nonkilling frost. Make sure the whole field is completely frozen down before grazing it again; it's usually safe after 48 hours following a killing frost. Don't graze crop residues that contain johnsongrass until it freezes down, since this weed is part of the sorghum plant family.

The best way to prevent this type of poisoning is to make sure hungry cattle never have access to toxic plants — especially sorghum species — when plants are drought stressed, immature, wilted, frostbitten, or growing rapidly after a period of stunting. Plants that have a potential risk for poisoning can only be safely fed (as hay or green chop) or grazed after they are more than 30 inches (76.2 cm) tall. If you suspect a potential for poisoning, test the hay or a pasture sample before you allow it to be eaten.

Nitrates

Nitrates are soil nutrients important for plant growth. Almost all plants contain detectable amounts of nitrates, but some (especially annuals) accumulate excess amounts when the uptake of nitrate occurs faster than the plant can use it for protein synthesis. Problems with nitrates occur in some forage plants when they have less-than-ideal growing conditions. Plants growing in normal moisture conditions contain nitrates but not in toxic quantities. When a plant is stressed, however, high concentrations may occur.

Nitrate poisoning may occur because animals ingest toxic concentrations in hay or pasture plants that were stressed by drought or hot, dry winds; dry plants that have a sudden growth spurt after a rain; or plants stressed by a long period of cool, cloudy weather without enough sunshine. Anything that inhibits or retards normal photosynthesis, including cloudy or cold weather, damage by hail, frost, plant disease, and spraying, can lead to excess nitrogen storage in plants because nitrogen is not being converted into protein. If the plants are allowed enough time to recover before being grazed or harvested, nitrate levels return to normal. If the plant is harvested or dies before it can use up the extra nitrates, however, the accumulated nitrate stays in the plant.

Some plants are more likely to cause nitrate problems than others. Oat hay can be toxic under certain conditions. Immature green oats, barley, wheat hay, Sudan grass, rye, and corn can also contain toxic amounts of nitrates when grazed as pasture, as can some annuals that often grow in pastures. Annuals, perennials, and legumes can all develop high nitrate levels under certain growing conditions. Excessive fertilization with nitrogen can also lead to abnormally high nitrate levels in plants.

Nitrate poisoning increases during drought years, because crops are often salvaged as hay or cattle feed when not suitable for grain harvest. Those crops usually are fertilized for grain production, and this creates excess nitrate accumulation in the drought-stunted crop. A serious problem for livestock occurs when an irrigated cornfield hasn't had enough water and nitrate levels are high.

The nitrate concentration is greatest in the lower part of the plant and can affect grazing animals eating summer annuals or grazing a pasture that's too short. Stalks have the highest nitrate, followed by leaves, then seed heads. The lowest 6 inches (15.2 cm) of the stem contain three times more nitrate than the top of the plant. Young plants have greater potential for nitrate accumulation than more mature plants. Filaree, which is normally a good forage plant, may develop high concentrations of nitrogen during fast periods of growth.

Cattle can also be poisoned by nitrates in water runoff from feedlots (due to the high nitrogen content in manure) or freshly fertilized fields. Nitrates and nitrites are also found in some water sources, such as wells or springs. Some species of algae produce nitrates. If cattle are consuming plant nitrates and drinking contaminated water, the cumulative amount may be toxic.

Young growing animals are at less risk for nitrate poisoning than adults. The most dangerous situation is to feed high-nitrate hay to pregnant cows during the last 3 months of gestation. This may cause abortions or birth of weak calves.

Symptoms

Nitrates convert to *nitrites* after being eaten. The latter compound ties up *hemoglobin,* the oxygen-carrying part of blood. Nitrite ions attach to hemoglobin (creating *methemoglobin*) at the same points as oxygen does, preventing hemoglobin from carrying oxygen. Heart rate increases, and mucous membranes and skin become blue instead of pink, due to lack of oxygen.

The most common signs of nitrite poisoning are respiratory distress and suffocation. Other symptoms may include drooling, watering eyes, nervousness, muscle tremors, incoordination, convulsions, diarrhea, and abortion. Cattle that are anemic for some reason (such as when infested by lice or worms, see chapter 7) are more readily affected by nitrate poisoning. Acute poisoning may occur within a few

Ruminants Are Most at Risk

Nitrate eaten by cattle is rapidly converted to nitrite by rumen bacteria and then to ammonia. Nitrite is about 10 times more toxic than nitrate. Nitrite is a building block of protein, but if excess nitrate is eaten, the extra nitrites begin to accumulate in the rumen because bacteria can't convert it all into ammonia, and some of the nitrate and nitrite are absorbed into the bloodstream.

Simple-stomached animals like horses or pigs are not as susceptible to nitrate toxicity because they don't have the microbes that make rapid conversion of nitrates to nitrites. They convert nitrate to nitrite in the intestine, near the end of the digestive tract, where there is less chance for nitrites to be absorbed into the bloodstream.

hours of ingesting the feed, and unless you are continually observing the animals, they may be found dead (with evidence of a short struggle) before you notice any symptoms.

Even if a cow doesn't eat enough nitrates to visibly affect her, low oxygen levels in her body may kill her fetus and cause abortion. Calves may be born 1 to 4 weeks early and die within the first day of life. Calves that survive may have seizures. Nitrates can also interfere with implantation of the fertilized egg in the uterus at the start of pregnancy. Elevated nitrate levels that are not high enough to be fatal may reduce weight gain and milk production.

Treatment and Prevention

Because poisoning is often acute, treatment should be given immediately after symptoms are noticed. Death from lack of oxygen can occur within minutes, especially if the animal exerts herself or becomes excited. Animals can sometimes be saved if given an IV injection of methylene blue to reverse the chemical change. This product is not readily available and may have to be compounded by your veterinarian. Discuss this with your vet ahead of time, in order to have an emergency plan in case of poisoning.

It's always better to prevent poisoning than to try to deal with the aftermath. It's safer to make risky forage into silage than hay; at least half the toxicity of these plants is eliminated by silage fermentation. The only safe way to feed high-nitrate hay is to dilute it by mixing it with other hay so cattle don't eat large quantities of the portion that contains excessive nitrates. In some instances the feed must be chopped and mixed together so the animals won't sort it and consume too much of the high-nitrate forage. Feeding grain can help dilute the nitrogen content of forage and also provide more energy, which seems to help with the conversion of nitrate to ammonia.

To avoid toxic concentrations of nitrate in hay after a long dry spell (or a long cloudy period), don't cut hay for at least 10 days to 2 weeks after the abnormal weather ends. Then there will be less chance for toxicity. If you suspect a possibility for nitrate problems, test some hay samples to see if it's safe to feed. Don't feed Sudan, sorghum, or oat hay without a chemical analysis. Samples can be sent to any lab that does forage testing. The cost of feed testing is less than the value of one animal lost to poisoning. Your county Extension agent can tell you how to collect and send samples. If hay is less than 5,000 parts per million (less than 0.5 percent of the dry weight of the forage is nitrate), it is fairly safe, especially if you dilute it by feeding other hay along with it. If forage has extremely high concentrations of nitrate, however, the only safe alternative may be to burn or bury it so livestock won't have access to it.

Frequent feeding of small amounts of high-nitrate feed is safer than feeding a lot at once. Consuming small amounts at a time increases the total amount of nitrate that can be safely eaten without toxic effects, and the animals adapt better to the higher level. Don't feed damp hay; it becomes more toxic when wet. Some of the nitrate is already converting to nitrite in wet feed.

On pasture with suspected high nitrate levels, adjust cattle gradually. Get them full by feeding a safe hay before putting them in the offending pasture. Turn them out in the afternoon after they are already full and when nighttime nitrate accumulation in plants has decreased. If possible, limit grazing time for the first 6 to 8 days, gradually increasing the amount of time allowed in the pasture. For instance, let cattle graze for 1 hour the first day, and increase the grazing time by 2 hours per day for 6 days, finally leaving them in the pasture. Rumen bacteria that convert nitrate to nitrite and then to ammonia adapt gradually to the increase and become more efficient in the conversion process as they increase their ability to survive in the changed rumen environment. Abrupt changes in feed or pasture, such as rotational grazing with moves to new pasture or a sudden change in winter feeds containing different nitrate levels, are risky.

Another method, if you can't round cattle up every day to adjust them gradually, is to feed them something else several times a day to disrupt their grazing and add rumen fill to dilute the nitrates and decrease the rate of pasture consumption. Adding a high-energy supplement to the diet can also help reduce nitrate problems. Feeding 2 to 3 pounds (0.91 to 1.36 kg) of corn per animal per day can help, as will feeding extra vitamin A (about double the recommended amount). Vitamin A must be in the feed or mineral mix (ingested, not injected) so it will get to the rumen. These measures, used in conjunction with diluting the hay with unaffected hay, can often head off a disaster and prevent nitrate poisoning.

Pesticides and Chemicals

Some types of pesticides are harmful if cattle accidentally ingest them in feed or water or receive an overdose when treated for parasite infestations (see chapter 5). Insecticides are usually more damaging than herbicides if the animal ingests or inhales them or absorbs too much through the skin.

Insecticides

Poisoning and death can occur if cattle consume harvested feed that had an overapplication of certain pesticides used to control insects that damage crops or if a crop was harvested too soon after pesticide treatment.

Livestock may be poisoned when grazing in areas where crops or orchards were recently sprayed, if spray is carried on the wind into pastures or if pesticides contaminate water sources. Poisoning also occurs if sprays designed to kill flies on barn walls or flies and maggots in manure are used on animals by mistake or if old insecticide containers are used for holding feed or water.

Poisoning occurs occasionally if certain livestock pesticides are applied in overdose when treating cattle for lice, grubs, worms, and other parasites. Signs of poisoning may include slobbering, watering eyes, nasal discharge, restlessness, difficult breathing (with audible grunting) or cough, diarrhea, frequent urination, muscle stiffness, and staggering. If poisoning is from overdose of an *organophosphate,* immediate treatment with large doses of atropine may reverse the condition.

Care should always be taken when using insecticides on crops. Always follow label directions and proper rates of application when applying pesticides. Discuss emergency treatments ahead of time with your veterinarian, to be prepared if toxicity occurs.

Herbicides

These products are usually less toxic to cattle than insecticides, but directions for use should be properly followed. In many instances the application of an

herbicide makes plants more palatable, and if cattle are allowed access to treated plants, they may consume toxic plants that they would otherwise avoid.

Different types of herbicides vary widely in toxicity. Some cause an increase in metabolic rate, resulting in restlessness, fever, sweating, rapid respiration, and collapse. The common weed killer 2,4-D is fatal to cattle in large doses. Signs of 2,4-D poisoning include salivation, rumen shutdown, fast heart rate, muscle weakness, and inability to get up. Instances in which an animals consume a large dose are rare.

Lead

Arsenic, mercury, copper, strychnine, and a number of other inorganic poisons are toxic to livestock, but the most common is lead. Calves are most often poisoned because they are curious and tend to sample everything in their environment. They may ingest toxic levels of lead if they have access to crankcase oil, batteries, paint cans, ashes where painted boards have been burned, or other waste materials containing lead. Cattle will readily sample oil; chew on peeling paint, batteries, or other discarded objects; or lick machinery grease. Lead particles may settle in the reticulum and are gradually converted to soluble lead acetate. Pastured cattle with access to rubbish dumps may consume lead and other toxic materials. Lead poisoning may also occur if pasture

Ammonia in Hay

Cattle may be poisoned when eating grass hay or straw that has been treated with too much anhydrous ammonia, which is used to improve the protein level and digestibility. In this type of overdose, cattle (and calves nursing cows that consumed the overly ammoniated forage) develop nervous disorders. Signs of poisoning include restlessness, dilation of pupils, impaired vision, rapid blinking, ear twitching, trembling, frequent urination and defecation, fast respiration, excessive salivation and drooling, bellowing, and sweating.

or forage crops are contaminated with nearby industrial lead sources or are near an oil field or a busy highway where vehicles constantly pass, belching lead-containing exhaust fumes.

Symptoms

Large doses of lead affect the nervous system, with signs appearing quickly after ingestion. Staggering, muscle tremors, chewing motions and chomping, rolling eyes, frothing at the mouth, and bellowing are common signs. The animal is blind and may charge into fences and other obstacles or press her head against a wall or fence. The frenzied movements may be mistaken for rabies. The animal eventually falls down and goes into convulsions and dies, generally within 12 to 24 hours.

If poisoning is subacute, the animal may be dull, blind, off feed, incoordinated, and staggering, with muscle tremor and grinding of teeth, but remains alive for 3 to 4 days. Death may be the result of walking blindly into a hazard or becoming trapped between trees. In other instances the animal dies quietly after getting to a point where she can't get up.

If a moderate dose of lead has been ingested, symptoms may merely involve the digestive tract and not the brain; the rumen stops working, and the animal passes very little manure, later followed by diarrhea. The protozoa in the rumen are killed off, and digestion is severely impaired. If lead poisoning is cumulative (small doses ingested over long periods of time), the animal typically suffers nerve damage and anemia.

Treatment and Prevention

Most animals die in spite of treatment, but sometimes poisoning can be reversed by IV administration of calcium versenate and thiamin hydrochloride. These chemicals remove lead directly from some of the tissues and help increase the elimination of lead from the body, but this requires multiple treatments. Your veterinarian may sedate the animal to halt convulsions.

The best way to avoid lead poisoning is to prevent access to garbage, used batteries, motor oil, and lead paint. Garbage should always be dumped or burned in a safe, fenced-off place or buried. Used batteries and oil should be stored or disposed of safely, without spilling. Cattle should be kept out of barnyards and areas where vehicles are parked or serviced. Use only lead-free paint on surfaces where livestock have access. Inspect every pasture before cattle use it. Make sure cattle have an adequate and well-balanced diet. Even though curious calves will check out strange things, proper nutrition may help reduce the incidence of animals licking and chewing.

CHAPTER EIGHTEEN

Accidents, Injuries, and Wounds

CATTLE ARE HARDY AND TOUGH, but they are also sometimes curious when they should be cautious and are clumsy in awkward, even dangerous situations. They occasionally make mistakes in judgment or have unexpected accidents that cause serious injuries. Wounds obtained from even minor mishaps can become infections that put their health at risk.

When raising cattle you discover that they can get themselves into some unusual predicaments! And just as with any creature in your care, you'll want to know how to treat or repair any resulting injury.

This chapter is just a sampling of predicaments and accidents that occasionally occur, with a few case studies and anecdotes hailing from our Idaho ranch. If you have owned cattle for any length of time, you doubtless will have encountered other problems as well. If you're new to raising cattle, you'll come to realize that some troubles will be easy to resolve and others will be baffling or extremely challenging. In many situations you'll need help from your veterinarian for proper diagnosis and treatment or advice on appropriate nursing care to help the animal recover.

Porcupine Quills

Any curious animal that gets too close to a porcupine may end up with a face full of quills. These are painful and often hinder the animal's ability to eat or drink, especially if there are quills in the mouth. A stockman always hopes to catch this situation right away, as quills tend to work in deeper, due to muscle movement, or get broken off and become harder to locate. The black portion of the quill is covered with a layer of sharp, microscopic barbs shaped like fish scales. The shape of these barbs facilitates inward movement of the quill but make removal quite painful for the animal.

A Very Sharp Fellow

Porcupines are timid, bark-eating rodents with a unique method of self-defense. Being slow of foot, a porcupine protects himself against predators with sharp spines that grow as part of his hair coat. He has about 30,000 multibarbed quills that regrow if lost or broken off. When frightened, he bristles with needle-sharp quills that he can raise or flatten at will. He curls into a ball to protect his face, belly, and the underside of his tail, which have no quills.

The quills are loosely attached to his skin and easily become embedded in the flesh of other animals. If pestered by a dog or a curious cow, he may swat with his tail, driving quills deep into his tormentor's flesh. He can't shoot his quills (as some people think); a quick slap of the tail is enough to stick them into any animal that gets too close.

We've had many instances in which one of our cattle got a face full of quills, especially in our upper fields where our bulls spend the winter. One of our young bulls had more than 80 quills; he must have tried to ram the porcupine with his head. The main reason we built a corral up there in 1985 was so we could capture and pull quills from any animals in those pastures without having to herd them 2 miles down to the corrals in our barnyard. Here's the best way to remove the quills:

1. Immobilize the animal in a squeeze chute, or if he's a small calf, one or two people can hold him while a third removes the quills.

2. Get a good grip on one quill with needle-nose pliers and give a straight, quick jerk. Don't pull to the side or the quill will break off and be hard to get out. With thick clusters of quills, you can sometimes get 3 or 4 at once. Otherwise it's best to take each one individually; you'll get a straighter pull, and the quill won't be so likely to break off.

3. Once you get them out, feel the skin to see if there are any broken-off quills you may have missed, perhaps hidden in the hair. (Rubbing the skin where quills were pulled will ease the pain and is often appreciated by the animal.)

4. Feel inside the mouth and around the lips and gums, in case more quills are hiding in these spots.

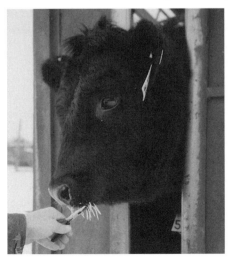

When a porcupine wandered across the pasture, one of our yearlings got too close out of curiosity. Lynn had to pull the quills out with needle-nose pliers.

If a porcupine wanders through pasture or barnyard on his way to and from the trees and shrubs he chews on, this slow-moving creature intrigues a curious cow or calf. A calf may approach the animal, and his mama may butt the porcupine with her head if she thinks it's too close to her calf.

There are several myths about removing quills. Some people claim you should trickle vinegar over the face of the suffering dog or cow in order to soak the quills in the acidic liquid to soften them so they'll pull out easier. Others think quills are filled with air and would be easier to pull out if cut in two—thinking that a collapsed quill, with the air let out, will come out better. Still others say you should twirl the quill as you pull it.

But these methods are counterproductive. Twirling a quill causes more pain for the animal, since the tiny barbs are caught in the flesh. Cutting a quill may make it more difficult to grasp and pull out; the part stuck in the animal (the shaft) is solid, so snipping it in two with scissors just leaves a shorter shaft to try to grasp. And if this short quill goes in deeper, with nothing showing above the skin, it may become impossible to locate. Broken quills below the skin surface are almost impossible to remove. As for soaking quills in vinegar, a mild acid will merely serve to soften the part above the skin surface, making it more likely to break off when you grasp it.

Usually, if you can remove quills soon after they become embedded, they won't be in too deep, very few will be broken off yet, and they will be easier to get out. Even broken quills can be grabbed with needle-nose pliers if the animal can be held still enough so you can get a good hold. Sometimes, however, quills may be broken off flush with the skin surface or so deeply embedded that they are hard to get. Keep track of quills you pull out, and get rid of them. Don't leave any lying around where they might poke into something else or end up in hay or feed where an unsuspecting animal may eat them. Quills ingested by an animal can have serious consequences.

Snakebite

There are several kinds of poisonous snakes in the United States and Canada; including the copperhead and water moccasin, both found in the East and Southeast; and the southern (from Texas and to the east) coral snake; but the rattlesnake is, by far, the most common. There are many subspecies of rattlesnake found in every part of North America except Northern Canada, and they vary in size and length. A cow or calf bitten by these may or may not be at risk for serious consequences, depending on circumstances and the location of the bite.

The rattlesnake is a *pit viper*, a poisonous snake type that includes the water moccasin and the copperhead. The potency of a bite from these snakes depends on the amount of venom injected. A large snake that hasn't eaten for a while has a full pouch of unused venom and is more deadly than a small snake or any snake that has recently killed prey. The rattlesnake bites small rodents, and the venom affects the prey's nervous system so it can't get away.

The venom of a pit viper contains two types of toxin, a *neurotoxin* and a *hemotoxin*. The latter creates severe and rapid swelling at the bite site. The neurotoxin paralyzes and poisons a small animal such as a mouse or chipmunk, and it dies within minutes, enabling the snake to eat it. The poison's effect is directly related to the size of the animal. The bite may be fatal to a small dog, a cat, or a small child, whereas a cow will survive the bite unless serious infection develops or swelling on the face results in suffocation due to constricted air passages.

Symptoms

The bite causes pain, tissue damage, and swelling. Neurotoxins in the venom will cause a small rodent to go into convulsions, causing muscle paralysis, and subsequent death because the muscles needed for breathing stop working. In a large animal the damage is local; the poison isn't strong enough to get very far. If there's a lot of venom, however, the circulatory system may carry it quite a way through the body, and this is why a bite victim should be kept quiet. Increased blood circulation due to exertion can spread the poison.

Bites on the legs of an animal are not nearly as dangerous as bites on the face. Venom from a bite on the lower leg rarely gets into the circulatory system. There may be local pain and swelling or few symptoms at all if the fangs strike the leg bone and venom does not get into soft tissues. The worst danger from

---

SNAKEBITTEN CALF

OVER THE PAST 41 YEARS we've had several dogs, a cat, one horse, and numerous cows and calves bitten by rattlesnakes. Fortunately, the snakes in central Idaho are small — the largest are only 3 feet long — and their bites are not as deadly as that of the large diamondbacks and sidewinders that live farther south. Those large snakes can inject much more venom.

About 15 years ago one of our calves was bitten on the face. It happened in August, when the calves were 6 to 7 months old and out on summer range with their mothers. My daughter and I found the calf while riding to check cattle. The calf was lying under a tree in the shade, struggling for breath. Swelling around her muzzle made it hard for her to breathe, and we were afraid to move her or even to try to catch her for treatment. The extra exertion and need for oxygen that would accompany any movement might have killed her. We hoped she would survive the night and rode back again the next day to check on her.

When we found her, we saw that she had traveled several hundred yards down the mountain to a water trough, where she was standing by the in-flow pipe, trying to sip cold water from the pipe. Her throat was nearly swollen shut, and though she couldn't nurse her mother, she had managed to swallow a little water. We left her alone, and that's where she still was the next day. The swelling on her face was reduced, thanks in some part to the cooling effect of the water she had been trying to drink for more than a day on the swollen tissues. She survived and recovered.

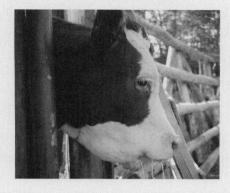

This snakebitten calf has her swelling around the bite on the lower jaw. We were able to bring her home for treatment because her breathing was not impaired.

snakebite in a large animal is when she is bitten on the face. Unless found and treated quickly, a cow bitten on the nose may suffocate within a few hours because the swelling can close the air passages.

Treatment

There are two things to worry about in a snakebitten animal: swelling and infection. Swelling can shut off air passages, and the dirty (contaminated) bite may create infection. Necrotic (dead) tissue at the bite site can send infection all through the body under certain conditions, creating fever and *blood poisoning*.

Snakebite should be suspected if you find an animal with sudden swelling and pain. If the hair coat is not too thick at the site of the bite, you may be able to see fang marks in the swollen skin. If you suspect snakebite, the animal needs immediate medical attention, especially if the bite is on the head. Prompt treatment can make a big difference and turn a potentially serious problem into a minor one.

Antivenin (obtained from your vet) is sometimes used and if given soon enough can reduce tissue reaction. It's expensive, however, and not used as much today as in the past. Cleaning and disinfecting the bite area can help. Your vet will probably advise you to put the animal on antibiotics until the danger of infection is past (see below) and can recommend the best products to use.

Reduce snakebite swelling with application of ice packs or cold packs, if you can keep them in place. DMSO (dimethyl sulfoxide) reduces swelling and inflammation and can be rubbed over the swollen area. If the animal was bitten on the face and is having trouble breathing, DMSO can also help keep air passages open. Apply it to the nose and face or give it orally, mixed with a little water and squirted into the mouth with a syringe, where it is readily absorbed into the throat tissues and helps prevent swelling.

Swelling also responds to treatment with furosemide (Lasix). This diuretic draws fluid out of body tissues, to be excreted in urine. The effects of this drug are temporary but fast acting, and it can help keep down the sudden swelling that can be so dangerous. Dexamethasone will reduce swelling and inflammation but should not be given to a pregnant cow, especially during the last trimester of gestation, or she may abort.

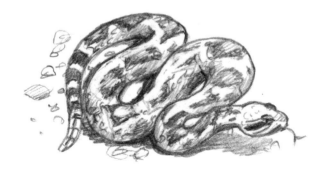

Northern Pacific rattlesnake

If Air Passages Are Constricting

In an emergency, when you don't have an appropriate drug, you may be able to save the cow by cutting two sections of garden hose about 8 inches (20 cm) long, lubricating the ends with water or petroleum jelly, and inserting them up each nostril far enough to get past the soft tissues that are swelling. If you can do this before the airways are compressed by swelling (still allowing passage of the hoses), these will keep the airways open so the animal can breathe. If a garden hose is too large in diameter for a calf, smaller tubing, such as pieces of a nasogastric tube, can be used.

As a last resort in severe and acute cases of swelling on the head in which the animal is having trouble breathing and is in danger of suffocating, you can perform a *tracheostomy*. This involves making a horizontal incision through the skin and into the windpipe. Make the cut a few inches below the jawbone, at the front of the windpipe. Carefully cut between the firm ridges of cartilage with a sharp, clean knife. It's similar to cutting between the rings of a vacuum cleaner hose.

The animal can breathe through this slit. Keep it open with any small, clean tube (like the cap of a ballpoint pen with the closed end cut off) until the vet arrives and can put a stainless-steel tracheal tube into the hole to keep it open. After the swelling that closed off the airway has gone down with anti-inflammatory drug treatment, the tube can be taken out and the hole stitched shut.

Infection

Snakebites often become infected, and this type of infection can be potentially more dangerous than the bite itself. It may start in the swollen tissue as a result of bacterial contamination that entered with the fangs. The dying tissue makes an ideal place for bacteria to multiply and send toxins into the bloodstream. This blood poisoning may cause death unless it's treated promptly. Even if the animal does not become ill from infection, there will be local abscessing. If the bite is several days old by the time it's discovered, the infected swelling should be lanced and flushed out with an antiseptic solution.

Antibiotic injections are recommended and should be continued until any infection is controlled.

A tetanus shot is also a good idea, in some instances. Ask your vet. If the animal is ill or in shock by the time you find her, fluids should be given intravenously or by stomach tube.

If the bite is on the head and subsequent pain and swelling make it difficult for the animal to eat or drink, treatment should include fluids and nutrients until the animal can eat and drink again. A calf can be force-fed milk or milk replacer via stomach tube. Give a more mature animal several gallons of water daily via stomach tube. A long, flexible tube inserted into the nostril, to the back of the throat where the animal swallows it, down the esophagus, and into the stomach, is the safest way to give fluids to a cow. Putting a tube down the throat presents more risk for fluid backing up into the windpipe, and then going down into the lungs. See chapter 2 for step-by-step guides to oral treatment.

If the cow won't eat for several days, propylene glycol is a good energy source and can be given by stomach tube. If her ability to eat is impaired for more than a few days, add some nutrients to the water, by soaking feed pellets until they create a "mush" that can be stirred and diluted with more water to pour down the tube and into the stomach. Good nursing care can sustain the animal until she can eat and drink again.

Fallen Cows

Cows are not as athletically agile as horses and are more at risk for getting stuck on their backs if they fall into a gully or roll into a ditch. They suffocate quickly when on their backs or when lying with the back slightly downhill because the large rumen puts pressure on the lungs. If a cow is on her back, she can't belch. When cows can't pass gas, they bloat, which increases the size of the rumen , the pressure on the lungs, and thus the speed at which they run out of air.

Over the years we've lost five animals in ditches. Irrigation ditches are necessary in our dry region, but they're a hazard for cattle. The ditch bank is often a dry, inviting place to sleep or get out of the wind, as it may have tall grass left by haying equipment running alongside it. If a cow lies next to the dry ditch and reaches her head around to lick her side, she may get off balance, roll into the ditch, and find herself stuck on her back. Unless you find her quickly, she dies.

Bloating begins almost immediately when a cow is on her back and resolves almost as fast as it began if you get her upright and belching before she dies.

Broken Bones

Cows have thick, strong bones and rarely suffer a break except in unusual situations, such as being run

WHEN THEY LIE DOWN IN DITCHES

YELLER FELLER, a heavily pregnant young cow, rolled onto her back in a shallow depression left by a vehicle driving through our calving pen. She died before we discovered her predicament. Our neighbor similarly lost a cow that got stuck in a small gully on the range.

Some stranded cows we were lucky enough to find in time. Funny Hornless was down on her back and bloating in a very shallow ditch one morning when we drove to our lower field to feed. She was barely breathing when we rushed to her and put a makeshift halter of baling twine on her head to pull her back to an upright position.

Huckle was a heifer that we couldn't locate until we searched with flashlights and finally saw her in a deep dry ditch. She wasn't completely on her back, which probably saved her, but she was quite bloated by the time we found her and got her out.

A heavily pregnant cow with a large belly is most at risk because she is more awkward and less agile. When our daughter, Andrea, hiked out through the cows to check them in the middle of the night, she found Tivvy in serious trouble on her back in our sloping maternity pen. She was bloated and barely breathing, with her legs waving feebly in the air.

Andrea yelled for us to come, and we jumped out of bed, threw our coats on over our pajamas, and rushed outside. But Andrea had already saved Tivvy — no small feat for a young teenage girl. Desperation and adrenalin had given her strength to push that 1,100-pound (499 kg) cow upright again.

into by a vehicle. The only broken bone in an adult animal in our herd was a cow shot in the hind leg by a hunter; the bullet shattered the bone between her hock and fetlock joint. She was lame when I found her but was still able to travel, so I brought her 3 miles to the corral. We could tell the bone was broken but didn't realize what had happened until we butchered her and examined the leg, and found the bullet.

In some instances bones may be weak and brittle from nutritional deficiency. Copper deficiency in calves (see chapter 16) can lead to broken bones. We suspect this may have been the reason for a fractured front leg bone in one of our weaned heifers during the winter of 1995, before we started supplementing our herd with copper. The best solution was to butcher her, as it's difficult to treat a broken leg successfully in an animal this large.

Baby calves sometimes suffer broken bones when adult cattle step on them. A broken bone in a young animal is not as life threatening as that in an adult, since young calves heal quickly and have less body weight to stress the healing bone. If a calf is stepped on or suffers a broken bone, contact your veterinarian for his or her take on various limb immobilization and mending methods.

Junk Hazards

Cattle are good at getting into trouble, and many farms and ranches have plenty of hazards, such as old, falling-down fences; junk piles; broken-down machinery; and other potential traps. Cattle have been known to walk through dumps and get a can stuck on a foot or strangle themselves in old wire. Even though we try to keep baling twine picked up and fences repaired, there are times an animal gets something caught around a leg. We've used electric wires along some fences, and if they get broken by wildlife or by cattle rubbing when they're not turned on, the wires may get strung out through the field before we get a chance to gather them.

On several occasions we've had to run an animal into the corral to capture him and take off a loop of wire. One calf got a foot caught in a loop of wire from a range fence that had been knocked down by wildlife and was dragging a piece of wire around. We had to bring that calf 5 miles (8 km) home to a corral

FOR 29 YEARS we leased the ranch next to the one Lynn and I own. It had some old buildings and a barnyard area that the cattle grazed in conjunction with one of the pastures. A small potbellied woodstove with the bottom rusted out sat next to one of the sheds.

One day my husband was checking cows and calves in that pasture and found a steer calf walking around with that stove on his head like a huge bonnet. He'd stuck his head down through the stovetop's missing lid, got his head caught, and pulled backward, bringing the stove with him as it came loose from its bottom. The other cows rushed up to look at the calf — an alien monster — with curiosity and alarm. The calf was wandering around blindly, trying to find his mother, who definitely did not recognize her child!

Lynn tried to sneak up to grab the stove and pull it off but was laughing so hard that even though the calf couldn't see him, he could hear the laughter and moved out of grabbing range. So Lynn came home to get me to help him. (The only thing I regret is that I didn't take a camera with me!)

As we began to sneak up on the bewildered calf to rope him, a jet flew over, and the noise of the jet drowned out additional sounds. Lynn was able to walk up and grab the stove. The startled calf rushed backward, and the stove popped off his head. The calf ran off, shaking his head, to find Mama and console himself with a vigorous stint at the udder.

so we could get the wire off. One old cow, Frankie, was not so lucky. The wire wrapped around her foot was so tight it cut off circulation, and the foot was gangrenous and beyond saving.

One of our neighbor's cows was luckier. She got a hind leg caught in a coyote snare someone had secured to one of our range fences; her foot was tied to the fence. My daughter and I were riding to check cattle and found her there, thin and thirsty. She'd been without feed or water for several days. Andrea quietly crept up behind the cow and undid the snare from the fence; the cow was too weak to get very excited or kick her. We gently herded her to the creek, where she drank and drank, then brought her to our corral so our neighbor could haul her home and get the snare off.

Getting Stuck

Sometimes cattle put their heads where they shouldn't and get caught. Unless someone finds them, they may die of thirst or starvation or from injuries sustained during a struggle to get free.

In 1989 we lost a 2-month-old calf that crept under an old horse-drawn freight wagon parked along the fence. He got underneath it for shelter during a spring blizzard, and while lying under it put his head between the wooden spokes of one of the

BARBED-WIRE HAZARD

Stockmen often roll up old barbed wire when a fence is taken down or repaired and sometimes hang a coil of the wire over a post. If an animal happens to put his head through the loops to scratch his face or neck and then gets caught and pulls back, the wire may strangle him if it tightens around his neck.

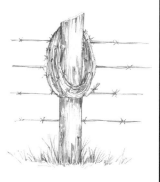

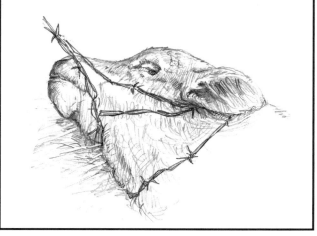

QUICKSIE IN A FIX

WHEN QUICKSIE WAS 8 YEARS OLD, she was missing one morning when we fed the herd. I hiked through the brush along the edges of the field and found her standing in the trees with her head caught. Piles of manure behind her told me she'd been there all night. Her calf must have been with her (until he joined the rest of the herd for morning hay) because she was completely nursed out. Her neck was between two huge trees, and her head was too big to pull out.

Apparently she'd been rubbing her head or neck on the trees, down next to the roots; the trees were a little farther apart at the bottom. When she raised her head, she was caught. She couldn't get free and had given up trying. She didn't realize that the only way to get free was to lower her head to the ground again where there was room to pull out. I tried to push down on her head to lower it, but she fought against my pushing. I was afraid we'd have to saw down one of the trees but also feared she might be injured if we tried that.

I hiked back to the feed truck, where my husband and young son were finishing the feeding, and we drove to the grove of trees and tried to lure her head downward with a flake of hay. She was suspicious and wouldn't lower her head, so the three of us tried to push her head down, but she was stronger than we were. The trees were slightly farther apart higher up, so we tried to make her stand on big limbs we gathered and put under her front feet, but we couldn't get her head quite high enough.

We drove back to the barnyard and got a block and tackle to try to pull the trees farther apart. We hooked one end of the pulley to the smallest tree (about 18 inches thick), which looked the weakest and most likely to bend, and the other end to the base of a huge tree several yards away. We started winching and the tree began to creak and finally moved a few inches away from its original position.

I pushed on Quicksie's nose, but she wouldn't back up; she'd resigned herself to being stuck and had given up on pulling back. I poked her nose, and suddenly she freed herself and stood there a moment in surprise. She shook her head and snorted — as if to blame us for all her troubles — then trotted off to find the rest of the herd and some hay to eat.

wheels. We found him dead the next morning. He'd apparently tried to pull free, got upside down in his struggles, and suffocated.

We were luckier with other calves that got caught by their heads. One morning at feeding time we were short a calf. We went searching and found him standing in a grove with his head stuck between two trees. He'd been able to push between them but could not pull his head back out. Fortunately, we were able to lift his head higher to the space where it was wider between the trees and freed him. It's always wise to take a head count (or check off ear-tag or brisket-tag numbers in a pocket notebook) every time you feed or check cattle, to make sure all of them are there and healthy.

In a field next to a hay yard we have tall mesh elk panels around the stack to keep deer and elk from jumping over and eating hay. We never had any young calves stick their heads through the mesh in earlier years when we calved in January; there was nothing on the other side except snow or frozen ground. But in the past several years we've sold more of our cows to our son and his wife and they now use our summer range permit. We've been calving our smaller herd later in the season and using our home pastures. Now the cows and calves are in the field next to the haystack in April, and green grass on the other side is a temptation. A cow's head is too large, but a calf can reach through the mesh.

One morning when I went out to do chores, I saw a calf lying by the fence, with legs flopping. I ran up there and found that she'd gotten her head stuck reaching for grass, had fallen down in her struggles, and nearly choked herself to death. She was a small calf, so I was able to get her back on her feet and force her head diagonally to get one ear back through the mesh, and then she could pull free. A few days later a bigger calf got stuck, and the only way we could get him out was to cut the mesh with bolt cutters. Fortunately we found both calves before they killed themselves. Not wanting to take any more chances, we put an electric fence along the elk panels to make sure no more calves got that close to them.

Hoof Injuries

Occasionally an animal gets a foot caught and damages the hoof. The worst hoof injuries we've encountered were horn shells pulled off. The first instance was a big calf named Lucy who got her foot stuck on the tipping apparatus when we turned her loose from the calf table where she'd been restrained for branding and vaccinating. The horn shell of one claw ripped right off, leaving her with a bloody bone. We disinfected it and put her and her mama out in a clean grassy pasture instead of turning them out on the range, and before summer's end she'd grown a new horn shell.

Starlight had a tougher case. She was a 3-year-old cow who got a hind foot caught in a cattle guard. She not only pulled off the hoof shell, she also broke the bone. It was a dirty, bloody mess, so we hauled her to one of the new vets in town. He said it likely wouldn't heal, but we wanted to give her a chance and insisted he treat it. He disinfected the damaged, exposed bone and wrapped it.

We brought her home and put her and her calf in our backyard, where it was clean and grassy and she didn't have to walk much. The goal was to keep her foot clean, with no mud or manure to contaminate the broken bone. Every 3 days we put her in the chute, took off the old bandage, flushed the area, and disinfected the bone again, rewrapping it with stretchy *vet-rap* and covering it with water-repellent adhesive tape.

She hobbled around most of the summer with a bandage on her foot. New hoof horn started growing down from the coronary band, and by fall the foot had healed enough so she could go without a bandage. The bone healed, though it wasn't perfectly straight, and she had a healthy foot again. She stayed in the herd and had seven more calves.

Facial Paralysis

One of the more unusual injuries we've witnessed was when Doreen, one of our crossbred cows, started having trouble eating hay one winter. On closer inspection we noticed that she was slobbering out one side of her mouth. The whole side of her face was droopy; her ear was down, her eye watered, and her muzzle was sagging. She seemed to have trouble moving her tongue around to position her feed, and food dropped out that side of her mouth.

Our vet told us this condition was due to nerve damage. She may have suffered a blow on the side of her head that affected nerves on that side of her face. If the damage wasn't too great, it would eventually heal, and the nerve would regenerate. Otherwise she might have a droopy face forever.

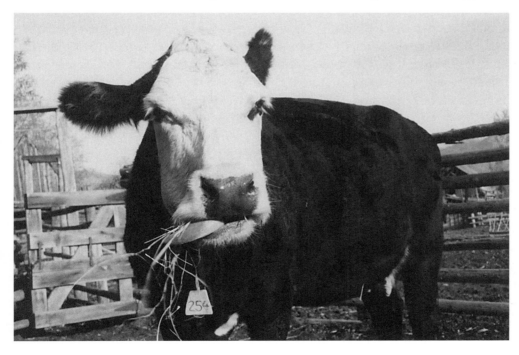

Doreen's facial paralysis caused her to have a droopy ear, droopy upper lip, and swelling along her jaw. She had trouble eating, with lack of control of the muscles on that side of her face.

We brought her down to a corral where we could supervise her and provide plenty of feed and water, and she would not have to compete with the other cows for food. She ate slowly but managed to keep eating. After a few weeks her face was less droopy, and by the time she calved a few months later it was back to normal.

Hernia

A *hernia* is an abnormal opening or separation in the muscles of the abdominal wall that allows inner tissues to bulge through. The muscle separation may be present at birth or caused by injury. In adults rupture of the abdominal wall may be due to a severe blow, such as a horn gore. These can sometimes be surgically repaired.

Umbilical Hernia

Most calfhood hernias are discovered early in life because the problem is generally due to a congenital weakness, separation, or gap in the abdominal wall that allows protrusion of abdominal contents through the opening. Most common is an *umbilical hernia;* a loop of small intestine drops down through a too-large hole in the navel area. In many cases this merely produces a bulge in the skin at the navel. If you press it, you can tell it is fluid that has come through the hole. A small opening will generally close up over time, with no correction needed.

If it's a large bulge, however, check to see if there's a loop of intestine down through the hole. If so, the hernia should be repaired. A large opening needs surgery, but a small one in a newborn calf can often be corrected by placing an *elastrator* rubber band, typically used for banding and castrating bull calves, over the navel cord area. After you have gently pushed the loop of intestine back up through the hole in the abdominal wall, the rubber band holds everything inside and closes the gap. With the tissues pressed together in this manner, the split in the muscle tissue will grow together, eliminating the hole.

Sometimes, however, intestines herniate through the navel cord at birth and come out of the body. This is a life-threatening condition that must be dealt with immediately. If discovered right away when the calf is born, there is a chance to save him if you wrap a clean, wet towel around the mass of exposed intestines so they won't get dirty and rush the calf to a veterinary clinic for surgery. Keep him upside down, so no more intestines will fall out. Your vet can disinfect and replace the intestines, cover them with antibiotic medication, and surgically close the opening. The calf will survive unless the intestines are contaminated with soil, manure, or straw or were stepped on and bruised.

On occasion the herniated loop of intestine will be enclosed within the umbilical cord tissues. You'll notice a large, sausagelike bulge in the cord stump soon after birth. The loop of intestine may not drop down till the calf gets up to nurse; he may seem normal until you check on him a few hours later. His intestines may have fallen out, or a loop may be encased in the umbilical stump.

If a section of intestine is encased in the umbilical stump, you can correct this with the following simple steps:

1. Put the calf on his back
2. Have a helper hold him very still
3. With clean hands, gently squeeze the intestine back up out of the navel cord and into the belly
4. Place an elastrator band (or something else that constricts the tissues) over the naval cord and snug against his belly to tightly close the hole

This emergency repair enables the opening to close up on its own, without surgery. Keep the calf on antibiotics for at least a week and closely monitored to make sure he does not get an infection, which would show up as local swelling or fever and other signs of illness.

Scrotal Hernia

Scrotal hernias are sometimes encountered in male calves. A weakness or separation in the muscle wall allows a loop of intestine to drop into the scrotal sac. Depending on the size of the hole or separation, this may or may not be life threatening. With a small hernia, there's protrusion of fluid or fatty tissue, but there isn't room for a loop of intestine to come through. If the hole is larger, a piece of intestine may drop down and become trapped and strangulate, cutting off the blood supply, which would kill the calf.

A small scrotal hernia might never be noticed, especially if the intestines have not come through and the calf is castrated by banding. The rubber band placed above the testicles would pinch the tissues together, closing the separation in the abdominal wall. A large hernia will look like an oversized *scrotum* (bulging with a loop of intestine within it) or will be discovered when you band the calf. You'd see and feel more than the testicles inside the scrotal sac. Your vet should surgically correct a large scrotal hernia if it's too large to be corrected by banding.

Emergency Surgery

A scrotal hernia may not be noticed unless a calf is "cut" for castrating, slitting the sac with a knife to remove the testicles. This creates a risk for abdominal tissue to fall through the opening you've created. Intestines may pop out through the slit scrotum while you are castrating the calf because his struggling is increasing the pressure and forcing the intestines out of the hole, or they may fall out after he gets up.

This is a life-threatening emergency. You must have your vet come immediately or take the calf to a vet for surgical repair. Put the calf upside down so no more intestines will fall through, and keep a clean, wet towel over exposed intestines to keep them from getting dirty. A small calf can safely stay on his back longer than an adult animal without suffocating since he does not have a large gut to put pressure on his lungs. A bigger calf is more at risk if he must be on his back for long.

If You Cannot Reach a Vet in Time

If intestines start coming out while a calf is being castrated on the ground or on a calf table, put a clean, wet towel over the area and try to keep him quiet until the vet arrives. If this is not feasible, repair the hernia yourself if you have someone to hold the calf while you work:

1. Rinse the exposed loops of intestine with clean water and Nolvasan, and gently replace them back through the hole, being careful not to bruise them. This can be tricky, since more loops may come out if the calf struggles.

2. Once they are back in, use a sterile surgical or sewing needle to close the hole. Be careful to put the needle just through the skin for the stitches,

and no deeper. Dental floss can be used if you don't have surgical thread.

Keep the calf on antibiotics for at least a week after the repair, to guard against infection. The stitches can be taken out a couple of weeks later, after the tissues have grown together.

A FAILED ATTEMPT

OUR ONLY EXPERIENCE with scrotal hernia was in 1973 when we were branding, castrating, and vaccinating our calves. At that time we castrated them with a knife. As soon as my husband started castrating Troilus (Cressida's calf), intestines began pushing out through the slit sac. Opting for a professional repair, I ran to the house to call the vet while my husband and a friend (who was helping us work cattle) held the calf still. I brought clean towels to cover and wrap the exposed intestines while we waited.

Our vet did not come, however. He sent his young assistant who crammed the intestines back into the abdomen and quickly stitched the hole. Our friend asked him how he could be sure he wasn't poking the needle too deep, and the young vet said he was doing it by feel.

Afterward we put the calf and his mama in our barn so we could monitor Troilus and keep him on antibiotics for a while. He seemed a little dull and didn't want to nurse. By evening we fed him by stomach tube since he was still not nursing. By the next day we could tell he was in trouble because he wasn't passing manure. We kept that poor calf alive for more than a week, feeding him fluids, but we knew he had a complete blockage; his abdomen kept getting bigger, and he was totally constipated.

Finally we put him out of his misery and cut him open — and found that one of the young vet's hurried stitches had gone through a loop of intestine, which had grown or sealed together. We realized we'd have been better off if we had done the stitching ourselves because we'd have been a lot more careful and cautious! We never had another problem with scrotal hernias, however; after that we changed to banding bull calves to castrate them, rather than cutting them with a knife.

Dehorning Complications

Dehorning is always easier on an animal if done at an early age when horn buds or horns are small. Newborn calves up to a few days of age can be dehorned with a caustic paste that eats away the horn buds. This works well if you make sure the cow doesn't lick it off and you can keep the head dry for a few hours — rain may wash the paste off and possibly into an eye, which could damage the eye. Calves up to several months of age can be dehorned with an electric dehorner that burns the tissue and kills the horn-producing cells. Larger calves' and adult horns must be removed by cutting them off with horn clippers or a horn saw (for adult cattle), or a wire saw (an abrasive wire/cable with handle on each end wrapped around the horn and then pulled swiftly back and forth to cut through the horn).

The bigger the horns, the more risk for serious bleeding, since the arteries feeding the horns are much larger. Steps must be taken to halt bleeding, since in some instances the animal could bleed to death. Some people use forceps to grasp and pull arteries after sawing the horns off. The spurting artery is grabbed and crushed with the forceps. The pulled and crushed arteries don't bleed as profusely, and the blood will clot faster.

A method that works to immediately halt bleeding requires the use of baling twine to create a tourniquet effect by tying the twine tightly around the poll under the lip of each sawed-off horn and putting pressure on the arteries under the skin surface. The loop can be pulled even tighter by putting another piece of twine underneath (over the top of the head) to pull the first twine tighter against the lips of the sawed off horns. If pulled tight enough, this pressure will halt the bleeding completely. This won't work, however, if you've sawed the horns off flush with the head, leaving no edge for anchoring the twine.

Sinus Problems

There is a risk for sinus-tract infection when dehorning a large animal. After taking the horns off, there is a very large hole that opens into the sinuses. If dehorning in warm weather, the open area must be protected from flies, or they will lay eggs in these openings, and the tissue will be infested with maggots before it can heal.

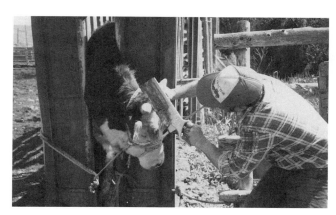

Sawing off large horns with a horn saw

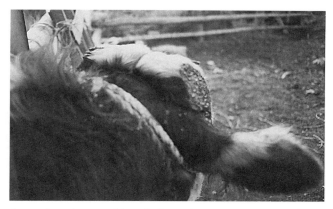

A tourniquet is created from baling twine to put pressure on the large arteries that feed the horn. Pressure on the skin under the lip of the horn stump stops the spurting blood.

If dehorning in cold weather, the exposed tissue may be stressed, and the animal may "catch cold" in those sinuses. In some instances the animal may develop an infection, which may put pressure on surrounding tissues and give the animal a headache before it breaks and drains. The animal will be dull and may carry the head at an odd angle. Treatment with antibiotics and anti-inflammatory medication (to help relieve the swelling, pain, and pressure) may be necessary. Consult your veterinarian.

The best way to avoid complications is to dehorn before or after fly season (or use fly repellant daily on the area until is heals) and before weather gets extremely cold.

Wounds

Compared to horses, cattle have a very thick hide and can go through barbed wire without being cut.

But they may still suffer lacerations or punctures on occasion (from colliding with vehicles or sharp obstacles) or need treatment or antibiotics following a surgical wound (such as a C-section). If the skin has been completely torn away or opened up, consult a veterinarian for advice on treatment.

Predators such as coyotes, wolves, or cougars sometimes inflict serious injuries. Calves are often more vulnerable than adults, but on occasion coyotes have chewed into the hindquarters of cows or heifers lying down in labor, unable to get up and defend themselves. A pack of wolves can easily kill adult cattle.

If you interrupt a predator attack and are able to save the animal, she may need medical treatment to clean and repair the wounds. If the wounds are in superficial tissues or muscles, the animal may have a chance for survival, but if a predator has torn into the abdominal cavity and disemboweled the animal, there's no hope for recovery.

Digestive-Tract Injuries

Cattle are tough and rarely suffer the types of digestive-tract problems or colic encountered by horses. But occasionally accidents compromise the tract.

In 1978 one of our cows suffered a bruised rumen when a herdmate horned her in the belly. Prue went off feed and stopped passing manure, so we called our vet. He examined her and said her rumen had stopped working and gave her laxative boluses and a gallon of mineral oil by stomach tube. We continued the treatment, giving her mineral oil and laxatives periodically over the next few days, and listened to her belly with a stethoscope, trying to hear any signs of renewed activity. Finally there was some action, and Prue started moving things through. The bruised tissue healed, and she recovered fully.

In another instance of shutdown digestion, we were not so lucky. In April 1985 Donnabelle stopped eating and seemed dull, so we brought her and her 3-month-old calf to the corral. We gave her antibiotics, mineral oil, and fluids by tube and tried to entice her to eat, but she only picked at food and was not passing manure. Finally she died, and we cut her open to discover she had a twisted intestine (a loop had flipped over on itself), completely blocking the tract. We were never sure how she did this, since cows don't roll like horses do. Maybe she had been fighting or had rolled down a hill, we surmised. We raised her calf, Danielle, on pasture and grain, and she grew up to replace her mama.

Back Injuries

Cattle are sometimes injured if a larger animal mounts and "rides" them. If a large bull tries to breed a small cow, she may be injured, especially on slippery or boggy footing if her hind legs collapse and she falls down with hind legs out behind her. On occasion a cow is seriously injured while being bred, and the only solution is slaughter. One of our cows suffered an injured back when a bull mounted her in a muddy corral and knocked her down. We tried to get her up, with ropes to steady her, and then realized her hind legs were paralyzed.

This also happened with a big steer one fall. Sometimes steers and bull calves try to mount in-heat cows, and the cows may try to ride them. This steer had an injured back, and his hind legs were nearly paralyzed. We were able to bring him home from range, even though he would occasionally drag his hind legs. There was no hope for his back to heal, however. We let him graze with his mother in one of our pastures for a few days until he was past the stress of the difficult trip home, and then we butchered him.

We were luckier with Angel Eyes, the injured cow my kids and I located on the far side of our range pasture, about 6 miles from our corrals. It was midsummer, and she was already pregnant, so we knew it wasn't a breeding injury (there were no bulls on the range); she probably fell down a mountainside. She was dragging her hind toes and having trouble walking. We started the long trek home slowly and carefully, because her hind legs were so wobbly and uncoordinated. The tricky part was getting her down out of the canyon without her falling off the trail into the deep draw. Once we got to flatter terrain, it was easier, but we had to let her stop often to rest.

A mile from home she could go no farther and lay down. I left the kids with her and rode home to get an injection of anti-inflammatory, painkilling medication. When I got back, she was still lying down. I got off my horse and was able to approach

TRANSPORT TRAGEDY

THE WORST SITUATION we ever experienced with back injuries involved a trailerload of big steers we were hauling to market. Several neighbors were helping us with their trucks and trailers, taking the calves to a scale to be weighed and put on a semi. On one particular trailer, the door latch popped open going down the rough dirt road from our ranch, and all 24 steers came out. My husband, my daughter, and I were following in our truck and could only watch in horror and helplessness as the steers tumbled out. The driver didn't realize what was happening until it was too late.

The steers next to the door suffered the worst injuries; most of them fell out backward, landing on their backs. One was killed outright, and three others had broken backs and could not move their hind legs. We had to humanely kill and butcher them. The other 20 had varying degrees of injury; some jumped out (instead of falling) and were unharmed. Our daughter and neighbors field-dressed the four with broken backs, and I herded the survivors back up the road a mile to our corral. We were able to send the uninjured ones on the load of calves we were shipping, but the ones that were bruised and lame we treated with painkillers and anti-inflammatory medication and kept them a couple of months longer until they were fully healed.

and give her the injection. She lurched to her feet as I finished, and we let her stand a while, then brought her and her calf on home.

We treated her with painkillers and anti-inflammatory medication for several weeks. Her back eventually healed to the point where she could get around fairly well. We didn't put her on the range the next summer, thinking she'd be safer on flatter ground, but after that she was fine — except for slightly impaired action that made her clack the dewclaws of her hind legs together as she walked. She stayed in the herd, raising eight more calves.

Hind-Leg Paralysis

The most common cause of hind leg paralysis is calving. Sometimes when a very large calf puts excessive pressure on his mama's pelvic nerves as he comes through, the force temporarily paralyzes one or both hind legs of the cow. Usually, once the calf is delivered and the pressure is gone, the cow regains the use of her leg muscles if she is able to get up. She may need help to stand the first time she tries to get up and may be wobbly and unsteady on the affected leg for a few hours or days, but she soon recovers.

If she can't get up, make her comfortable where she is, and help her get up, several times a day. In some instances it may be necessary to hoist her up so she can put some weight on her legs. Chances for recovery are always more favorable if you can get her up as soon as possible. A hip hoist (which hooks onto her hip bones) can be used to support her rear end if necessary. See the companion volume for this book, *Essential Guide to Calving* (Storey Publishing, 2008), for a complete discussion of the topic and a diagram of how to use the hoist.

Other situations in which hind-leg damage may temporarily impair a cow's ability to stand include slipping on ice or a concrete barn floor and tearing or pulling the hind-leg muscles. Swelling and nerve damage may make it impossible for her to get up. We've had two instances in which cows slipped on ice and ended up on their bellies with hind legs splayed out, unable to rise.

Hornless Fatty was a Hereford cow who spent a cold December night stranded on an ice flow on one of our upper fields in 1972. She'd fallen near the top of the field and slid all the way down the slope, nearly to the creek. We found her the next morning when we went to feed. We tried to reposition her hind legs and help her get up, but the legs wouldn't work; in her one brief effort, her legs splayed out to the sides again. We drove back home and searched under the snow for an old hay slip — a board platform on wooden runners, which we used to pull behind a pickup or tractor when gathering bales of

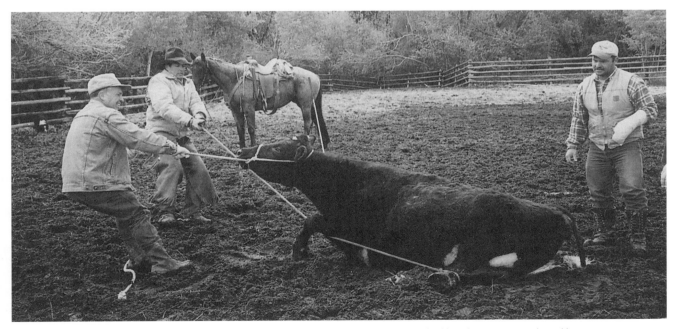

Trying to get an injured cow (Gargle) back on her feet in a boggy corral after a bull knocked her down trying to breed her.

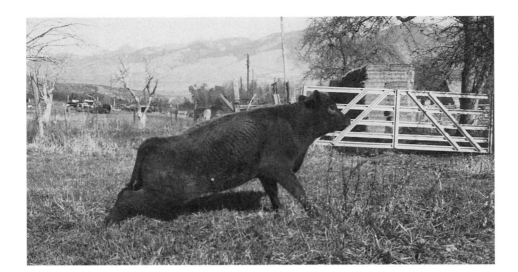

Texas Tim was a steer with an injured back. We were able to bring him home from the range to this pasture, but he occasionally had trouble walking, dragging his hind legs.

hay off our fields in the 1950s. The boards were only a few inches off the ground, and we thought it might work as a sled.

We pulled it behind our jeep up the snow-packed road two miles (3.2 km) to our upper field and drove on the ice as close to Hornless Fatty as possible. It took a lot of effort for the two of us to roll that 1,200-pound (544 kg) cow onto the hay slip. We brought ropes, a halter, and a wide pulley belt off our old baler. We put the belt around her shoulders like an oversize breast collar, tied it to the hay slip in six places, and tied her head with a halter. She resigned herself to the sled ride behind the jeep, only seeming alarmed when we had to go straight down off a bank to get across the creek, with a burst of speed to make sure the loaded sled wouldn't outrun the jeep going down the bank. As the front hung out over space for a split second before plummeting over the edge, her eyes got big as saucers.

We got her home, pulled the slip into an old shed, and rolled her off onto straw bedding. She was chilled after spending so much time on the ice, so we hung a propane heater above her from the rafters. We consulted our vet, who suggested we let her lie quietly for a couple of days before trying to get her up, to let the damage to her muscles start to heal. Following his instructions, we hobbled her hind legs together (about 12 inches [30.5 cm] apart) with a rope, so they could not splay again if she tried to get up on her own. To prevent "bedsores" we turned her over twice a day so she wasn't always lying on the same side. We gave her antibiotics for several days to ward off pneumonia and medication to reduce swelling and inflammation in the damaged muscles.

We encouraged her to eat and drink, with food and water within reach of her head. After 2 days' rest, we got her on her feet with a lot of pulling, pushing, and steadying. The hobbles kept her hind legs from splaying out. She swayed unsteadily, panting from the effort, then lay down. After that we got her up several times a day. It was a week before she was able to stay on her feet very long.

We were afraid she might have trouble calving after all this trauma, but 3 weeks after her accident she gave birth to a big bull calf named Figero. Mama was almost as wobbly as baby, but she managed to lick him dry and suckle him. After that she no longer needed the hobbles to keep her legs steady, and we were soon able to put the pair out in a field with other cows and calves.

Sixteen years later we resorted to the same method to rescue another cow. Dayo, a 3-year-old crossbred cow, was down at the creek getting a drink from a water hole chopped in the ice and slipped or got pushed out onto the ice by another cow. When we went to check the waterhole, we found her helpless on the ice with her hind legs out to the sides. Unable to get her up, we went home for a sled. Our old hay slip was long gone (rotten and disintegrated), so we made a sled with two poles and part of an old truck rack. Thanks to Hornless Fatty's sled ride earlier, we knew we could get Dayo safely home. She recovered and had nine more calves. But she never forgave us for saving her; she probably associated her pain

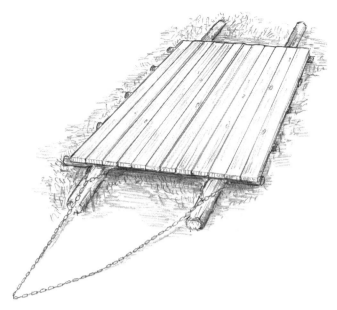

This improvised sled was created using two big poles for runners under an old truck rack to bring Dayo home. We made her comfortable on a thick bed of fluffy straw until she could get up again.

and temporary paralysis with our intervention. She always had a snorty attitude and was an aggressive ornery mama at calving time.

Burns

Animals trapped in fires (in a barn or in forest or range fires on pasture land) are sometimes killed or injured by smoke inhalation or burns. In some instances the injured animal must be humanely destroyed; consult your veterinarian for prognosis on a case-by-case basis. If burns are superficial or only small areas of the body are affected, the animal may survive with good nursing care. Skin may slough off and raw areas need antibiotic salve. Feet may be badly burned if the animal had to walk through hot ash and coals. The hoof may separate from the coronary band and seem quite loose, but some of these damaged hoofs will heal; other victims may lose their feet.

Lightning

When struck by lightning, most cattle are killed, since four-legged animals are so well grounded. Cattle standing under trees, next to metal fences, or in water are most at risk during a lightning storm. Tall trees may be struck, killing animals that have taken shelter beneath them. Metal fences and water carry electricity, and damp ground may also carry it a distance from the actual strike. Electrocution or electric burns may occur if power lines go down or if animals come into contact with faulty wiring.

If the animal is not killed outright by high voltage, she may be knocked unconscious or suffer superficial burns at the point of contact or along the flow of electricity through the body from point of contact to the ground. The animal may fully recover after regaining consciousness or may be temporarily blind with varying degree of paralysis that may or may not resolve over time. If the animal is burned, those areas may need treatment. Consult a vet.

Frostbite

In severely cold or windy weather, cattle may suffer frostbite. Usually ears, tail, teats, and feet are most severely affected by the condition. Calves are most vulnerable, especially if circulation is already impaired by scours and dehydration.

Windbreaks and bedding for the herd and shelter for young calves during cold can reduce risk (see chapter 3). If affected parts of the body can be warmed and circulation increased, damage may not be permanent. Tail tips and ear tips may be lost. Skin over frozen feet and legs may slough off. If the raw area doesn't extend up the leg much farther than just above the feet, it can be treated with antibiotic ointments and bandaged for several days until it begins to heal.

CHAPTER NINETEEN

Miscellaneous Diseases

Previous chapters in this book have touched on common — and some uncommon — cattle diseases and health problems, but there are others that should not be ignored. Some diseases are seen infrequently, but stockmen need to be aware of these rarities so that if theirs is one of the herds experiencing the ailment, they will recognize it. Others are foreign livestock diseases we hope never to see in this country but which should be mentioned because they exist in countries that export livestock to the United States and Canada. We need to know the facts about these frightening diseases in case an infected or exposed animal is found in our midst.

Cancer

Cancer refers to an abnormal growth of cells that multiply without any particular arrangement or control. The technical term is *neoplasm,* which means new growth. The most common cattle cancer is cancer of the eye, which can be readily cured if discovered early (see chapter 9). Other types of tumors may not be discovered in time to remove them, such as cancers located in the digestive tract or other internal organs.

Tumors can occur in any tissue or organ, and may be *benign* (slow growing or remaining localized) or *malignant* (spreading to adjacent tissues or traveling via the bloodstream to create problems in other parts of the body). Benign growths rarely come back

if removed. Malignant growths may eventually kill the animal unless removed before they spread. A neoplasm may start growing from any type of body cell (such as blood, bone, or muscle), but most of the cancers seen in humans, such as those of the reproductive tract and mammary glands, are rare in cattle.

Cattle cancers include *carcinomas,* which are malignant new growths made up of *epithelial cells* in tissues that line internal and external body surfaces. Carcinomas tend to infiltrate the surrounding tissues and metastasize to other areas of the body. Squamous cell carcinoma commonly affects skin tissues. *Sarcomas* are another type of tumor, usually arising from connective tissue, and most of them are malignant. Papillomas are growths, often initiated by a virus, that are most often benign.

Bovine Lymphosarcoma

The bovine leukemia virus (see chapter 5) spreads from one animal to another by blood exposure to infected white blood cells. This can happen when contaminated tools are used on multiple animals for dehorning, castration, or other procedures, or when biting flies carry blood from one animal to another. Susceptibility and resistance depend on the genetic makeup of the animal. Many cattle are exposed to (and infected by) the virus, but only a small percentage actually develops cancerous growths.

The incubation period for lymphosarcoma is usually 4 to 5 years; thus, the cancerous form is rarely seen in animals less than 2 years old and most commonly appears in adults 4 to 8 years old. Lymphosarcoma is the terminal stage and is always fatal but only occurs in about 1 percent of infected cattle. Cows with great genetic potential for milk production are more susceptible to persistent infection with the virus than cows with lesser genetic potential, and this is probably why lymphosarcoma is seen more commonly in dairy cows.

Symptoms

In adult cattle almost any organ can be affected by the cancerous lesions, which develop in various sites at various rates in different animals. These growths are never benign; they keep growing and spreading and eventually kill the cow, though the rate of growth and the duration of the disease may be short or prolonged over several months before the animal succumbs and dies.

The abomasum (first stomach), heart, and abdominal and peripheral (near the surface) lymph nodes are the most common sites in adults, while calf spleens, livers, and abdominal lymph nodes are most typically affected. Growths in the abomasum wall result in impaired digestion and persistent diarrhea, which may be mistaken for Johne's disease (see chapter 4). Tumors in the digestive tract may cause chronic, moderate bloat. When the heart wall is affected, the result is congestive heart failure. If growths occur in nerve tissue, the primary lesion spreads along the nerves to the lining of the brain and spinal cord, which eventually results in gradual paralysis of the hind legs. In some instances involvement of spinal nerves may be mistaken for rabies. The skin and reproductive tract are often affected. Thickened areas between the layers of the skin produce lumps. Enlarged lymph nodes next to the esophagus in calves may result in an inability to swallow food.

These growths are malignant and quickly metastasize, spreading widely through the body. Tumors may develop rapidly at many body sites, producing varying signs. In 5 to 10 percent of cases, the course of the disease is short. The affected animal may die suddenly without prior evidence of illness. Death may be due to involvement of the adrenal glands, rupture of an abomasal ulcer, or a damaged spleen with internal hemorrhaging. More often the animal survives for several months, with a poor appetite and weight loss, pale membranes, and weakness. Usually after illness becomes evident and the tumors are detectable, the animal goes downhill rapidly and dies within two to three weeks.

Enlargement of superficial lymph nodes (lumps seen and felt on the body surface) occurs in a majority of cases and is often one of the earliest symptoms of lymphosarcoma. If enlarged nodes are inside body cavities, however, they are not detected unless they put pressure on other organs, such as the intestines or nerves, and create other symptoms. In advanced cases it may be easy to feel those enlargements with rectal palpation.

There is no effective treatment.

Digestive-Tract Tumors

Growths in the mouth of cattle are sometimes viral papillomas but may also be caused by eating bracken fern (see chapter 17). These tumors are usually squamous cell carcinomas on the gums and may interfere with chewing. They appear most often in older animals. Growths in the throat area and esophagus are generally papillomas (caused by a virus); the resultant swelling may interfere with swallowing. Sometimes these relatively benign growths develop into carcinomas in older animals.

Squamous cell carcinomas sometimes occur in the rumen. A growth may obstruct the area between rumen and esophagus, causing chronic bloat. *Lymphomatosis* in the wall of the abomasum may cause chronic diarrhea. Occasional tumors in the intestine may interfere with digestion, causing chronic bloat or intermittent diarrhea.

Cancer of the Bladder

Tumors in the bladders of cattle are usually associated with eating bracken fern, but occasionally other types of growths are involved. Signs of bladder tumors include weight loss, difficulty urinating, blood in the urine, and secondary inflammation of the bladder.

Bone Cancer

Osteosarcomas are malignant and fairly common in dogs and cats but rare in cattle. Most bone tumors in large animals occur in the skull.

A STRUGGLE WITH CANCER

MOST CASES OF CANCER in our herd are eye problems. We've only had a couple of incidents of growths in the abdomen, in older cows. One cow lost weight as she neared calving in 1978. We put her in a pen by herself and tried to entice her to eat alfalfa hay and grain to keep her alive until she calved. She calved several weeks prematurely, but we saved the tiny calf. He lived in the house for a couple of weeks, and then we raised him on another cow. Our vet diagnosed the old cow with abdominal tumors, and we ended her life.

A 13-year-old cow, Jamaican Janet, went off feed December 10, 2001. We found her lying down, reluctant to get up, not interested in food. Her manure was very firm and scanty. We hauled her to our corrals, took her temperature (which was normal), gave her antibiotics and a magnet, and put her in a corral with straw for bedding and some good hay to eat.

Still Janet wouldn't eat, so the next day we had a vet check her. Her rumen was working, so he suspected something wrong in the rest of the tract. He gave her mineral oil and stool softener, vitamin B, Banamine, and dextrose and took blood samples. By the third day she ate a little and passed soft manure.

We kept treating her, but by the fifth day she was eating less and passing less manure. Though her blood counts were normal, she continued to do poorly, in spite of all our efforts. We gave her more glucose by IV, probiotics, and our best hay. Several times a day I made her stand up, and she'd stand for 30 minutes to an hour, eating. The weather was cold — down to 10 below zero by Christmas — so we kept her well bedded with straw and gave her warm water to drink, but she wasn't drinking or eating much.

The vet came back December 28, gave her more injections, and pumped propylene glycol into her stomach to give her energy, in hopes it might help her digestive tract function better. The next 2 days my husband and I gave her dextrose, more propylene glycol, mineral oil, and several gallons of water by stomach tube, since she was no longer eating or drinking. She was due to calve February 5; we wanted to keep her alive long enough to get the calf out, but she was becoming weak.

On the morning of January 1, our vet came to do a C-section and take the calf out. He was very tiny and didn't start breathing very well, and though we carried him right into the house to dry and warm him by the stove, he continued to have breathing problems and lived only a few hours. While the vet had Janet's abdomen open, he felt around in there and discovered the cause of her problem; she had several large grapefruit- to cantaloupe-size tumors on her intestine, which he didn't dare remove. He stitched her up anyway, in hopes she might do better for a while with the calf out of her. By the next morning she was chewing her cud for the first time in 3 weeks. She did better for a few days, then got diarrhea and died a week later.

We've had only one case of cancer in a calf. He developed golf-ball-size lumps all over his body at about 4 months of age, so we hauled him to the vet clinic for diagnosis. Our vet told us he had a rare type of cancer. It was not treatable, so we opted to have the vet euthanize him.

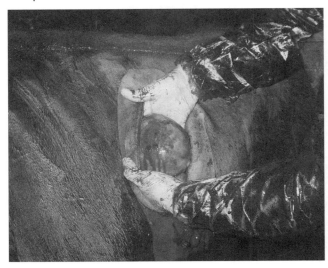

One of the tumors is pulled into view after taking Jamaican Janet's calf out by C-section. After the vet removed Janet's calf, he felt around on her intestines and found several large grapefruit-size tumors attached to her intestines.

Lung Tumors

Tumors that originate in the lungs are very rare in cattle, and metastatic tumors (that originate somewhere else and spread to the lungs) are uncommon. Symptoms include a decrease in lung capacity, and over time the animal has more difficulty breathing and develops a cough. There is no fever, and the cancerous growth may be mistaken for a chronic abscess. The most common type of lung growth in cattle is due to lymphosarcoma (see page 322), but it usually puts pressure on the heart as well as the lungs, resulting in congestive heart failure.

Kidney Tumors

Carcinomas that originate in the kidney are unusual in cattle. The typical sign is enlargement of the kidney. Most growths in the kidney are due to metastatic neoplasms that spread to the kidney from other areas of the body, generally due to lymphosarcoma. The problem is generally not detected until it is quite advanced and may only be detected at slaughter.

Skin Cancer

Squamous cell carcinoma can occur anywhere on the skin or in the mouth. Cancer eye is the most common type, appearing on the eyeball or eyelids (see chapter 9). Growths sometimes occur on the vulva but most often on unpigmented areas of skin (as on light-skinned cattle), rather than on pigmented vulvas. If discovered early, these growths can be surgically removed.

Cancer of the horn core sometimes occurs in cattle. This is a squamous cell carcinoma arising from the lining of the frontal sinus and invading the central area at the base of the horn. This problem is most frequently seen in older, light-colored cattle and mainly affects breeds from India. An early sign is discomfort. The animal may be observed shaking her head or rubbing her horns against solid objects. There may be a bloody discharge from the base of the horn or from the nostril on the affected side, since the sinus cavity is involved, and the animal may hold her head to one side. The horn becomes loose and falls off, leaving the tumor exposed and vulnerable to infection and flies.

Cattle branded with hot irons or freeze branding occasionally develop a warty growth at the site. Most of these growths are due to chronic inflammation and are not considered cancerous, but sometimes they develop squamous cell carcinoma.

Melanomas sometimes afflict dark-skinned cattle, but unlike human melanomas, these skin-surface growths are usually benign in cattle and horses. Other types of skin cancer in cattle include *cutaneous angiomatosis,* which is characterized by periodic profuse bleeding from small lesions along the back. These small lesions are generally seen only in adult dairy cows and are benign. They can be surgically removed. Skin lumps in cattle can also be due to lymphosarcoma (see page 322) and in these instances are generally accompanied by lesions in other organs. *Mast-cell tumors* (tumors of the connective tissue cell) may occur in cattle, appearing as rapidly growing nodules between layers of skin. They are malignant (but only spread to other areas of the skin), and may recur and spread if removed, but they do not metastasize internally.

Nervous System Tumors

Squamous cell carcinomas (cancers that begin in skin tissues) and lymphomas metastasize in later stages and may travel to other body locations, including the brain or spinal cord. These may cause abnormal function and behavior and are not usually diagnosed until after death.

Udder Cancer

Cancerous growths in the udder are rare in cows. Growths on teats are more common, and these can usually be surgically removed.

Mycoplasma bovis

This bacterium was discovered in 1961 as a regular inhabitant of the nose, throat, lungs, and reproductive organs of healthy and sick cattle. Illness caused by *M. bovis* was recognized in the mid-1970s, but it has only recently gained the attention of veterinarians and stockmen. One of the problems with this disease is the difficulty of differentiating between it and other respiratory illnesses.

Because most antibiotics are designed to kill bacteria with cell walls, and because *M. bovis* belongs to a group of bacteria that have no cell wall, it is difficult to treat. It's also hard to produce an effective vaccine for the disease because it's so adept at mutating. These bacteria are some of the smallest and simplest organisms on earth and can change their protein profile to evade the action of antibiotics.

M. bovis is usually an opportunist. During periods of stress it expands its territory from where it benignly lives in the nose and throat or moves into tissues after they are damaged by another pathogen, such as the BVD virus. This bacterium is so small it can pass through membranes. Different strains affect cattle in different ways. Cows may abort. Weaning-age calves or feedlot animals may develop pneumonia, *arthritis* (inflammation and infection in the joints), and a condition called *chronic pneumonia polyarthritis syndrome (CPPS),* which has become a common cause of feedlot deaths. Stressed animals are most susceptible.

These bacteria are found nearly everywhere but cause disease only sporadically. Researchers are wondering if only a certain strain may be involved in disease or if other pathogens are needed to suppress the immune system before *M. bovis* can cause illness. Infected animals that get sick can spread the bacteria for months or years if they don't die. In a feedlot situation, they may spread it to the next group of calves that come into the yard.

Symptoms
Disease in weanling or yearling cattle starts with fever. The animal looks dull, goes off feed, and may have a clear nasal discharge. The illness progresses to pneumonia, and eventually the leg joints start to swell. Often several joints, such as the knee, elbow, hip, or fetlock are affected at once. The animal has trouble getting up and may lie down with legs out straight because it is too painful to flex the joints.

The animal becomes thin and dehydrated. Death may occur after 2 or 3 weeks. The most common scenario is pneumonia and lameness occurring about 2 weeks after a group of calves is brought together from several sources, with the sick ones not responding very well to treatment. Most death losses occur 3 to 6 weeks after the calves arrive, and then the outbreak stops. If your vet does a postmortem on an animal that dies, there will be huge abscesses in the lungs with very little healthy tissue left. The animal

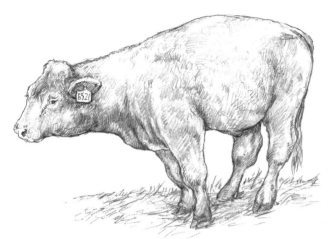

Steer with pneumonia and painful, swollen joints due to Mycoplasma bovis *infection.*

may also have swollen, abscessed leg joints and tendon sheaths.

Treatment and Prevention
Any cattle with signs of respiratory disease should be treated quickly and with the proper antibiotics. Delaying treatment may enable *M. bovis* to take over and invade the lungs.

Prevention involves good management, keeping cattle well protected from other diseases with vaccination and a healthy environment, reducing stress, and avoiding mixing purchased cattle from different sources. There are two vaccines for *M. bovis* currently on the market, but some veterinarians question their effectiveness. If you plan to vaccinate, do it before weaning. Once the animals are stressed, it is usually too late.

Vesicular Stomatitis

Vesicular stomatitis (VS) is a foreign-animal disease caused by a virus. It commonly occurs in warm regions of South and Central America but sometimes spreads north into the United States during the summer months. A serious outbreak in 1995 began in New Mexico and affected many western states, causing quarantines of farms and halting interstate travel of livestock. Millions of dollars were lost due to cancellation or postponement of livestock sales, county fairs, shows, and rodeos. Additional losses resulted from the costs of transporting feed to animals quarantined in pastures with no remaining forage.

Monitoring the Disease

VS enters the United States sporadically and causes a great deal of hardship and concern. Even though it's not a fatal disease, health officials in the United States work diligently to prevent its spread because symptoms are so similar to those of foot-and-mouth disease (FMD). FMD (see page 328) is a much more serious foreign disease of cloven-hoofed animals and was eradicated from the United States in 1929. Officials are vigilant and take great care to prevent the reappearance of FMD. Clinical signs of VS are also similar to swine vesicular disease, another serious foreign illness. The only way to tell them apart is by laboratory tests.

Even though VS is not as serious as FMD, the USDA's Animal and Plant Health Inspection Service (APHIS) wants to keep VS from becoming established in the United States because of its adverse affect on livestock production. Animals with VS lose weight and drop in milk yield. VS is also a threat to human health, and state and federal authorities must be notified if VS is suspected. Many countries that import livestock and animal products from the United States would impose restrictions if VS were allowed to exist here.

Veterinarians don't become as worried if VS is found in a horse, but discovering an affected cow is a different story. VS can be devastating for beef and dairy production, but vets also have to make sure it's not foot-and-mouth disease, which is actually worse. Sheep, cattle, and goats can get FMD, which could wipe out our livestock industries.

Spread of the Virus

Vesicular stomatitis has been recognized for more than 80 years. The virus occurs year-round in central Mexico and sometimes moves north into the United States in the spring, being spread by biting insects, such as sandflies and blackflies (some of which act as mechanical vectors, and some transmit the virus as infected carriers), and by the movement of livestock.

Insects traveling on wind currents can carry the virus, allowing it to leap many miles at a time to infect susceptible livestock. Fairs, livestock sales, or other events that congregate animals from wide areas increase the risk for spreading VS. An outbreak that began in 1982 affected 14 states, infecting many herds of cattle and horses.

Transmission occurs when a healthy animal comes in contact with saliva or fluids from an infected animal or ingests infected material. It can travel through a herd via direct contact or exposure to saliva on other objects. Transporting infected animals, lack of sanitation (not cleaning out vehicles used in transport), and contact between infected and noninfected premises are ways in which the virus can be spread. Blister fluid or saliva in water troughs or buckets can also infect susceptible animals.

Animals can be protected by avoiding contact with other animals. Good sanitation, along with quarantine of any affected animals can usually keep VS from spreading until the insects that transmit it die in the fall with the onset of cooler weather.

Symptoms

VS is rarely fatal, but it causes blisters in the mouth and on the dental pad, tongue, lips, nostrils, teats, and feet of cattle. The blisters swell and break, and the skin sloughs away, leaving painful, raw ulcers. Pain causes animals to stop eating and drinking, so they lose weight. Blisters at the coronary band may cause lameness and occasionally the loss of a hoof.

The most common signs are drooling and high fever. The incubation time from exposure to blister formation is 2 to 8 days, sometimes longer. Excessive saliva production and drooling is often the first thing you notice about the animal; then its temperature begins to rise about the same time blisters appear in the mouth. If there are no complications due to secondary infection, the affected animal usually recovers in 2 to 3 weeks.

Since VS mimics FMD, there must be a proper diagnosis to rule out FMD. Sometimes toxic plants, allergic reactions, or exposure to insecticides can

---

ANIMALS TO HUMANS

VS can affect cattle, pigs, and horses, and occasionally sheep, goats, and llamas. Many species of wildlife can also get VS, including deer, bobcats, raccoons, and monkeys. Humans may become infected when handling sick animals.

cause similar symptoms. Your vet must make a diagnosis based on clinical signs or blood-test results or by isolating the virus from a tissue sample. There is no specific treatment for VS except to try to prevent secondary infection where blisters have broken and raw tissue is exposed. Mild antiseptic mouthwashes and ointments can help alleviate the pain.

Preventing and Limiting VS

If a case of VS occurs on your farm, take the following measures to prevent further spread.

▶ **Quarantine the sick animal** as far away from other animals as possible, preferably in a barn where there's less risk of insects taking the virus to nearby animals. Livestock on pasture are more frequently infected; isolating a sick animal in a barn stall reduces the risk. Isolate any newly infected animals for at least 21 days before putting them with your healthy cattle.

▶ **Do not move any of the other animals** from the premises (unless they go directly to slaughter). They should be kept where they are for at least 30 days after the last sick animal's blister lesions have healed.

▶ **Keep animals in dry lots** instead of on pasture, where there are more insects, and use insecticide ear tags or apply insecticide daily. Insect control can help prevent the spread of VS. Most outbreaks occur near water or wet areas with high insect populations and in animals not treated with insecticides.

▶ **Disinfect equipment** used on the animals and all work areas such as chutes and head catchers with disinfectants containing chlorine bleach or chlorhexadine (Nolvasan) to kill the virus.

▶ **Don't use the same equipment** for quarantined animals that you use for other livestock. Use separate feeding, cleaning, and health-care equipment. If it must be shared, clean and disinfect it for at least 10 minutes between uses. Clean and disinfect all feed bunks and water sources daily.

Use protective measures when handling infected animals to prevent human exposure. Don't touch infected-animal body fluids such as saliva and blister seepage. Protect your hands with rubber gloves, and don't let infected fluids come in contact with mucous membranes such as eyes or mouth or open wounds. *Caution:* The virus can be transmitted to humans through the skin and respiratory system. VS in humans may be misdiagnosed; it causes acute illness with fever, muscle aches, headache, and general discomfort. Blister lesions appear only rarely.

▶ **Shower and change clothing and boots** when moving between the quarantined animals and the main herd. If possible, the care for isolated animals should be done after handling the other cattle to avoid any chance for contamination.

▶ **Consult your veterinarian;** he or she may have additional tips for protecting your herd and your family, as well as helpful treatment methods.

A farm or area that has had even one sick animal cannot be considered free of VS until at least 30 days after the affected animal's lesions heal. For more information, contact the USDA Animal and Plant Health Inspection Service (APHIS). Information on VS is also available at any state veterinarian's office or state Department of Agriculture.

Foot-and-Mouth Disease (FMD)

This dreaded foreign-animal disease is caused by a virus that has seven main types, and each type has several subtypes. It affects all cloven-hoofed animals and also affects camels and llamas to a lesser degree. Some researchers think this is the oldest and most contagious virus known to affect livestock. Infected animals exhale the virus into the air, and it can be carried considerable distances by the wind.

Many countries have had or are presently having problems with this serious disease; in the past decade there have been outbreaks in countries such as Great Britain, Ireland, Argentina, Brazil, and France. The only continents presently free of FMD are North America, Australia, and Antarctica. This disease was eliminated in the United States in 1929. South America has had FMD for a very long time; it is not a new disease. But care must be taken to make sure that it is not brought to North America again.

Some people confuse foot-and-mouth disease with bovine spongiform encephalopathy, often called "mad cow disease," but these two diseases are very different. FMD is not a human health or food-safety issue; it does not affect humans. It does, however, severely impact the health of livestock and could devastate our livestock industries if it ever comes into this country again. This is the reason for concern and for biosecurity measures to try to prevent the import of animals or animal products that might possibly bring this disease.

Preventing the Spread of FMD

FMD is very fast spreading. If one animal in a herd gets it, almost every animal in the exposed herd becomes sick, and many of the young animals die. The disease is highly contagious and can be spread by exposed animals, feeding utensils, vehicles, clothing, chutes and corrals, and other equipment contaminated with the virus. FMD is not a threat to humans, but people can carry the virus in their nasal passages for up to 28 hours. Thus anyone who has been in contact with the virus can spread it to susceptible animals.

The FMD virus can also be carried in raw meat, animal products, or milk from affected or exposed animals. A few years ago in Japan, where FMD had not occurred since 1908, the virus arrived on straw imported from China. An outbreak in South Africa began after food scraps containing raw meat were taken from an international ship anchored offshore and fed to a farmer's pigs.

Officials from the USDA fear that a traveler coming from an infected country will bring the disease here on clothing or footwear, or in meat, unpasteurized dairy products, or other food contaminated with the virus. Because the disease is so devastating to livestock production, the occurrence of even one case of FMD in a previously disease-free country results in an immediate ban on export trade from that country to the United States. And if the disease were to become active here, other countries would respond in kind.

Researchers at Plum Island Animal Disease Center (the US lab for foreign animal diseases), off the tip of Long Island, New York, try to monitor all FMD outbreaks around the world because there are different strains to contend with. Because this virus

---

International Travel Risks

Any travelers going to a country that has FMD must be very careful if they have occasion to visit a farm. They need to be aware that clothing, boots, and shoes can carry the virus. Someone visiting an area or attending an event where there are livestock may bring the disease home just by walking where cattle, goats, or other animals might have been.

Anyone coming from an FMD-infected foreign country to visit one of our farms or attend a livestock event may inadvertently bring us the disease. If people come to North America from infected countries, it's best if they haven't been on any livestock premises for at least 2 to 3 weeks before they visit a farm or attend a livestock event.

If you have foreign visitors, they should avoid all animal facilities in their own country before they come, launder all their clothes, and thoroughly clean their shoes by wiping them with a bleach solution (5 teaspoons [24.6 cc] of bleach in a gallon [3.8 L] of water) just prior to travel. After arrival here, they should avoid contact with livestock and wildlife for 5 days.

When they come to your farm, provide them with clean protective clothing and require them to wear it. They should wash their hands prior to entering any livestock facility. The virus is not long-lived, but it is very easily transported and transmitted.

---

can mutate and change, officials continue to make vaccines and keep them on hand in case of a catastrophic emergency. Vaccination is limited by the fact that there is no cross-protection from one type or subtype of the virus to another.

To prevent spread of the disease, the policy of most governments, including that of the United States, is to destroy all animals exposed to the virus. There is a vaccine for FMD, but its use is limited to outbreaks only. It just gives temporary protection for about 6 months. Any vaccinated animal must then be slaughtered before international trade can be resumed.

Symptoms

Affected animals may start showing signs within 24 to 48 hours of being exposed to the virus. FMD is characterized by fever and creates blisters and sores in the mouth, on the tongue and gums, and on the teats and between the toes, making it difficult for the animal to eat, drink, or walk. It causes mastitis in dairy cattle. When the symptomatic blisters break, the skin comes off the affected area. Hooves may fall off, and affected animals may lose weight rapidly. They can recover but remain severely debilitated, with poor performance.

No Treatment

Treatment is not attempted. In cooperation with Canada and Mexico, the United States has a vaccine bank. In the event of an outbreak in North America, 300,000 doses of vaccine can be sent immediately to an infected area and 2.5 million doses within 1 week, but the vaccine is only effective against certain types of the virus. Animals exposed to FMD can be vaccinated, then sent to be processed for human consumption, since there is no risk to humans.

Care should be taken when bringing food products into this country from other countries that have FMD, however. After slaughter the pH in muscle tissue drops enough to kill the virus, but it may still survive in organs and bone marrow. The last outbreak of FMD in Canada in 1952 was caused by sausage from Germany, fed to a hog in Canada. If a food product containing the virus is not heated sufficiently to kill the virus, it may be a potential source of infection for cloven-hoofed animals.

Mad Cow Disease

An aberrant (mutated) protein molecule called a *prion* causes mad cow disease or *bovine spongiform encephalopathy (BSE)*. The prion contains DNA and is highly resistant to chemical or physical agents that usually inactivate viruses. Boiling or freezing does not destroy the prion, and it survives for several years in dead tissues. Steam sterilization at a high temperature (269.6°F [132°C]) is required to totally destroy it. BSE belongs to a group of very slow-developing diseases, which include *scrapie* in sheep and goats, wasting disease in deer and elk, and transmissible encephalopathy in mink.

All of these related diseases are caused by a prion — a unique protein — rather than by viruses, bacteria, or other pathogens, and the body does not produce an immune or inflammatory reaction against it. In cattle the protein is almost always in the brain, spinal cord, and *retina* tissue (in the eye) of infected animals. It affects the central nervous system, causing

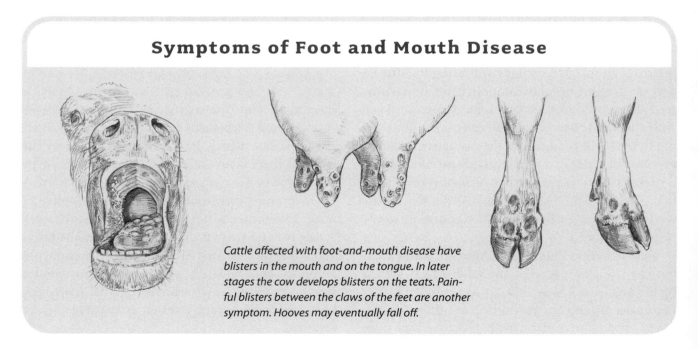

Symptoms of Foot and Mouth Disease

Cattle affected with foot-and-mouth disease have blisters in the mouth and on the tongue. In later stages the cow develops blisters on the teats. Painful blisters between the claws of the feet are another symptom. Hooves may eventually fall off.

nervous or aggressive behavior, abnormal posture, lack of coordination, and weakness. Typically the animal goes down and is unable to get up.

How BSE Is Spread

Cattle are exposed through consumption of contaminated feeds, which happens most readily if rendered animal parts (from animals with scrapie or BSE) have been used as a protein source in a feed mix. BSE is not contagious from animal to animal, and the prion causing it is not found in blood or muscle tissue. The main way an animal can get this disease is by ingesting brain and spinal cord tissue. This would never happen under natural conditions, but during the past century stockmen in many countries inadvertently made this transmission possible by feeding bone meal and other protein supplements derived from dead animals. Humans cannot get BSE from cows; however, humans that eat brain or spinal tissue from an infected animal may be at risk for Creutzfeldt-Jakob disease (CJD), which is similar to BSE.

Meat meal and bone meal are manufactured by the rendering industry from tissues discarded at slaughterhouses and from dead animals or those that are down and can't get up and have to be destroyed. Food value in these tissues and carcasses is often salvaged by rendering plants to utilize as a source of protein for livestock feeds. BSE first appeared in England and then spread to Europe because the UK continued to export feed containing tainted bone and meat meal.

BSE was first diagnosed in cattle in England in 1986 and developed into an epidemic by 1988, at which time the feeding of ruminant-derived protein sources was banned. BSE was found mainly in dairy cattle and only sporadically in beef cattle, probably because dairy calves are more commonly fed concentrate feeds that might contain bone meal. Other ungulates seem susceptible to BSE; it has been found in seven species of animals in zoos or wildlife parks in Great Britain after they were fed meat meal. The annual incidence of BSE cases in the UK peaked in 1992 and then began to decline. More than 170,000 cases had been reported in Great Britain by 1998. The reduction in cases after 1992 was attributed to the feed ban.

In 1989 the USDA banned importation of any cattle and feed from England or any other country with known cases of BSE, and efforts were made to trace and identify all cattle imported between 1981 and 1989. Of 499 cattle imported into the United States from England during that period, almost all were accounted for and examined, re-examined every 6 months, then checked for BSE when they were culled for slaughter. All were found to be free of BSE. The United States began testing for BSE in 1990 and was the first country to do so, even though BSE had never been found here.

In 1997 the ban on importations of cattle was expanded to include all European countries, whether or not BSE had been found in them. In August 1997 the U.S. Food and Drug Administration banned the use of ruminant-derived protein in the manufacture of feed products in the United States intended for cattle and other ruminants.

Eating Mad Cow Meat

It's still not certain if BSE in cattle can be transmitted to humans. There is fear that humans consuming animal products might later develop Creutzfeldt-Jakob disease. Even if this is the case, the prion causing BSE is only in brain, spinal cord, and eye tissues; meat from the animal is safe to consume.

Symptoms

It may take 2 to 8 years after the animal is exposed for signs of BSE to become apparent. The abnormal protein slowly and silently travels through various tissues and lymph glands before the brain is affected. The changes in the brain and the onset of symptoms occur at about the same time. The long incubation period makes it difficult to know how the animal became infected. Once signs appear, however, the animal will generally deteriorate within 2 weeks to 6 months and then die.

The animal shows a change in temperament, behavior, posture, and gait, becoming progressively uncoordinated. Nervousness, hypersensitivity to sound and touch, weight loss, drop in milk yield, and reluctance to go into a barn or pass through a gate are typical signs. The animal may be disoriented and stare at imaginary objects. Ears and muscles may twitch. If the head or neck is touched, the animal may throw her head sideways or give a vigorous shake of the head and neck. She may avoid other animals by leaving the herd or become aggressive and charge at herdmates or humans when confined. Soon the hind legs become weak, with a shortened stride or swaying gait, knuckling, stumbling, or falling, especially when turning. The animal becomes progressively weaker and eventually can't get up.

Since BSE affects the central nervous system, animals act in strange ways, and this may be mistaken as a symptom of rabies (chapter 5). Today, most animals checked for rabies are also screened for BSE. Diagnosis for both diseases is made by postmortem examination of brain tissue. For diagnosing sheep, one test uses a biopsy from the third eyelid of live sheep to identify incubating scrapie. Lymph nodes are affected before the brain in sheep, but this is not the case with cattle.

Prevention

There is no treatment. Even though symptoms may be variable, the disease is always fatal. The best prevention is to make sure livestock are never given feeds or supplements that contain animal parts. There is a ban in the United States on manufacture or sale of these types of feeds.

In order to protect human health in Great Britain, suspect animals (and their milk) are not allowed as human food. Certain tissues (brain, spinal cord, eyes, tonsil, thymus, spleen, and intestines) from slaughtered animals over 6 months of age are prohibited for use as human food.

In countries that do not have BSE, such as the United States, officials have found that the best preventive measure to ensure the safety of the meat supply is to ban imports of live animals and animal products from any country that has BSE. They have also enacted policies that ensure the elimination of rendered products in cattle feed. In the US, cattle that die with suspicious symptoms are tested for accurate diagnosis and differentiation between BSE and other neurological diseases.

The average stockman generally doesn't worry about foreign-animal diseases, but in our global economy the symptoms and effects of these maladies must be kept in the backs of our minds so that we can quickly address any problem that arises.

Testing for Mad Cow Disease

Testing for BSE focuses mainly on cattle 30 months of age and older who exhibit behavior that might be caused by neurological disease and any "downer" cattle that cannot get up. Animals younger than 30 months of age that are sent to slaughter are considered free from BSE because there has not been enough time elapsed for this disease to affect the brain and spinal cord tissue. There is no way their body parts could transmit BSE.

Epilogue

Cattle are strong and hardy, yet vulnerable to a wide variety of ailments and diseases. As their caretaker, you can usually prevent most health problems by conscientious management and care. Diligent observation will help you to know your animals' personality traits and recognize their normal behavior, and can also enable you to know, early on, when one of them encounters a problem.

I have tried to learn all I could about cattle care in times of both health and illness in the herd and for individual animals. This education has been ongoing, since the cattle are always teaching me something new. Anyone who owns cattle has the same opportunity for "continuing education" in the art and science of cattle health care. It is my hope that this book will serve as a helpful reference tool along the way.

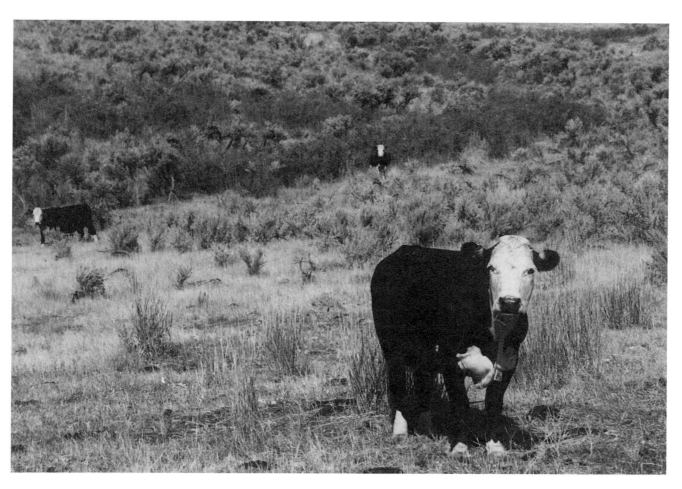

Appendixes

A. Determining Age of Cattle by the Teeth

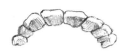

AT BIRTH TO 1 MONTH
Two or more of the temporary incisor teeth are present at birth. Within the first month, you can fully see the 8 temporary incisors.

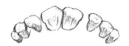

2 YEARS
As a long-yearling, the animal's central pair of temporary incisor teeth is replaced by the permanent incisors. At 2 years, the central permanent incisors are fully developed.

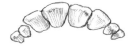

2½ YEARS
The animal cuts his permanent first intermediates, one on each side of the centrals. Usually, these are fully developed at 3 years.

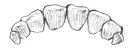

3½ YEARS
The animal cuts his second intermediates or laterals. They are level with the first intermediates and begin to wear at 4 years.

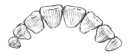

4½ YEARS
The immature corner teeth are replaced by permanent versions.

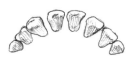

5 OR 6 YEARS
The animal usually has the full complement of incisors, with fully developed corners. The permanent centrals are leveled, both pairs of intermediates are partially leveled, and the corner incisors show wear.

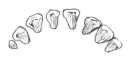

7 TO 10 YEARS
At 7 or 8 years, the centrals show noticeable wear; at 8 or 9 years, the middle pairs show noticeable wear; and at 10 years, the corner teeth show noticeable wear.

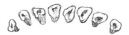

12 YEARS
The arch is nearly straight. The teeth are triangular, distinctly separated, and show wearing to stubs. These conditions become more obvious as the animal gets older.

B. Disease Characteristics

Many diseases have symptoms that are similar to other types of illness, which can make diagnosis confusing. You should always have your veterinarian help you arrive at a proper diagnosis, but it is helpful to be aware of various possibilities when confronted with a specific symptom, such as labored breathing, fever, or diarrhea.

DISEASES CHARACTERIZED BY RESPIRATORY DISTRESS	
DISEASE	**DESCRIPTION**
Anaphylactic shock	Severe allergic reaction
Brisket disease	Pulmonary and heart failure, high altitudes
Diphtheria	Bacterial infection in throat
Emphysema	Fluid in lungs due to change from dry to green feed
Infectious bovine rhinotracheitis (IBR)	Viral disease of respiratory tract
Nitrate poisoning	Reduction in oxygen-carrying capacity of blood
Pneumonia	Lung infection

DISEASES CHARACTERIZED BY DIARRHEA

DISEASE	DESCRIPTION
Bovine viral diarrhea (BVD)	Mucosal BVD impairs digestive-tract function
Coccidiosis	Protozoal infection in intestine
E. coli scours	Highly infectious disease of young calves
Indigestion	Disruption of microbes in rumen
Internal parasites	Heavy worm loads damage intestine
Johne's disease	Chronic bacterial disease with weight loss
Salmonellosis	Bacterial disease; may also cause septicemia

DISEASES CHARACTERIZED BY NERVOUS SYSTEM DISORDERS

DISEASE	DESCRIPTION
Botulism	Acute bacterial disease that usually kills the animal
Grass tetany	Metabolic disorder caused by magnesium shortage
Lead poisoning	Brain damage, blind staggers
Listeriosis	Bacterial; "circling disease"
Polioencephalomalacia	Thiamine deficiency and brain swelling
Rabies	Viral; abnormal behavior, coma and death
Salt poisoning	Abnormal behavior, staggering
Thromboembolic meningoencephalitis	Affects brain

DISEASES CHARACTERIZED BY FEVER

DISEASE	DESCRIPTION
Anaplasmosis	Rickettsia; spread by insects, causes anemia
Anthrax	Bacterial; highly fatal
Blackleg	*Clostridia* bacteria in young animals, highly fatal
Bluetongue	Viral; causes ulcers on tongue and skin
Bovine viral diarrhea (BVD)	Viral; causes abortion, diarrhea
Diphtheria	Bacterial; affects mouth and throat, usually calves
Infectious bovine rhinotracheitis (IBR)	Viral, respiratory
Leptospirosis	Bacterial; affects kidneys, causes abortion
Listeriosis	Bacterial; affects brain
Lyme disease	Bacterial; spread by ticks, causes lameness
Malignant edema	Clostridial bacterium; wound entry, highly fatal
Navel ill/joint ill	Bacterial; may cause septicemia and lameness
Pasteurellosis (shipping fever)	Bacterial; respiratory
Redwater	Clostridial bacterium; fatal
Salmonellosis	Bacterial; diarrhea (mainly in calves)
Tetanus	Clostridial bacterium; wound entrance, affects brain
Thromboembolic meningoencephalitis	Bacterial; affects brain
Vesicular stomatitis	Viral; affects mouth and teats

C. Anatomy of the Cow

RIGHT SIDE

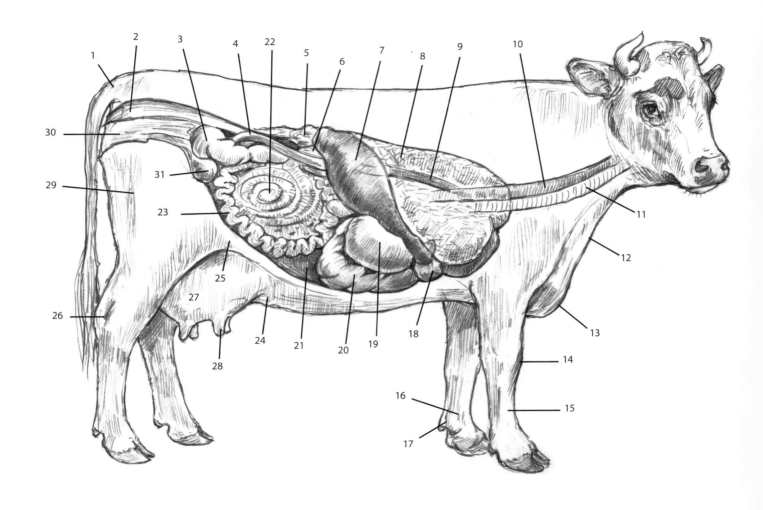

1 tail head		**17** dewclaw	
2 rectum		**18** reticulum	
3 cecum		**19** omasum	
4 duodenum		**20** abomasum	
5 right kidney		**21** rumen	
6 pancreas		**22** colon	
7 liver		**23** intestines	
8 right lung		**24** milk vein	
9 aorta		**25** flank	
10 esophagus		**26** hock	
11 trachea		**27** udder	
12 brisket		**28** teat	
13 dewlap		**29** buttock	
14 knee		**30** vagina	
15 cannon bone		**31** bladder	
16 fetlock joint			

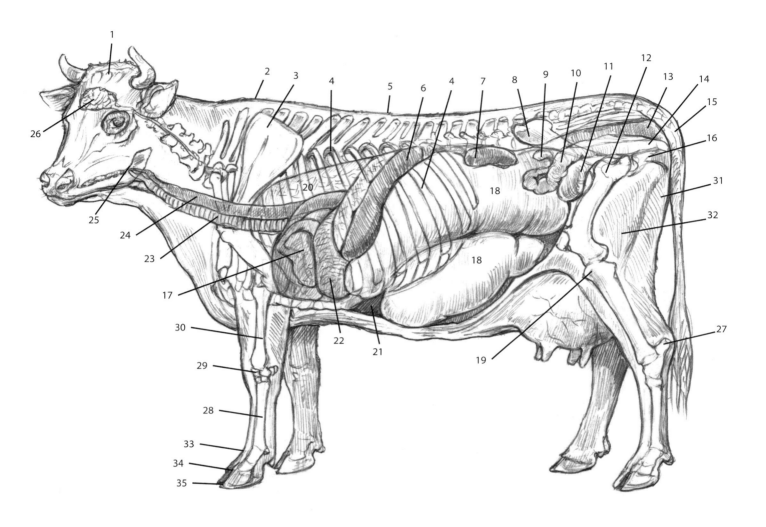

1	poll	19	stifle joint
2	withers	20	left lung
3	shoulder	21	abomasum
4	ribs	22	recticulum
5	back	23	trachea (windpipe)
6	spleen	24	esophagus
7	kidney	25	larynx and pharynx
8	hipbone	26	brain
9	left ovary	27	point of hock
10	uterus	28	cannon bone
11	bladder	29	knee
12	hip joint	30	forearm
13	rectum	31	buttocks
14	vagina	32	thigh
15	tail head	33	pastern
16	pin bone	34	coronary band
17	heart	35	toe (claw)
18	rumen		

D. Reproductive Tract of a Bull

1 backbone
2 rectum
3 anus
4 urinary bladder
5 seminal vesicular gland
6 prostate
7 balbo cavernosus muscle
8 spermatic cord
9 vas deferens
10 distal sigmoid flexure of penis
11 retractor penis muscle
12 head of epididymis
13 body of epididymis
14 tail of epididymis
15 testis (testicle)
16 glans penis

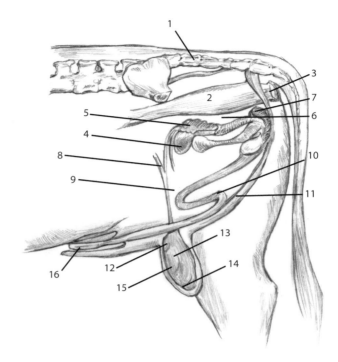

E. Illnesses That Can Be Passed from Cattle to Humans

Anthrax is a rare, but highly fatal, bacterial disease transmitted when humans handle infected or dead cattle, or come in contact with bacterial spores.

Brucellosis (Bang's Disease) causes undulant fever in humans and in 1954 the federal government, individual US states, and livestock producers began a program to eradicate this bacterial disease in US cattle, and to keep it from being imported with foreign animals. Among other symptoms, the disease causes rising and falling fever, sweats, muscle weakness, and fatigue. Today most states are free of the disease.

Cowpox is a skin disease that is transmitted from animals to human handlers via contact with infected udders. Humans develop small red blisters and are immune to smallpox after recovery.

Cryptosporidiosis is a protozoal disease that causes diarrhea in calves and humans.

Leptospirosis is a bacterial disease that causes "seven day fever" and Weil's disease in humans. Symptoms include enlargement of the spleen, jaundice, and nephritis. It is commonly transmitted when water contaminated with infected animal urine comes in contact with breaks in human skin.

Rabies is a fatal viral disease spread to humans via infected animal saliva.

Ringworm, a fungal infection named after the typically ringlike appearance of the condition on the skin of humans and animals.

Salmonella is a bacterial disease that causes diarrhea and "food poisoning" symptoms in humans.

Tuberculosis can be brought into the US with infected cattle and spread to humans via milk and animal respiratory discharge. There are well-established federal regulations, which seek to control and eradicate this bacterial disease that lodges in the lungs of both cattle and humans.

Vesicular Stomatitis is a flu-like viral disease transmitted when humans fail to follow proper biosafety methods around sick cattle or horses.

Glossary

A

abomasum. True stomach (fourth stomach) of a ruminant animal.

abortion. Expulsion of embryo or fetus before it is mature enough to be viable outside the uterus.

abscess. Accumulation of pus in infected tissue.

acetonemia. *See* ketosis (acetonemia).

acidosis. Change in the acid-base balance of the body, in which the tissues become too acidic. Also, digestive disorder caused by rapid production and absorption of acid in the rumen, from overfeeding on grain.

Actinomyces bovis. A type of bacteria that causes bony lump jaw.

Actinomyces pyogenes. A type of pus-forming bacteria that often causes abscesses in mouth and cheek tissues.

actinomycosis. Bony lump jaw; an infection that settles in the jawbone.

active immunity. Defense created by the immune system in response to an antigen (in contrast to passive immunity from an outside source).

acute. Appearing quickly and severely.

adjuvants. Aluminum hydroxide, oil, or other chemicals and substances added to a vaccine to enhance its effectiveness.

adrenal gland. One of two ductless glands sitting atop each kidney, secreting a number of hormones, including adrenalin and cortisol.

adrenalin. *See* epinephrine.

aerosol. A substance sprayed into the air.

aflatoxin. Toxic compound produced by *Aspergillus* fungi.

AI. *See* artificial insemination (AI).

AIP (atypical intestinal pneumonia). *See* emphysema.

albendazole. Oral deworming drug that also kills liver flukes.

alfalfa. Legume forage plant often used as hay; when harvested at optimum time, alfalfa hay contains more protein (as well as more of certain vitamins and minerals) than grass hay.

alkali disease. "Bob-tail disease"; loss of tail, hoofs, and other parts due to selenium toxicity.

alkaline. Base (as opposed to acid); caustic substance that has a pH of more than 7.

alkaloid. Compound of plant origin with druglike properties; many alkaloids are toxic.

ammonia. Alkaline gas with sharp odor that stings the eyes and nose.

amprolium. *See* Corid (amprolium).

anaphylaxis. Acute hypersensitivity reaction that may lead to collapse and death.

anaplasmosis. Protozoan disease that affects red blood cells, spread by biting flies or by use of hypodermic needles or surgical instruments on more than one animal without sterilizing them; also called yellow fever.

anemia. Shortage of red blood cells.

anthrax. Acute disease acquired by ingestion of bacterial spores from infected pastures or carcasses. It can also be spread to humans by contact with infected animals or their discharges.

antibiotic. Chemical substance produced by a microorganism that has the ability to kill or inhibit the growth of other microorganisms.

antibodies. Protein molecules in the blood or lymph system that fight a specific antigen.

antidote. A remedy for counteracting a poison.

antigen. Any foreign substance invading the body that stimulates production of protective antibodies.

antihistamine. A drug that counteracts the action of histamine in the body, usually given to help reverse an allergic reaction.

anti-inflammatory. Medication to relieve pain, swelling, fever, and inflammation.

antimicrobial. Drug used to combat microbe pathogens.

antioxidant. Element of diet such as vitamin A or E or selenium that protects body cells from damage during the metabolic processes that produce energy (oxidation).

antiseptic. Disinfectant; substance that inhibits the growth and development of microorganisms.

antitoxin. Antibody that counteracts a bacterial toxin.

antivenin. Antiserum containing antibodies against specific poisons in the venom of a biting animal or insect.

anus. Rectal opening through which feces pass.

A180. An antibiotic product similar to Baytril (enrofloxacin).

arachnid. Arthropod with four pairs of walking legs, such as spiders, mites, and ticks.

artery. Blood vessel delivering blood to the body (pulsing with every beat of the heart).

arthritis. Inflammation of a joint.

arthropod. Invertebrate animal with segmented body and jointed legs, such as insects and spiders.

artificial insemination (AI). Inserting semen (collected from a bull) into the cow's uterus via a pipette.

aspergillis. Type of mold on feed or forage plants that can be pathogenic, often causing abortion in pregnant cows.

aspiration pneumonia. Infection of the lungs caused by irritation from fluid or foreign material, such as milk, feed, or medication given by drench, getting into the windpipe and down to the lungs, enabling pathogens to become established.

atropine. Poisonous alkaloid (belladonna) found in deadly nightshade, sometimes used medicinally in certain conditions or as an antidote for other poisons.

atypical interstitial pneumonia (AIP). See emphysema.

autogenous vaccine. Vaccine produced using antigens from the animal's own body.

avermectin. Chemical produced by soil microbes, effective against parasites (internal and external) that feed on blood. Includes the ivermectin and moxidectin classes of endectocides.

B

bacteremia. Presence of bacteria in the bloodstream.

bacteria. One-celled organisms that sometimes cause disease.

bacterin. Killed bacterial product that stimulates immunity against a specific type of bacteria.

bacteriocidal. A drug that kills bacteria.

bacteriostatic. A drug that hinders bacterial growth.

balling gun. Long-handled tool for placing a bolus or pill at the back of the throat for a cow to swallow.

Banamine (flunixin meglumine). Nonsteroidal anti-inflammatory drug, given to reduce pain, inflammation, and fever.

Bang's disease. See brucellosis.

Baytril (enrofloxacin). Antibiotic for cattle, often used in treating respiratory disease.

BCS (body condition score). See body condition.

benign. Harmless, such as a slow-growing tumor that remains localized.

bicarbonate. Alkalizing agent, often used to reverse acidosis.

biopsy. Tissue sample to examine, generally under a microscope, for help in diagnosis.

biosecurity. Protecting the animals on a farm or ranch from outside diseases by minimizing exposure to other animals with use of quarantine measures, fence maintenance, and immunization.

biotin. One of the B vitamins, important to healthy hoof horn.

biotype. A variant strain of a bacterial or viral species, differing in its identifiable physiologic characteristics from the other strains.

bismuth. A metal, the salts of which are astringent, antacid, and mildly germicidal; often used in treating diarrhea.

biting lice. Tiny external parasites that feed on the skin; also called chewing lice.

black disease. A highly fatal clostridial disease of cattle.

blackflies. Small gnatlike flies that feed on cattle.

blackleg. Highly fatal disease of young cattle, caused by a clostridial bacterium.

bladder stone. See calculi, urinary.

blister beetle. Small flying insect that feeds on legume blossoms, coming into alfalfa fields in swarms. Certain species have high levels of toxin in their bodies, which can cause indigestion or fatal poisoning of animals that consume dead beetles in hay.

bloat. Distension of the rumen with gas or frothy fluid.

blood glucose. Blood sugar.

blood poisoning. Infection that gets into the bloodstream.

blue nose disease. See photosensitization.

bluetongue. Viral disease of ruminants, transmitted by biting gnats.

B lymphocyte. A type of white blood cell responsible for humoral immunity; precursors of antibody-producing cells.

bob-tail disease. Selenium toxicity, resulting in loss of tail or hoofs.

body condition. Amount of flesh covering. The standard scale for measuring body condition of cattle is 1 to 9, with 1 being emaciated and 9 being obese. Optimum body condition for good health and reproduction is BCS (body condition score) 5 or 6.

bolus. Soft ball of chewed food or a large, oblong pill.

bomb fly. Gadfly or warble fly that lays eggs on the hairs of cattle; the hatching larvae penetrate the skin and migrate to the back, where they overwinter under the skin.

bony lump jaw. Infection that settles in the jawbone.

booster. Another dose of vaccine, to stimulate the immune system to build an immune response — to increase or renew the effect of an earlier injection.

Bos indicus. Humpbacked cattle from India, Asia, and Africa.

Bos taurus. Species of cattle originating in Europe.

bottle jaw. Edema (fluid) between the lower jawbones, which causes swelling beneath the lower jaw.

botulism. Toxic condition affecting the nervous system of animals that eat feed contaminated with *Clostridium botulinum*.

bovine leukemia. Disease in which the animal has an abnormally high white-blood-cell count, with many immature cells. *See also* lymphosarcoma.

bovine leukosis. *See* bovine leukemia.

bovine respiratory disease (BRD). Disease syndrome that may be a combination of viral and bacterial infection; also called shipping fever.

bovine respiratory syncytial virus (BRSV). Respiratory virus that causes severe, acute respiratory disease, mainly in young cattle.

bovine spongiform encephalopathy (BSE). "Mad cow" disease; slow developing disease that affects the brain, caused by a prion (aberrant protein) rather than a virus or bacterium and transmitted by feeding ruminant animal parts containing brain and spinal tissue to other ruminants.

bovine viral diarrhea (BVD). Viral disease that causes numerous problems, including abortion, damage to the digestive tract and immune system, and calf deformities.

brackenfern. A type of fern that causes poisoning when eaten

brain stem. Stalklike base of the brain connecting with the spinal cord.

Brahman. Breed of zebu (*Bos indicus*) cattle.

BRD. *See* bovine respiratory disease (BRD).

brisket. Area between the front legs, covering the front of the breastbone.

brisket disease. Lung insufficiency and right-heart failure that affects some cattle at high altitudes, resulting in edema (swelling) of the brisket.

broad-spectrum antibiotic. Drug effective against both gram-negative and gram-positive bacteria.

broken mouth. Condition in which some of the front teeth are missing.

bronchial tubes. Two main branches of the trachea (windpipe) that each enter a lung and then split into smaller branches.

brown stomach worm. Internal parasite that lives in the abomasum and small intestine of cattle.

BRSV. *See* bovine respiratory syncytial virus (BRSV).

brucellosis. Bacterial infection resulting in abortion; also called Bang's disease.

BSE. *See* bovine spongiform encephalopathy (BSE).

buffalo gnat. Small fly that feeds on cattle.

burdock. Tall plant with burrs that stick to hair and clothing; the tiny seed "slivers" from shattered burrs can cause eye inflammation if they get caught under an eyelid.

BVD. *See* bovine viral diarrhea (BVD).

C

cake. Hard, painful swelling in the udder before calving.

calcium. One of the major minerals needed by the body, which must be supplied in feed.

calculi, urinary. Bladder stones or kidney stones, formed when certain minerals in the urine precipitate out of solution and clump together.

calf table. Small "chute" for calves that can be tipped after the calf is caught by the head, restraining the calf in a lying-down position at a level that makes it easy to work on him for branding, vaccinating, castrating, and dehorning.

campylobacteriosis. *See* vibriosis.

cancer. Any malignant growth or tumor due to abnormal division of body cells.

cannon bones. Bones between knee (or hock) and fetlock joint.

cannula. A tube or catheter that is inserted into a blood vessel or body cavity to hold it (or a hole into it) open.

cantharadin. Lethal toxin found in blister beetles.

capillary. Smallest blood vessel; capillaries connect the small branch ends of arteries and veins. Their semipermeable membranes facilitate interchange of fluid and other substances between the blood and the body tissues.

carcinoma. Malignant growth in epithelial tissue that lines an internal or external body surface.

carotene. Yellow pigment present in many plant and animal tissues, stored in the liver, to be converted to vitamin A.

carrier. An animal that appears healthy but harbors pathogens or parasites that can be shed or passed to other animals. Also, fluid or substance that keeps a vaccine stable.

cast. Held down on the ground, unable to get up.

castor oil. Thick oil from castor beans, used as a laxative and purgative.

castrate. To remove the testicles of a male animal.

cataract. Opacity on the lens of the eye that impairs vision.

catheter. A flexible tube inserted into the body or into a vein to withdraw or insert fluid.

cellular immunity. Cell-mediated immunity facilitated by T lymphocytes that recognize and destroy altered or damaged cells.

cephalosporin. Broad-spectrum antibiotic, related to penicillin in structure and mode of action; destroys the cell walls of bacteria that have cell walls.

cerebrocortical necrosis. *See* polioencephalomalacia.

cerebrospinal fluid. Fluid surrounding the brain and spinal cord.

cerebrum. The front part of the brain.

cervix. The opening between uterus and vagina. In the cow it remains closed and sealed except when she is in heat or giving birth to her calf.

chaff. Small piece of hay or straw.

chelated. Combined; a chemical compound in which a metallic ion is firmly bound into the chelating molecule. Mineral supplements for cattle often contain chelated products that make the mineral more available to the body as a nutrient.

chewing lice. *See* biting lice.

Chlamydia. A certain type of gram-negative bacteria that multiplies only within the host body cell.

chlorhexidine. General disinfectant solution (Nolvasan).

chlorophyll. Green coloring matter in plants that produces food energy via photosynthesis.

chlortetracycline. Broad-spectrum antibiotic.

choke. To have an obstruction at the back of the throat.

chokecherry. Shrub or tree (wild cherry), the leaves of which may contain poisonous hydrocyanic (prussic) acid when damaged by frost or wilted.

Chorioptes. A type of mange mite.

chronic. Persisting for a long time.

chronic pneumonia polyarthritis syndrome (CPPS). A combination of pneumonia and septic arthritis due to infection with *Mycoplasma bovis*.

chute. Facility for restraining cattle. A running chute is a narrow alley where cattle are restrained single file, usually with a squeeze chute at the end for individual restraint.

cilia. Tiny hairlike structures lining the windpipe, moving in waves to sweep pathogens and foreign material up to the back of the throat to be swallowed or coughed out.

circling disease. *See* listeriosis.

CL. *See* corpus luteum (CL).

cleft palate. Birth defect consisting of a hole in the roof of the mouth and the bottom of the nostril; often due to exposure to toxic alkaloids in lupine ingested by the dam in early pregnancy.

clinical signs. Evidence of illness; obvious symptoms.

closed herd. A term for a herd with no new cattle coming onto the farm.

clostridial. A term used to describe a group of fatal diseases caused by various species of spore-forming clostridial bacteria (which include blackleg, malignant edema, black disease, redwater, enterotoxemia, tetanus) that can survive indefinitely in the environment.

coccidia. Pathogenic protozoa that cause coccidiosis.

coccidiosis. Intestinal disease and diarrhea caused by a certain type of pathogenic protozoan.

coccidiostat. Drug that inhibits multiplication of coccidia.

coccobacillus. Oval-shaped bacterium.

cocklebur. Low-growing plant with oblong burrs that stick to hair and clothing. The plant can be toxic if eaten by livestock.

colic. Acute abdominal pain.

colostrum. First milk after a cow calves, containing high-energy fat and antibodies that give temporary protection against disease.

coma. Deep unconsciousness that often precedes death.

comatose. In a coma.

composite. "Breed" or type of cow created by mixing two or more breeds in a uniform system so that all the individuals of that breeding system are similar in characteristics.

conceptus. The new living creature, from the time of fertilization of the egg until birth.

conduction. Movement of heat from an animal to a cooler solid surface, such as the ground.

congenital. Acquired before birth, such as a birth defect.

conjunctiva. Membrane covering the eye; also, the inner lining of the eyelid.

conjunctivitis. Inflammation of the conjunctiva, the membrane lining the inner eyelid and eyeball.

convection. Movement of air over the body, taking body heat with it.

convulsion. Seizure; involuntary spasms or muscle contractions.

copper. Trace mineral, important in diet; crucial to a healthy immune system.

Corid (amprolium). A drug used for prevention or treatment of coccidiosis.

cornea. Transparent outer covering of the front part of the eye.

coronary band. Fleshy tissue just above the hoof at the hairline, where horn-growing cells produce new hoof tissue.

coronavirus. Virus that causes diarrhea in young calves.

corpus luteum (CL). Glandular mass that forms on the ovary in the spot where a follicle has matured and ovulated. The CL produces progesterone and keeps the cow from coming back into heat.

corticosteroid. Adrenal hormone. Synthetic steroids are often used as anti-inflammatory drugs.

cortisol. Hormonal steroid produced by the adrenal glands during stress, regulating the immune system and affecting metabolism.

cowpox. Related to smallpox; now eradicated in the United States; also called milkmaid's disease.

CPPS. *See* chronic pneumonia polyarthritis syndrome (CPPS)

critical temperature. The temperature below which an animal must increase its rate of heat production to stay warm, needing more food to do so.

crossbred. Animal created by crossing two or more breeds.

cryosurgery. Killing and removal of tissue by freezing.

cryptosporidia. Pathogenic protozoan that causes cryptosporidiosis.

cryptosporidiosis. Protozoal disease that causes diarrhea in calves and humans.

cud. Wad of partly digested food, burped up by a ruminant to be more thoroughly chewed.

cull cows. Cows removed from the herd and sold due to poor production, infertility, or some other problem.

culture. Growth of microorganisms in a laboratory.

cutaneous angiomatosis. A type of skin cancer resulting in small lesions along the cow's back that tend to bleed readily.

cyanide. A highly toxic poison.

cyanogenic glycosides. Compounds found in certain plants and shrubs; toxic to cattle when converted to hydrocyanic acid or cyanide when the plant is damaged.

cyst. Fluid-filled lump of tissue, often containing a parasite larva.

cysticercoid. Infective form of tapeworm egg.

cytopathic. Viral strain of BVD that can alter and kill tissue cells in the body, as opposed to noncytopathic strains that infect but do not kill cells and remain longer in the body.

D

dally. To wrap a rope around something rather than tie it.

dam. Mother of a calf.

death camus. Poisonous plant found on arid rangelands.

Deccox (decoquinate). Drug used as a treatment or preventive for coccidiosis.

deerfly. Large fly with painful bite that feeds on blood; closely related to horseflies.

dehydration. Shortage of fluid in body tissues.

demodectic. A type of mange mite that lives within the hair follicle.

dental pad. Hard pad at the top and front of the mouth of ruminant animals, against which the lower incisors press for eating and biting, since these animals have no top incisors.

dermatitis. Inflammation of the skin.

dewclaw. Vestigial digit; horny protuberance at the back of the lower leg, behind the fetlock joint.

dewlap. Flap of skin hanging below the brisket.

dexamethasone. Synthetic steroidal anti-inflammatory drug.

dextrose. Simple sugar, often given to sick calves or cows as a source of instant energy.

diaphragm. Strong muscle used in breathing that separates the chest cavity from the abdominal cavity.

diarrhea. Loose, watery feces.

digits. Toes.

diluent. A diluting agent.

dimethyl sulfoxide (DMSO). Powerful solvent used in veterinary medicine as a topical anti-inflammatory and also for certain conditions in which tissue swelling must be reduced, such as snakebite and diphtheria.

diphtheria. Bacterial disease causing swelling in mouth or throat; also called necrotic laryngitis.

diuretic. Drug that draws fluid from body tissues.

DMSO. *See* dimethyl sulfoxide (DMSO).

dose syringe. Syringe for administering oral fluid medication.

downer cow. A cow that can't get up.

Draxxin (tulathromycin). Antibiotic product that lasts 8 to 10 days in the tissues; often used for treating respiratory disease.

drench. To administer fluid or medication via the mouth, forcing the animal to swallow it.

dry. A term used to refer to a cow that has weaned or lost her calf; not lactating.

dumb rabies. A form of rabies in which the animal is lethargic and uncoordinated.

dummy calves. Calves that are lethargic and "retarded" at birth, due to oxygen shortage during the birth process or to disease.

dung beetle. Beetle that lives in and feeds on manure.

E

ear notch. Small skin sample taken from the ear to send in for testing for certain diseases, such as BVD.

E. coli (Escherichia coli). A type of bacteria that causes disease in cattle, including scours in newborn calves.

edema. Swelling; fluid in the tissues

elastrator. Tool for putting a strong rubber band or ring up over the testicles, to constrict the tissue above them and halt blood flow to them; used for castrating calves.

electrolyte. Part of a salt that disperses in water, breaking into its separate ions, which conduct electricity; part of the normal makeup of body fluids.

ELISA. *See* enzyme-linked immunosorbant assay test.

embryo. Conceptus in early stages of development, up to 45 days of pregnancy.

emphysema. Impairment of the lungs due to breakdown of the small air sacs, caused by an allergic reaction to a certain compound created in the rumen from an amino acid found in lush green forage. Most often occurs when animals are moved abruptly from dry forage to lush green pasture.

encephalitis. Inflammation of the brain.

encysted. Enclosed in a sac or cyst.

endectocide. Product effective against both internal and external parasites.

endemic. Always present in a geographic area or population.

endophyte. A plant that lives within another plant, such as a fungus living inside the cells of a grass plant.

endotoxemia. Endotoxins in the bloodstream.

endotoxin. Toxin produced by the outer covering of certain gram-negative bacteria as they die, including various bacteria that cause severe diarrhea and sometimes shock.

enteric. Pertaining to the small intestine.

enzyme-linked immunosorbant assay (ELISA) test. Laboratory test used to measure or detect an antigen or antibody.

enterotoxemia. Inflammation or infection caused by bacterial toxins in the intestine. The term often refers to disease caused by *C. perfringens.*

enzymes. Complex protein molecules that promote biochemical reactions in other substances.

epidemic. Sudden outbreak of disease, with the number of cases much higher than what would normally be expected.

epinephrine. Hormone released in response to stress; synthetic preparations are used in cattle to help reverse effects of shock or severe allergic reactions to injections; adrenalin.

epithelial cells. Cells that form a covering layer, such as skin.

ergot. Type of toxic fungus that grows on certain grasses and grain plants in wet conditions; ingestion impairs blood circulation to the extremities.

ergovaline. Toxic alkaloid produced by a fungus that lives within the cells of fescue grasses.

Escherichia coli. *See E. coli.*

esophageal feeder. Metal or plastic probe tube inserted into the mouth and down the throat and esophagus, with a container attached for holding fluid; used for force-feeding baby calves.

esophageal groove. Fold of tissue that routes milk directly to the true stomach, bypassing the rumen, when a calf nurses the cow.

esophagus. Passage between the mouth and stomach.

Excede. Ceftiofur; antibiotic product often used for respiratory disease; has a long-lasting effectiveness.

exotoxin. Toxin created while bacteria are still alive, produced as they multiply.

extra label. Off-label use; using a product in a manner not specified on the label (different dosage, different timing, or in a different species than intended).

F

face fly. A type of fly that feeds on eye secretions and spreads pinkeye bacteria from cow to cow.

false negative. Test result that comes up negative even though the animal does, indeed, have the disease. Conversely, a false positive is a test result that indicates a disease condition when the disease is not present.

false sole. Separation (by infection) of the layers of the sole, as an abscess travels under the surface.

fecal sample. Sample of manure to test for presence of pathogens or parasites.

feces. Manure.

feeding efficiency. The amount of feed it takes to maintain or put weight on an animal. Some animals are more feed efficient than others, taking less feed to gain the same amount of weight.

fenbendazole. White-paste oral deworming drug.

fescue. Group of grasses, some species of which are popular pasture grasses, in spite of the fact that a high percentage of the most popular variety is infected with an endophyte fungus toxic to livestock.

fescue foot. Lameness and swelling due to loss of blood circulation to the foot, caused by effects of fescue toxicity.

fescue toxicosis. Term covering all the toxic effects in cattle that consume endophyte-infected fescue grass.

fetlock joint. Joint at the end of the lower leg bone, just above the pastern, with dewclaws at the rear.

fetus. Unborn calf, from 45 days of gestation (when the embryo becomes a fetus) until birth.

fever. Body temperature above normal.

flank. Rear part of the abdomen and belly, just ahead of the hind leg and above the udder.

flanking. Putting a calf on the ground by lifting him by the flank skin and front leg to get him off his feet.

flexor tendons. The major tendons at the back of the lower leg, which flex the joints.

fluorescein dye. A harmless dye put into the eye to help locate any scratches or ulcerations on the surface of the eye.

fluoroquinolone. A type of broad-spectrum antibiotic that includes floroxacin and ciprofloxacin.

FMD. *See* foot and mouth disease (FMD).

foggage. British term for lush pasture-grass regrowth.

foot and mouth disease (FMD). Highly contagious and very serious foreign-animal disease, caused by a virus, that affects cloven-hoofed animals, causing blisters in the mouth and on teats and feet and sometimes loss of the feet.

foothill abortion. Disease spread by ticks in certain areas of the West; causes abortion in cows.

foot rot. Acute bacterial infection in the foot; causes severe pain and lameness.

forceps. An instrument with two blades and a handle, used to grasp tissues during a surgical operation.

founder. Damaged hoof wall and dropped sole due to inflammation of the hoof attachments; laminitis.

full mouth. A mouth with no teeth missing.

fungi. Group of primitive plants that includes molds and yeasts, some of which can cause disease.

fungicide. Chemical that kills fungi.

furious rabies. Form of rabies in which the animal is aggressive.

Fusobacterium necrophorum. Type of bacteria that causes foot rot, diphtheria, liver abscesses, and navel ill.

G

gadding. Frenzied activity of cattle when trying to evade heel flies or gadflies.

gadfly. *See* bomb fly.

gangrene. Death and decomposition of body tissues due to lack of blood circulation.

genotype. The type species of a genus; a term used in describing a certain type within a bacterial genus and species, for instance.

gentian violet. Purple skin-tinting medication with antifungal and antibiotic properties; sometimes added to topical pinkeye treatments or used to treat skin disease.

gestation. Pregnancy; period of development of the conceptus — from the time of conception until birth.

girth. Circumference of the body just behind the front legs.

glucose. Dextrose; blood sugar, the main source of energy in the body.

glycerin. A clear, syrupy, slippery fluid.

gnat. Small, two-winged biting fly.

goiter. Enlarged thyroid gland.

gram-negative bacteria. Bacteria with thin (or no) cell walls.

gram-positive bacteria. Bacteria with thick, well-defined cell walls.

granuloma. Small nodule.

grass staggers. *See* grass tetany.

grass tetany. Nervous system and muscle malfunction due to low levels of magnesium in the body.

gristle. Connective tissue.

ground hemlock. Yew (ornamental shrub); poisonous to livestock.

grub. The larva of a fly.

gut. Digestive tract.

H

Haemophilus somnus. Bacterium that causes respiratory, nervous, and reproductive disease.

hairy heel warts. *See* heel warts.

halogens. Nonmetallic elements (such as chlorine, fluorine, and iodine) that form compounds, such as sodium chloride, by simple union with a metal.

halogeton. Poisonous plant.

hardware disease. Peritonitis caused by a sharp foreign object's penetrating the stomach wall.

harrowing. Breaking up manure pats by dragging a pasture — pulling a toothed frame or some other type of "drag" behind a tractor or vehicle.

head catcher. Frame with movable sides or bars by which a cow can be caught by the head for restraint.

heat index. Combination of humidity and temperature.

heel fly. Fly that lays eggs on the leg hairs of cattle, causing cattle to run frantically in efforts to avoid the fly; the larvae burrow through the skin and migrate to the animal's back, spending the winter in a cyst (warble) under the skin of the back.

heel warts. Painful infection or growths at the back of the foot, sometimes with strawberry-like appearance, caused by a spirochete bacterium.

heifer. Young female bovine before she has a calf.

hemlock. One of several types of poisonous plants. Water hemlock is a perennial in the carrot family and is more deadly than poison hemlock, which is a biennial in the parsnip family.

hemoglobin. Oxygen-carrying component of red blood cells.

hemorrhagic bowel syndrome (HBS). Massive hemorrhage in the small intestines, caused by *C. perfringens* type A.

hemotoxin. A toxin, as in snake venom, that destroys red blood cells.

hepatitis. Inflammation of the liver.

herbicide. Chemical that kills plants.

herbivorous. A term referring to animals that feed on plants; grazing animals.

hernia. Bulging of tissue or an organ through a defect in the wall of a body cavity.

herpes virus. A group of viruses that cause a number of serious diseases in humans and animals, including IBR in cattle.

heterosis (hybrid vigor). A crossbred individual showing qualities superior to those of both parents, especially in traits such as hardiness, growth rate, fertility, disease resistance, and longevity.

high mountain disease. *See* brisket disease.

hives. Lumps in the skin due to allergy.

hock. Large joint halfway up the hind leg.

honda. Small loop on a lariat through which the end is threaded to create the throwing loop.

hookworm. Parasite that enters the body via ingestion or through the skin.

hormone. Chemical substance produced by an organ or gland that has a specific regulating effect on the activity of various organs.

horn fly. Small fly that feeds on blood, spending most of its time on cattle.

horsefly. Large fly with slashing mouthparts that creates painful stab wounds; it then laps up the blood that flows from the wound.

host. Animal or plant that harbors or nourishes another organism.

host specific. Refers to an organism that completes its life cycle in only one kind of host.

humoral immunity. Antibody-mediated immunity.

hybrid vigor. *See* heterosis.

hydrocyanic acid (prussic acid). Poisonous substance found in wilted chokecherry leaves and some other plants under certain growing conditions or when there is damage to the plants.

hypothermia. Below-normal body temperature.

I

IBR. *See* infectious bovine rhinotracheitis (IBR).

IM. *See* intramuscular (IM).

immune system. Network of defense systems within the body that fights pathogens.

immunity. Ability to resist a certain disease.

immunoglobulin. Antibody; a serum protein that circulates in the blood and lymph to seek and destroy a particular antigen.

impaction. Constipation; blockage in the large intestine due to accumulation of hard, dehydrated feces.

incubation period. Time elapsing between when a pathogen enters the body and when the animal shows signs of disease.

infectious bovine keratoconjunctivitis (IBK). *See* pinkeye (infectious bovine keratoconjunctivitis).

infectious bovine rhinotracheitis (IBR). Viral disease causing respiratory signs and abortion; also called red nose.

inflammation. A local protective tissue reaction to injury or infection that destroys, dilutes, or walls off the injurious agent and affected tissue.

interferon. Protein that interferes with viral replication.

intramuscular (IM). Injection into the muscle, usually with a needle at least an inch in length.

intranasal vaccine. Vaccine product sprayed up into the nostril.

intravenously (IV). Into a vein.

iodine. Trace mineral; also a chemical disinfectant.

iodophor. Any of various compounds of iodine with certain types of carriers, used as a surface disinfectant or surgical scrub.

ionophore. Antibiotic class that includes monensin and lasalocid, which alters the activity of rumen bacteria and can help prevent bloat and acidosis, as well as improve feed efficiency.

IV. *See* intravenously (IV).

J

jaundice. Yellow color of mucous membranes — gums, whites of the eyes — resulting from a breakdown of red blood cells.

Johne's disease. Contagious, chronic, and usually fatal infection of the small intestine that takes years to develop; paratuberculosis.

joint ill. Infection, usually bloodborne and often entering via the moist navel of the newborn calf, that settles in the joints and causes damage and lameness; navel ill.

jugular vein. Large vein in the neck; one of the easiest veins to use when giving an intravenous injection.

K

kaelin. A type of hydrated aluminum silicate found in clay; often used with pectin as a treatment for diarrhea.

keratoma. Warty growth or rough area on the eyelid, which often becomes cancerous.

ketones. Acidic organic compounds, such as acetone, in the body that result from metabolism of fat.

ketosis (acetonemia). Energy metabolism disorder of cattle, caused by incomplete metabolism of fatty acids and shortage of glucose and glycogen in the body.

killed-virus vaccine. Vaccine created from antigens derived from killed viruses — stimulates immune reaction without danger of passing the actual disease to the animal.

Klebsiella. Bacteria commonly found on tree bark and sometimes transmitted to cattle from wood products used as bedding; causes mastitis, navel ill, and other ailments.

L

lactating. Term used to refer to cows who are producing milk.

lactation tetany. *See* grass tetany.

laminae. Interlocking interface between hoof horn and the inner sensitive tissues of the foot.

laminitis. Inflammation of the sensitive laminae in the hoof, sometimes resulting in separation of the hoof wall from the underlying structures (founder).

lance. To cut with a sharp knife or surgical blade, as when opening an abscess to allow drainage.

laparotomy. Incision through the flank.

lariat. Long, small diameter rope used for catching an animal by looping it over the head or around the foot.

larkspur. Poisonous wildflower; delphinium.

larvae. Immature stage of insects and worms.

larvicide. A product that kills the larval stage of an insect.

laryngitis. Inflammation of the larynx.

larynx. Voice box at the back of the throat, between the nasal passages and the windpipe.

lasalocid. *See* ionophore.

Lasix. A diuretic drug.

latent. Hidden, dormant.

LA-200. *See* oxytetracycline.

lead poisoning. Poisoning due to ingestion of lead; causes weight loss, constipation, anemia, nervous system disorders, and paralysis.

legume. Family of plants that includes peas, beans, and alfalfa.

leptospire. Spiral-shaped bacterium that causes leptospirosis

leptospirosis. Disease spread by rodents and many other types of animals. In cattle it causes abortion in cows and occasional cases of illness.

lesion. Damage or injury to the tissue.

lice. Small parasitic insect that feeds on skin or blood.

lime. Calcium oxide or calcium hydroxide, often used as a disinfectant, especially in barn stalls.

listeriosis. Caused by bacteria that may also cause abortion; also called circling disease.

liver fluke. A two-host parasite (requiring a snail and a grazing animal) that finishes its life cycle in the bile ducts of the liver.

locoweed. Poisonous legume that grows on arid rangelands and causes nervous disorders and sometimes abortion in cattle that eat it.

lump jaw. Abscess in the soft tissues of the mouth and cheek.

lunger. Cow with emphysema.

lung fever. See emphysema.

lungworm. Parasite that damages the small branches of the bronchial tubes during its migration through the lungs.

lupine. Wildflower that contains alkaloids that cause birth defects if consumed by the dam in early pregnancy.

Lyme disease. Bacterial disease in humans and animals, spread by ticks; causes recurrent fever, arthritis, and sometimes nervous and circulatory disorders.

lymnaeid snail. Small freshwater snail that serves as intermediate host for liver flukes.

lymph. Clear fluid found in the lymphatic system of the body.

lymph node. A small mass of tissue (gland) in the lymphatic system where lymph is purified and lymphocytes are formed.

lymphocyte. A white blood cell that forms in the lymph node.

lymphocytosis. Excess number of lymphocytes in the blood.

lymphomatosis. Development of multiple lymphomas (cancerous new growths) in lymph tissue.

lymphosarcoma. Malignancy in lymph tissue. Terminal (cancerous) stage of bovine leukemia virus infection. *See also* bovine leukemia.

M

mad cow disease. *See* bovine spongiform encephalopathy (BSE)

maggot. Larva of a fly.

magnesium sulfate. Epsom salts.

malignant. Cancerous; spreading to other tissues or traveling via blood or lymph to other parts of the body.

malignant edema. Highly fatal clostridial disease caused by *C. septicum.*

malnutrition. Unbalanced or inadequate nutrition.

mammary tissue. Milk-producing glands in the udder.

mange. Dermatitis (skin inflammation) and hair loss due to mange mites.

manyplies. *See* omasum.

mast-cell tumor. Rapidly growing nodule between the layers of skin (mast cells are connective tissue cells).

mastitis. Infection and inflammation in the udder.

melanoma. Skin cancer that sometimes occurs in dark-skinned cattle; usually benign.

meningitis. Inflammation and infection of tissues around the brain.

metabolic rate. Rate of metabolism.

metabolism. The sum of all the physical and chemical processes by which a living creature functions in which body cells are produced and maintained, including the transformation by which energy is made available for use of the body.

metabolize. Break down and change, as when a certain ingested substance is metabolized in the liver.

metalloid. Element in between metals and nonmetals in its physical and chemical properties.

metaphylaxis. Administration of a drug, such as an antibiotic, as an aid in both prevention and treatment.

metastasize. Spread to a new location in the body; for example, a malignant tumor spreading to adjacent tissues or traveling via the lymph system or bloodstream to other areas.

methemoglobin. Hemoglobin with nitrite ions attached and inhibiting the oxygen-carrying ability of the hemoglobin.

Micotil (tilmicosin). Antibiotic product effective against bacteria that cause bovine respiratory disease; this drug is fatal to humans if accidentally injected.

midges. Small biting flies.

milk fever. Acute lack of calcium in the body, affecting muscle function and resulting in inability of a cow to get up; usually occurs soon after calving.

milo. Sorghum grain.

mineral oil. Often used as a gut lubricant or laxative or to relieve bloat.

miracidia. Free-swimming immature liver flukes after they hatch from eggs.

mite. Tiny arthropod that feeds on the skin, causing mange.

modified live-virus (MLV) vaccine. Vaccine created by using live virus that has been altered or inactivated so it won't cause disease but can still stimulate strong immunity.

mold. A type of fungus, some of which are toxic.

molting. Shedding feathers, skin, or shell.

molybdenum. Element in soil that can tie up copper and make it inaccessible to the body, producing copper deficiency.

monensin. *See* ionophore.

mortality rate. Percent of animals in a group that die from a disease.

mountain sickness. *See* brisket disease.

mucosal disease. Highly fatal form of BVD that impairs proper function of the intestine, resulting in diarrhea.

mucous membrane. Moist, mucus-producing tissue that lines a body cavity.

mucus. Slimy lubricating substance secreted by mucous membranes.

mummification. Conversion into a state resembling that of a mummy, such as the shriveling and drying of a dead fetus that remains in the uterus rather than being expelled.

mummy. A dead, dry fetus within the uterus.

mycobacterium. A type of gram-positive, slow-growing bacteria that includes the pathogen that causes tuberculosis.

Mycoplasma. Type of gram-negative bacteria lacking a true cell wall, which makes this kind of infection more difficult to treat.

mycotoxins. Toxins produced by mold and fungi.

myoglobin. Red pigment in the iron-containing protein of muscles.

N

nasogastric tube. Long, flexible tube put into the nostril to the back of the throat, down the esophagus, and into the stomach.

natural beef. Meat grown without use of chemicals or antibiotics.

navel ill. Infection entering via the navel stump at birth, often causing problems elsewhere in the body, such as joints (joint ill).

Naxcel. Ceftiofur; short-acting antibiotic with minimal withdrawal time.

necropsy. Examination of an animal after death to determine the cause of death.

necrotic. Dead.

necrotic laryngitis. *See* diphtheria.

nematode. Worm.

neoplasm. New growth, such as a tumor.

neosporosis. Protozoal infection that can cause abortion in cows; spread by canine feces that contaminate cattle feed.

neurotoxin. A toxin that affects the nervous system.

neutrophil. Certain type of white blood cell.

nitrate poisoning. Highly fatal; due to consumption of plants with high nitrate levels (caused by abnormal growing conditions).

nitrite. Building block of protein, derived from nitrate via the action of rumen bacteria; highly toxic in excess.

nits. Lice eggs.

nodular worm. Parasite that lives in the rumen wall.

Nolvasan. See chlorhexidine.

nose flap. Antisucking device used in weaning calves while they are still with their mothers.

nose lead. Nose tongs.

Nuflor (florfenicol). Antibiotic drug effective against many of the bacteria that cause pneumonia and foot rot.

nymph. Immature stage of lice and mites.

O

off label. See extra label.

omasum. Third stomach; also called manyplies.

oocyst. Reproductive cell of protozoal organisms.

open cow. Cow that's not pregnant.

optic nerve. The major nerve between the eye and the brain.

oral. By mouth.

organic beef. Produced without the use of drugs or chemicals, including production of the feed — no chemical fertilizers, no pesticides.

organophosphate. A highly toxic class of insecticides.

osteosarcoma. Cancer in the bone.

overshot. A term for a jaw that protrudes farther forward than the opposite jaw.

oxalates. A salt of oxalic acid, found in certain feeds and excreted in urine; a diet high in oxalates may lead to urinary calculi (kidney or bladder stones).

oxfenbendazole. White-paste oral deworming drug.

oxytetracycline. Broad-spectrum antibiotic (some examples are LA-200, Biomycin, and Tetradure).

P

pajahuello tick. Tick that transmits the pathogens that cause "foothill abortion."

palpation. Feeling an organ or structure to determine its shape or characteristics.

papillae. Small nipple-shaped projections or elevated areas on a body structure.

papilloma. Plaque; for instance, a small growth on the eyeball (a precursor to cancer).

PAP test. See pulmonary arterial pressure (PAP) test.

papular stomatitis. Viral disease of young cattle, which causes small lumps on the muzzle and inside the mouth, lips, and nostrils.

papule. Tiny lump on the skin.

parainfluenza 3 (PI3). Viral respiratory disease.

parasite. Organism that lives inside or on another living organism that serves as its host.

parasitic wasp (predator wasp). Tiny wasp that lays eggs in manure; the larvae feed on fly larvae.

parathyroid gland. Small gland that sits beside the thyroid gland and secretes a hormone that regulates calcium levels in the body.

paratuberculosis. See Johne's disease.

parturient paresis. Milk fever.

passive immunity. Temporary immunity obtained from a source outside the body, such as via maternal antibodies in colostrum ingested by a newborn calf or from the antibodies in an antitoxin or serum.

passive transfer. Temporary protection against disease, such as given to a calf when he absorbs antibodies from his dam's colostrum.

pastern. Area between hoof and fetlock joint.

Pasteurella. Gram-negative bacteria that cause bovine respiratory disease (BRD) or shipping fever, a serious respiratory disease, generally following a viral infection.

pasteurization. Heating milk or some other liquid to a certain temperature that destroys most pathogens.

pathogen. Organism that causes disease.

PCR test. See polymerase chain reaction (PCR) test.

penicillin. Any of a large group of natural or semisynthetic antibacterial products derived directly or indirectly from strains of *Penicillium* mold (fungi) and other fungi that live in the soil, which kill or inhibit susceptible bacteria by having a negative effect on the bacterial cell wall.

peritoneum. Inner lining of the abdominal cavity.

peritonitis. Inflammation and infection inside the abdominal cavity.

persistently infected (PI). A term used to describe animals infected with BVD in utero during the first three months of gestation; they carry the virus for the rest of their lives.

pesticide. Product used to destroy pests of any kind, such as a fungicide, herbicide, insecticide, or dewormer.

pH. Measure of acidity or alkalinity. On a scale of 1 to 14, 7 is neutral, 1 is most acid, and 14 is most alkaline (base).

phagocyte. Blood or lymph cell capable of ingesting microorganisms such as bacteria.

pharynx. Throat; passage between the mouth (and rear part of the nasal passages) and the larynx and esophagus.

phosphorus. Essential element of diet, abundant in all body tissues and involved in almost all metabolic processes; a major component of bones.

photodynamic agent. Substance that can induce or intensify a toxic reaction to sunlight.

photosensitization. Abnormally high reactivity of the skin to sunlight, resulting in inflammation and death of the cells.

photosynthesis. Chemical combination caused by the action of light; the formation of carbohydrates and release of oxygen from carbon dioxide and water in the chlorophyll tissues of plants.

phylloerythrin. Photosensitizing agent; a metabolite of chlorophyll.

PI. *See* persistently infected (PI).

PI3. *See* parainfluenza 3.

pili. Filament-like appendages of certain bacteria that bind to tissues; pili are associated with antigenic properties.

pin bones. Extensions of the pelvic bone; bony part of the buttock.

pine-needle abortion. Abortion caused by the cow's eating ponderosa pine needles.

pinkeye (infectious bovine keratoconjunctivitis [IBK]). Infection of the eye caused by the bacterium *Moraxella bovis*; spread by face flies.

piroplasmosis. Infection with a certain species of protozoan, spread by blood-sucking ticks.

PI3. *See* parainfluenza 3 (PI3).

pit vipers. Group of poisonous snakes with a heat-sensing pit between the eye and the nostril by which they detect prey (warm-blooded animals).

placenta. Membranes surrounding the fetus and attached to the uterus, providing blood supply to the fetus via the umbilical cord.

plaque. Flat, raised precancerous lesion such as a growth on an eyeball.

pneumonia. Infection in the lungs.

polioencephalomalacia. Serious condition caused by softening (necrosis) of the gray matter in the brain.

poloxalene. A detergent antifoaming agent; the active ingredient in Bloat Guard.

polymerase chain reaction (PCR) test. A type of lab test, sometimes used for detecting the presence of a specific pathogen, such as the protozoan that causes trichomoniasis.

pox virus. A virus that creates small round lesions, such as on the teats.

preconditioning. Vaccinating and weaning calves before selling them, so they are less apt to become sick from the stress of transport to a new location.

prion. A unique type of aberrant protein, such as that found in brain and spinal-cord tissue of animals infected with BSE.

probang. Long, flexible rod with a ball on the end, for removing a throat obstruction.

probiotics. Products containing microorganisms needed in the gut for proper digestion.

progesterone. Hormone secreted by the corpus luteum (CL) in the ovary and by the placenta in a pregnant animal; it prepares the uterus for reception and development of the fertilized egg and maintains an optimum environment in the uterus for sustaining pregnancy.

prophylaxis. Preventive therapy; treatment aimed at preventing a certain disease.

propylene glycol. Clear, colorless, viscous liquid, sometimes given orally to provide a source of energy to a debilitated animal or one that is unable to eat.

prostaglandin. Any of a group of hormonelike compounds that have various effects in the body, such as stimulating uterine contractions; also released during inflammatory responses, causing fever and a higher sensitivity to pain.

protozoa. One-celled animals, some of which cause disease.

prussic acid. *See* hydrocyanic acid (prussic acid).

pseudocowpox. Viral infection of cattle producing lesions on the teats similar to those of cowpox (and in the mouth of suckling calves). It may be transmitted to humans during milking, producing milker's nodules (lesions on the fingers).

Psoroptes. A type of mange mite.

pulmonary. Pertaining to the lungs.

pulmonary arterial pressure (PAP) test. Test that measures pressure in the pulmonary artery, to check for brisket disease.

pulmonary hypertension. *See* brisket disease.

pupate. Become a pupa, the stage between larva and adult.

pus. Thick yellowish or greenish liquid produced by infected tissue.

pustular vulvovaginitis. Inflammation of the vulva and vaginal tissues.

pyrethrin. Active constituent of pyrethrum flowers, used in the manufacture of insecticides.

pyrrolizidine alkaloid. Alkaloid in certain plants that causes liver damage.

Q

quarters of the udder. Four compartments of the bovine udder.

quick-release honda. Release snap on the honda of a lariat that allows the loop to come apart in order to release the animal without having to pull the rope off its head or legs.

R

rabies. Fatal viral disease of mammals, transferred through the saliva of an infected animal when it bites another animal.

radiant heat. Heat radiating out from an object.

recrudescence. Reappearance; recurrence of symptoms; the disease breaks out afresh after a period of abatement.

rectum. Final portion of the large intestine.

red nose. *See* infectious bovine rhinotracheitis (IBR).

redwater. Acute and highly fatal clostridial disease, one sign of which is blood in the urine.

reservoir. Source of infection; host animals or species for a certain disease.

respiratory system. Nasal passages, windpipe, bronchial tubes, and lungs.

reticulum. Second stomach; often called the hardware stomach or honeycomb stomach.

retina. Membrane at the back of the eyeball that sends nerve impulses to the optic nerve.

rickettsia. Genus of gram-negative bacteria that multiply only inside the body cells of the host animal; spread by lice, fleas, ticks, and mites.

rigor mortis. The stiffening of a dead body.

ringworm. Fungal skin disease, so-called because of the ring-shaped nature of the lesions.

rotavirus. Viral disease that causes diarrhea in young calves; spread by feces.

roundworms. Certain type of internal parasite; nematodes.

rumen. Large first stomach of a ruminant.

ruminant. Cud-chewing animal.

ruminate. Burp up food and chew the cud.

ryegrass staggers. Incoordination due to toxic effects of an ergot fungus on ryegrasses.

S

salmonella. Bacteria causing intestinal infection and diarrhea.

salmonellosis. Severe illness caused by *Salmonella* bacteria.

salt. Sodium chloride; one of the most important element compounds needed by the body for proper function.

salt toxicity. Toxic effects, sometimes fatal, of ingesting too much salt.

sand cracks. Hoof cracks.

sand fly. Any of various two-winged small flies of the genus *Phlebotomus*.

sarcocystosis. Protozoan infection spread to cattle by predatory animals.

sarcoma. Tumor arising from connective tissue.

Sarcoptes. Mite that burrows inside the skin and causes scabies.

sarcosporidiosis. Tiny purple spots in the muscle tissue caused by sarcosystis protozoa.

scabies. Contagious dermatitis caused by the *Sarcoptes* mite; the egg-laying female digs into the upper layer of skin and creates burrows that cause tiny skin eruptions and intense itching.

sclera. The white of the eye.

scours. Diarrhea.

scrapie. Disease in sheep involving the central nervous system (and one of the first prion diseases discovered); related to BSE in cattle.

scrotal hernia. Hole in the abdominal wall at the scrotum, which may allow loops of intestine to fall into the scrotum.

scrotum. Sac enclosing the testicles of a bull.

secondary infection. Another pathogen moving in and taking advantage of the animal's lowered resistance following a primary illness.

seleniferous. A term that describes soils containing selenium.

selenium. Trace mineral needed in very small amounts in the diet; too much or too little can be harmful to good health.

self-limiting. A disease that runs a definite limited course with no need for treatment; the animal throws off the infection and recovers.

septic arthritis. Infection within the joints; causes crippling lameness.

septicemia. Infection that infiltrates the whole body via the bloodstream.

serotype. The category of a microorganism as determined by the antigens present within it.

sheath. Outer covering of the penis of the male animal when it is withdrawn into the body.

shipping fever. Bovine respiratory disease (BRD).

shock. Extreme circulatory and metabolic disturbance in the body, characterized by failure of the circulatory system to maintain adequate blood supply to vital organs.

silicates. Insoluble compounds that contain silica and occasionally create bladder stones.

sinuses. Cavities or channels, such as the nasal sinuses or the horn sinus in an adult horned animal.

slough off. Dead tissue coming away, separating from live tissue.

sodium. One of the crucial elements needed by the body; combines with chloride to produce table salt.

sodium chloride. Salt.

sodium iodide. Drug given IV to treat bony lump jaw and wooden tongue.

somatic cells. Body cells that may be indicative of infection, such as those found in milk when a cow has mastitis.

sord. "Sudden death"; swiftly fatal disease caused by *C. sordellii*.

speculum. Tube or instrument for holding a body cavity open; a short, rigid pipe used for passing a stomach tube down the throat, preventing the animal from chewing on the tube as it is passed through the mouth.

spinal stenosis. Pressure on the spinal cord caused by the narrowing of the vertebral column.

spirochete. Spiral-shaped bacterium.

spore. Reproductive element of fungi, protozoa, algae, and some spore-forming bacteria; spores are the dormant stage that can live for a long time until conditions are better for multiplication.

sporocyst. Cyst or sac containing spores or reproductive cells.

sporozoite. Mobile, infective stage of coccidia protozoa.

sporulate. Produce or liberate spores.

squamous cell carcinoma. Malignant new growth in epithelial tissue, initially localized and superficial, but in later stages invasive or metastasizing.

stable fly. Biting fly, about the size of a housefly, that feeds on blood, creating painful bites, often on the legs of cattle.

stanchion. Upright pair of bars or frame for securing a cow by the neck and holding her in place.

Staphylococcus. Genus of gram-positive bacteria, some of which can cause serious disease.

steroid. Hormone or hormonelike substance.

stifle. Large joint high on the hind leg by the flank.

stillborn. Born dead.

stomach tube. *See* nasogastric tube.

strawberry warts. *See* heel warts.

Streptococcus. Group of gram-positive bacteria that cause a variety of diseases, including mastitis and pneumonia.

subacute. Term used to describe a medical condition that develops less rapidly and with less severity than an acute condition.

subclinical. Showing no signs of illness; not obvious.

subcutaneously (SubQ). Under the skin, between the skin and the muscle.

sucking lice. Type of lice that attach to the skin and suck blood from the host.

sulfa. Any of the sulfanilamides, potent antibacterial compounds that were the first sulfonamides discovered.

sulfonamide. Sulfa drugs that inhibit certain gram-positive and gram-negative bacteria. Many of the earlier sulfa drugs have been replaced by more-effective and less-toxic antibiotics.

sulfur. A nonmetallic element.

summer slump. Term for reduction in weight gain experienced by cattle grazing endophyte-infected fescue pastures.

supplement. Feed additive that supplies something missing in the diet.

suture. Stitch, to sew up an incision.

systemic. Pertaining to the whole body.

T

tabanid. Family of large biting flies that include deer flies and horseflies.

tannic acid. Poisonous substance found in some types of trees, such as oak.

tannins. Complex organic compounds found in certain tree barks and other plants.

tapeworm. Internal parasite that requires a pasture mite as intermediate host.

taxine. Poisonous alkaloid found in yew.

TEME. *See* thromboembolic meningoencephalitis (TEME).

tetanus. Acute, fatal disease caused by clostridial bacteria that enter through a wound.

tetracycline. Any of a group of biosynthetic antibiotics, effective against a wide variety of pathogens.

Texas cattle fever. Serious disease caused by protozoa spread by ticks.

thermal load. Heat accumulation in the body.

thermo-neutral. Ideal weather temperature in which the body can stay comfortable with no extra energy necessary to heat or cool it.

thiaminase. Enzyme that destroys vitamin B_1.

thiamine. Vitamin B_1.

third eyelid. Movable membrane in the front corner of the bovine eye.

threadworm. Internal parasite that lives in the small intestine.

threshold number. The number of pathogens needed in order for disease to occur.

thromboembolic meningoencephalitis (TEME). Highly fatal infection with *Haemophilus somnus* bacteria that affects the nervous system.

thyroid gland. Large gland in the neck that secretes a hormone that regulates growth, development, and body metabolism.

tick. Parasitic arachnid that embeds its head in the skin of warm-blooded animals and feeds on blood. Some ticks transmit disease.

tick paralysis. Wasting disease caused by toxins secreted in tick saliva.

titer. Quantity of a substance required to produce a reaction with a certain volume of another substance, measured in blood tests to determine if the animal has been exposed to a specific disease, such as having a high titer for a specific antigen.

T lymphocyte. T cells; white blood cells originating from cells in bone marrow, and responsible for cell-mediated immunity.

topical. Applied on the body surface.

toxemia. Bacterial toxins circulating through the bloodstream.

toxins. Poisons; often refers to proteins produced by plants or certain pathogenic bacteria.

toxoid. Modified or inactivated bacterial toxin, used as a vaccine to stimulate immunity or protection against that bacterial toxin.

trace minerals. Important minerals needed in very small amounts for proper function of the body and good health.

trachea (windpipe). Tube between the nasal passages (back of the throat) and the lungs.

tracheostomy. Cutting into the trachea to create an opening through which the animal can breathe when upper airways are blocked.

trichomonads. One type of parasitic protozoa that causes trichomoniasis.

trichomoniasis. Protozoan disease spread by breeding, causing early embryonic death and infertility.

trimethoprim. Antibacterial drug, administered orally in combination with a sulfonamide because the two drugs work much better together to combat certain types of infections.

trocar. Sharp tool for stabbing a hole in the rumen to let out excess gas.

tryptophan. Amino acid found in lush green forage that can sometimes be changed by the action of rumen bacteria into a poison.

tuberculosis (TB). Infectious disease caused by mycobacterium and characterized by formation of tubules in various organs, such as the lungs.

tumor. Abnormal growth of tissue.

U

udder. Mammary glands and teats.

ulcer. Cavity or open sore on the surface of a tissue or organ.

ultrasound. Ultrasonography; visualization of deep structures of the body by recording the echoes of pulses of ultrasonic waves directed into the tissues.

umbilical hernia. Hole or separation in the outer wall of the abdomen (at the navel) that allows tissue to bulge through.

umbilical tape. Thick white cotton "tape."

underrun heel/sole. Terms used to describe weak, squashed-forward heel (and toes too long); no support at the back of the foot.

undulant fever. Brucellosis in humans.

ureter. Small tube from kidney to bladder.

urethra. Tube from the urinary bladder to the external opening to facilitate passage of urine.

V

vaccine. Product containing killed or modified germs (bacteria or viruses) or the antigenic proteins or DNA obtained from them, injected or sprayed into the body to stimulate production of antibodies and create immunity.

vagus indigestion. Any condition in which the cow can't belch to chew her cud.

vagus nerve. Major nerve with branches to the heart, lungs, and gut.

vector. Carrier of a disease; agent by which a disease is spread.

vein. Vessel that takes blood back to the heart.

vesicular stomatitis (VS). Foreign-animal disease caused by a virus that creates blisters in the mouth and on the teats and feet, with symptoms similar to but not as severe as foot and mouth disease.

vet-rap. Stretchy bandaging material that adheres to itself without being sticky.

vibriosis. A bacterial disease spread by breeding, causing death of the embryo or fetus and infertility; also called campylobacteriosis.

villi. Fingerlike projections on the intestinal lining that absorb fluid and nutrients.

viremia. Stage of a viral disease in which the virus is present in the blood; characterized by fever.

virus. Very tiny agent that can only replicate (multiply) in a living host.

VS. *See* vesicular stomatitis (VS).

vulva. External part of the female reproductive tract; the tissues that compose the opening into the vagina.

W

warble. Cyst under the skin of the back, containing a grub (larva of a fly).

warts. Skin growths caused by a virus.

waterbelly. Condition due to urinary stones that block the urinary tract and cause an enlarged or ruptured bladder.

white blood cells. Various large cells in the bloodstream that devour bacteria, produce antibodies, and fight infection.

white muscle disease. Fatal condition in which some of the heart-muscle fibers are replaced with connective tissue; due to selenium deficiency.

wind chill. Cooling effect of wind on exposed skin, producing the equivalent of a much lower temperature.

windpipe. *See* trachea (windpipe).

wireworms. Barber pole worms; large stomach worms.

withdrawal time. Length of time it takes for residues from an ingested or injected drug or vaccine to be eliminated from the body. Meat or milk from the animal cannot be used for human consumption until this time has elapsed.

withers. High point of the back, behind the neck and above the shoulders.

wooden tongue. Infection in the mouth/throat/tongue that makes the tissues hard and sore.

worms. Internal parasites that generally live in the digestive tract, though some may also migrate through other parts of the body.

Y

yeast. A type of fungi; some kinds are produced and involved with fermentation in the rumen, while other types may cause infection.

yellow fever. *See* anaplasmosis.

yew. Ornamental tree or shrub; highly poisonous.

Z

zebu. Humped cattle of India, Asia, and Africa; *Bos indicus* (a different species from the *Bos taurus* cattle of Europe and the British Isles).

Resources

Publications and Books

Blood, D. C., and O. M. Radostits. *Veterinary Medicine: A Textbook of the Diseases of Cattle, Sheep, Pigs, Goats, and Horses.* 7th ed. London: Balliere Tindall, 1989.

Blowey, Roger W., and A. David Weaver. *Color Atlas of Diseases and Disorders of Cattle.* 2nd ed. Philadelphia: Mosby/Elsevier, 2003.

Grandin, Temple. *Humane Livestock Handling.* North Adams, MA: Storey Publishing. 2008.

Haynes, N. Bruce. *Keeping Livestock Healthy.* 3rd ed. North Adams, MA: Storey Publishing, 1994.

Howarth, R. E., R. K. Chaplin, K.J. Cheng, B. P. Goplen, J. W. Hall, R. Hironaka, W. Majak, and O. M. Radostits. *Bloat in Cattle,* #1858E. Ottawa: Agriculture Canada, 1991.

James, L.F. *Plants Poisonous to Livestock in the Western States.* Agriculture Information Bulletin #415. Washington: United States Department of Agriculture, 1980).

Jeffers, Keith. *Management, Nutrition, and Medicine for Calves.* 5th ed. West Plains, MO: Quill Press, Inc., 1993.

Radostitis, O. M., C. C. Gay, D. C. Blood, and K. W. Hinchcliff. *Veterinary Medicine.* 9th ed. New York: W. B. Saunders Company, 2000.

Straiton, Eddie. *Cattle Ailments: Recognition and Treatment.* 6th ed. Ipswich, UK: Farming Press, 1993.

Thomas, Heather Smith. *Essential Guide to Calving.* North Adams, MA: Storey Publishing, 2008.

Thomas, Heather Smith. *Getting Started with Beef and Dairy Cattle.* North Adams, MA: Storey Publishing, 2005.

Thomas, Heather Smith. *Storey's Guide to Raising Beef Cattle.* North Adams, MA: Storey Publishing, 1998.

University of Idaho Cooperative Extension Service. *Cow-Calf Management Guide.* Moscow, Idaho: University of Idaho Cattle Producers Library, 2007.

Whittier, Jack C. (editor). *Cow-Calf Production: Resource Information and Research Updates.* Fort Collins: Colorado State University Extension, 1997.

Periodicals

These publications frequently feature articles on the topics of cattle health and management.

Angus Beef Bulletin
St. Joseph, Missouri
800-821-5478
www.angusbeefbulletin.com

Angus Journal
St. Joseph, Missouri
800-821-5478
www.angusjournal.com

Arkansas Cattle Business
Little Rock, Arkansas
www.arbeef.org

Beef
Minneapolis, Minnesota
952-851-4660
www.beef-mag.com

Calf News
Garden City, Kansas
620-276-7844
www.calfnews.com

Carolina Cattle Connection
Fuquay-Varina, North Carolina
www.nccattle.com

Cascade Cattleman
Klamath Falls, Oregon
541-885-4460
www.cascadecattleman.com

The Cattleman
Fort Worth, Texas
817-3323-7155
www.thecattlemanmagazine.com

Cattlemen
Winnipeg, Manitoba
204-944-5753
www.canadiancattlemen.com

Cattle Today
Fayette, Alabama
205-932-8000
www.cattletoday.com

Charolais Journal
Kansas City, Missouri
816-464-5977
www.charolaisusa.com

Countryside
Medford, Wisconsin
800-441-5691
www.countrysidemag.com

Cow Country News
Lexington, Kentucky
859-278-0899
www.kycattle.org

Dairy Herd Management
Lenexa, Kansas
913-438-8700
www.dairyherd.com

Dairy Today
Philadelphia, Pennsylvania
www.agweb.com

Drovers
Lenexa, Kansas
913-438-8700
www.drovers.com

Feedlot Magazine
Dighton, Kansas
620-397-2838
www.feedlotmagazine.com

Florida Cattleman
Kissimmee, Florida
800-460-2648
www.floridacattleman.org

Grainews (Cattlemen's Corner)
Winnipeg, Manitoba
204-944-5568
www.grainews.ca

Gulf Coast Cattleman
San Antonio, Texas
210-344-8300

Hereford World
Kansas City, Missouri
816-842-8878
www.hereford.org

Iowa Cattlemen
Ames, Iowa
515-296-2266
www.iacattlemen.org

Limousin World
Guthrie, Oklahoma
www.limousinworld.com

Midwest Beef Producer
Saint Paul, Minnesota
www.mwbeefproducer.com

Midwest Cattleman
Lowry City, Missouri
417-644-2993
www.midwestcattleman.com

Missouri Beef Cattleman
Kansas City, Missouri
816-471-0200
www.mocattle.org/MissouriBeefCattleman.htm

National Cattlemen
Centennial, Colorado
303-694-0305
www.beefusa.org

Nebraska Cattlemen
Lincoln, Nebraska
www.nebraskacattlemen.org

Nevada Rancher
Winnemucca, Nevada
866-644-5011
www.nevadarancher.com

Small Farmers Journal
Sisters, Oregon
541-549-2064
www.smallfarmersjournal.com

Tennessee Cattle Business
Murfreesboro, Tennessee
www.tncattle.org

Texas Longhorn Trails
Fort Worth, Texas
817-625-6241
www.tlbaa.org

Tri-State Livestock News
Spearfish, South Dakota
877-347-9100
www.tsln.com

Weekly Livestock Reporter
Fort Worth, Texas
817-831-3147
www.weeklylivestock.com

Western Cowman
Fair Oaks, California
916-362-2697
www.westerncowman.com

Western Livestock Journal
Greenwood Village, Colorado
303-722-7600
www.wlj.net

Western Livestock Reporter
Billings, Montana
406-259-4589
www.cattleplus.com

Cooperative Extension Service

For more information about cattle health care and management in your area, contact the Cooperative Extension Service in your state. This program is affiliated with the various land-grant universities and USDA and can provide publications and information on a wide range of cattle-care topics. Extension offices in your state and county can also give assistance if you have specific questions or problems. **To find the nearest Cooperative Extension office, contact:**
Cooperative State Research, Education, and Extension Service
United States Department of Agriculture
Washington, DC
202-720-7441
www.csrees.usda.gov/extension

Livestock and Veterinary Supply Companies

Acadia Agritech
Dartmouth, Nova Scotia
902-468-2840
www.acadianagritech.ca
Producers of Tasco, a feed supplement to reduce the toxic effects of fescue

Air-Tite Products Company, Inc
Virginia Beach, Virginia
800-231-7762
www.air-tite.com
Syringes, needles, and medical supplies

American Livestock Supply
Madison, Wisconsin
800-356-0700
www.americanlivestock.com
Animal health supplies, handling equipment, hoof care products, and vaccine

Animal Health Express
Tucson, Arizona
800-533-8115
www.animalhealthexpress.com
Animal health and livestock supplies

Animart
Beaverdam, WI
800-255-1181
www.animart.com
Livestock health supplies and Horn-stop dehorner for baby calves

Barnyard Health
Baltimore, Maryland
866-602-3486
www.barnyardhealth.com
Animal health products and equipment

Dominion Veterinary Laboratories, Inc.
Winnipeg, New Brunswick
204-589-7631
www.domvet.com
Veterinary pharmaceuticals, medicines, and cattle supplies

Horseline Products
Henderson, Tennessee
800-208-4846
www.horselineproducts.com
Flytraps

JDA Livestock Innovations, Ltd.
Saskatoon, Saskatchewan
306-262-6618
www.quietwean.com
Nose flaps for weaning calves

Jeffers
West Plains, Missouri
800-533-3377
www.jefferslivestock.com
Livestock equipment and health supplies

Koehn Marketing, Inc
Watertown, South Dakota
800-658-3998
www.koehnmarketing.com
Unique livestock equipment

Lambert
Fairbury, Nebraska
800-344-6337
www.lambertvetsupply.com
Cattle health care supplies

NASCO
Fort Atkinson, Wisconsin
800-558-9595
www.eNASCO.com
Farm and ranch supplies, livestock-handling equipment, and baby calf electric dehorners

Northstar (Farmers of North America)
Saskatoon, Saskatchewan
866-383-7827
www.fna.ca
Livestock-handling equipment and chutes

Omaha Vaccine
Omaha, Nebraska
800-367-4444
www.omahavaccine.com
Animal health supplies

SSI Corporation
Julesburg, CO
800-654-3668
www.ssihoofcare.com
Hoof care products

PBS Animal Health
Massillon, Ohio
800-321-0235
www.pbsanimalhealth.com
Cattle health care supplies

QC Supply
Schuyler, Nebraska
800-433-6340
www.qcsupply.com
Livestock equipment and supplies

Spalding Laboratories
Arroyo, California
800-955-4248
www.spaldinglabs.com
Source of predator wasps for fly control

Tractor Supply Company
Brentwood, Tennessee
615-366-4600
www.tractorsupply.com
Livestock supplies, feeds, health care and veterinarian supplies

Valley Vet Supply
Marysville, Kansas
800-419-9524
www.valleyvet.com
Cattle health supplies, medicines, and equipment

Western Ranch Supply
Billings, Montana
800-548-7270
www.westernranchsupply.com

Index

Page numbers in *italics* indicate photos or illustrations; page numbers in **bold** indicate charts or graphs.

intramuscular (IM) injection
(*continued*)

    how to give an, 43, *43*

    needle specifications for,
    41–42

intravenous (IV) medication, 40,
    46–48, *241*

    how to give an, 47, *47*

    IV catheter, 48

    needles, tips for, 46, *46,* 48

iodides, 240–41

iodine deficiency, *274,* 274–75

iodophors, 10

ivermectin, 140, 144

IV medication. *See* intravenous
    (IV) medication

Ixodes tick. *See* deer ticks

J

jaw. *See* mouth problems

Johne, Heinrich Albert, 96

Johne's disease (paratuberculosis),
    95–99, *96*

    contamination cleanup, 98

    four stages of, 96

    prevention, 98–99

    as stealthy disease, 98

    symptoms, 97

    transmission, 97

    treatment, 97–98

joint ill. *See* navel ill and joint ill

jugular vein, 47, *47*

junk hazards, 310–11

K

Kamloops Research Station, 169

ketosis, 251–52

    treatment and prevention,
    251–52

    wasting/nervous forms of,
    251

kicking. *See* restraints

Klebsiella, 258

L

LA-200, 34, 100, 191, 204

lameness. *See* foot problems

laminitis, 230–31, *231*

large stomach worms, 134

larvicides, 151–52

leptospirosis, 5, 80–81

lice, 141–45

    biting lice, 141, 142, *142*

    carriers of, 143

    delousing tips, 143–44

    evidence of, 142, *142*

    life cycle of, 142

    nits (eggs) of, 141

    rubbing and scratching from,
    141, 141

    sucking lice, 141, *142*

    treatment, *143,* 143–44

lightning, 321

listeriosis (circling disease),
    99–100, 101

    symptoms, 99, *99*

    treatment and prevention,
    100

liver flukes, 9, 87, 136–38, *138*

    harmful effects of, 138

    infection region, 139, *139*

    life cycle of, 137, *137*

    prevention and treatment,
    138

    symptoms of infestation, 138

liver malfunctions, 200–201

locoweed, 267, 268, *287*

Lone star tick, *156*

low-stress cattle handling, 20–22

lump jaw (soft tissue abscess),
    236–38

    causes, 236

    lancing and flushing of, 238,
    238

    treatment, 237–38

lung capacity, 212

lungworms, 134

Lyme disease, 159–60

    regions for, *159*

M

macrolides, 38–39

"mad cow disease." *See* bovine
    spongiform encephalopathy

magnesium deficiency. *See* grass
    tetany

malignant edema (*Clostridium
    septicum*), 86, 87

mange mites, *146,* 146–47

manure, 163

mastitis, 258–62

    antibiotic application for, 261,
    261

    in baby heifers, 262

    in beef/dairy cattle, 259, 261

    in one quarter, 260, *260,* 263

    prevention, 262

    symptoms, 259, *259*

    treatment, 259, 261

M. bovis. See *Moraxella bovis*

meat quality, 42. *See also* with-
    drawal times

medicine. *See* drugs

metabolic problems, 245–55

Micotil, 33, 215, 227

milk fever, 245–47

    calcium drop and, 245–46

treatment and prevention, 87
reproduction, 63, 101, 129. *See also* breeding; pregnant cow management
residue avoidance, 34–35
respiration rate, 30, 31
respiratory problems, 208–24
    diseases characterized by, **334**
    stress and infection, 219
    upper respiratory challenges, 209–12
restraints, 52–58
    flank rope, 54, *54*
    front leg restraint, 57, *57*
    on the ground, 56–57, *56–57*
    halters, 52–53
    hobbles, homemade, 257, *257*
    kick restraints, 54–55
    for lifting injured cow, 319
    against a post, 56, *56*
    rear leg restraint, 57, *57*
    rope restraints, 56–57
    stanchions as, 52
    tail head holding, 54
reticulum (second stomach), 163, *163*
    hardware disease and, 175, 176
ringworm, 206–7, *207*
Rocky Mountain wood tick, 156, *156,* 158
roller dung beetles, *154,* 154–55, *155*
rope halter
    how to make a, 52, *53*
    instant halters, 53, *53*
rope tying. *See* restraints
rotavirus, 6, 117, *117*
roughage. *See* forage

roundworms, *133,* 133–34
rumen (first stomach), 23, 162, 163, *163*
    gas production in, 164–65
    microbes in, 164, 183
    tannins and, 171
ruminants, 49, 95
    nitrate poisoning of, 301
    stomachs of, 163–64

S

Salmonella, 35, 94–95
salt, 64, 70, 168, 277
sarcocystosis, 127
scabies, 146
scours, 5, 182. *See also* diarrhea
scrotal hernia, 314–15
    emergency surgery and, 315
seasonal health, 59–76
secondary infections, 32
selenium accumulators, 267, 268
selenium levels, 232
selenium-related illness, 266–70, *270*
    deadly discoveries, 267
    prevention, 269, 270
    selenium distribution, 267–68
    selenium deficiency, 268–70
    selenium distribution, *267*
    selenium toxicity, 270
    vitamin E and, 269
septicemia, 80, 91, 92, *92,* 100. *See also* navel ill and joint ill
sexually transmitted diseases, 17, 81, 82
"shipping fever," 104, 218–19
sick animal treatment, 31–35, 40
sickness. *See* illness detection

skin problems, 199–207
    allergies, 204
    photosensitization, 200–204
    ringworm, 206–7
    sunburn, 207
    vaccination reactions, 206
    warts, 205–6
slaughter, withdrawal times, 17, 33
slow-release injections, 45, *45*
small intestinal worms, 134
snakebite, 306–9
    air passage constriction and, 309
    infection and, 309
    symptoms, *307,* 307–8, *308*
    treatment, 308–9
snow as water source, 76, 174
sodium chloride. *See* salt
sodium iodide, 240–41
soft-bodied tick, 160, *160*
sole abscesses, 229–30, *230*
solid feeding, 164
SORD (sudden death), 86–87
stable flies, 147, *148,* 148–49
    control of, 149
Staphylococcus, 91, 258
steroids, 20
stifle, *54*
stomach. *See* digestion
stomach and intestinal worms, 133–36
    "bottle jaw" from, 135, *135*
    prevention and treatment, 135–36
    roundworms, *133,* 133–34
    symptoms, 135
stomach tube, 89
Streptococcus, 213, 258

Other Storey Titles You Will Enjoy

Essential Guide to Calving, by Heather Smith Thomas.
Complete coverage on what to expect at every step of the calving process to
ensure healthy pregnancies, safe births, and thriving calves.
336 pages. Paper. ISBN 978-1-58017-706-1.
Hardcover. ISBN 978-1-58017-707-8.

Getting Started with Beef & Dairy Cattle, by Heather Smith Thomas.
The first-time farmer's guide to the basics of raising a small herd of cattle.
288 pages. Paper. ISBN 978-1-58017-596-8.
Hardcover with jacket. ISBN 978-1-58017-604-0.

Grass-Fed Cattle, by Julius Ruechel.
The first complete manual in raising, caring for, and marketing grass-fed cattle.
384 pages. Paper. ISBN 978-1-58017-605-7.

Keeping Livestock Healthy, by N. Bruce Haynes, DVM.
A complete guide to disease prevention through good nutrition, proper
housing, and appropriate care.
352 pages. Paper. ISBN 978-1-58017-435-0.

Livestock Guardians, by Janet Vorwald Dohner.
Essential information on using dogs, donkeys, and llamas as a highly effective,
low-cost, and nonlethal method to protect livestock and their owners.
240 pages. Paper. ISBN 978-1-58017-695-8.
Hardcover. ISBN 978-1-58017-696-5.

Oxen: A Teamster's Guide, by Drew Conroy.
The definitive guide to selecting, training, and caring for the mighty ox.
304 pages. Paper. ISBN 978-1-58017-692-7.
Hardcover. ISBN 978-1-58017-693-4.

Raising a Calf for Beef, by Phyllis Hobson.
A no-nonsense guide to choosing a calf, providing housing and nutrition,
and finally butchering.
128 pages. Paper. ISBN 978-0-88266-095-0.

Small-Scale Livestock Farming, by Carol Ekarius.
A natural, organic approach to livestock management to produce healthier
animals, reduce feed and health care costs, and maximize profit.
224 pages. Paper. ISBN 978-1-58017-162-5.

These and other books from Storey Publishing are available
wherever quality books are sold or by calling 1-800-441-5700.
Visit us at *www.storey.com*.